DATE DUE

SEP 2 6 1996	
JUL 23 1997	
APR 26 1998	
MAY 22 1998	
JUL 2 1999	

GAYLORD   PRINTED IN U.S.A.

Competing
Solutions

JOSEPH WHITE

Competing Solutions

American Health Care Proposals and International Experience

THE BROOKINGS INSTITUTION
Washington, D.C.

Copyright © 1995
THE BROOKINGS INSTITUTION
1775 Massachusetts Avenue, N.W., Washington, D.C. 20036

Library of Congress Cataloging-in-Publication data:

White, Joseph, 1952-
    Competing solutions : American health care proposals
and international experiences / Joseph White.

        p. cm.
    Includes bibliographical references and index.
    ISBN 0-8157-9364-2.—ISBN 0-8157-9363-4 (pbk.)
    1.   Medical care—Finance.   2.   Health care reform—
United States.   3.   Medical care—Finance—Case
studies.   I.   Title.
RA410.5.W47   1995
362.1—dc20   95-7675
                                                  CIP

9 8 7 6 5 4 3 2 1

The paper used in this publication meets the minimum requirements of American National Standard for Information Sciences—Permanence of Paper for Printed Library Materials,
ANSI Z39,48-1984

Typeset in Palatino

Composition by Harlowe Typography, Inc.
Cottage City, Maryland

Printed by R.R. Donnelley and Sons Co.
Harrisonburg, Virginia

ℬ THE BROOKINGS INSTITUTION

The Brookings Institution is an independent organization devoted to nonpartisan research, education, and publication in economics, government, foreign policy, and the social sciences generally. Its principal purposes are to aid in the development of sound public policies and to promote public understanding of issues of national importance.

The Institution was founded on December 8, 1927, to merge the activities of the Institute for Government Research, founded in 1916, the Institute of Economics, founded in 1922, and the Robert Brookings Graduate School of Economics and Government, founded in 1924.

The Board of Trustees is responsible for the general administration of the Institution, while the immediate direction of the policies, program, and staff is vested in the President, assisted by an advisory committee of the officers and staff. The by-laws of the Institution state: "It is the function of the Trustees to make possible the conduct of scientific research, and publication, under the most favorable conditions, and to safeguard the independence of the research staff in the pursuit of their studies and in the publication of the results of such studies. It is not a part of their function to determine, control, or influence the conduct of particular investigations or the conclusions reached."

The President bears final responsibility for the decision to publish a manuscript as a Brookings book. In reaching his judgment on the competence, accuracy, and objectivity of each study, the President is advised by the director of the appropriate research program and weighs the views of a panel of expert outside readers who report to him in confidence on the quality of the work. Publication of a work signifies that it is deemed a competent treatment worthy of public consideration but does not imply endorsement of conclusions or recommendations.

The Institution maintains its position of neutrality on issues of public policy in order to safeguard the intellectual freedom of the staff. Hence interpretations or conclusions in Brookings publications should be understood to be solely those of the authors and should not be attributed to the Institution, to its trustees, officers, or other staff members, or to the organizations that support its research.

---

*To Honor
the Memory of
Richard C. Parker*

Foreword

THE Clinton administration made reform of the U.S. health care system its preeminent goal. The president insisted not only that guaranteeing health insurance to all was a moral imperative, but that reform would help address such major problems as the international competitiveness of American firms, long-term federal deficits, and dependency on means-tested welfare programs. He showed his personal commitment by appointing the first lady, Hillary Rodham Clinton, to spearhead the health care reform effort. The proposed reform turned into one of the loudest and most confusing political debates in memory. In the end President Clinton's effort not only failed to result in legislation, but also, many believe, contributed to his party's loss of both houses of Congress for the first time in forty years.

In the wake of that political result, it is easy to focus on supposed political errors and to lose sight of the substance of the debate: the growing millions of Americans without health insurance, and the consequences of proposed means of controlling costs or expanding coverage. In *Competing Solutions: American Health Care Proposals and International Experience*, Joseph White illuminates the substantive reality behind the political furor.

White analyzes the experience of other countries to show that affordable health insurance with quality care for all Americans was not impossible. He describes the international approaches that guarantee access and control costs, while comparing the Australian, Canadian, French, German, Japanese, and British arrangements to show that the international norm does not require a one-size-fits-all approach.

Then White compares the international standard to the theory of managed competition. His analysis shows both the internal logic of many of the Clinton plan's choices and the difficulty of finding a compromise among competing plans. White concludes by discussing the choices faced after the collapse of the 1993-94 reform effort: Would any partial measures do much good without the full-fledged reform that proved so frightening? What kind of comprehensive health care reform would be best for the United States?

Joseph White is a Research Associate in the Brookings Governmental Studies program. In preparing this book he benefited from consultations with many scholars and practitioners. He wishes especially to thank persons who reviewed discussions of individual countries: Peter Botsman, John C. Campbell, Laurent Chambaud, Dr. Pascal Chevit, Stephen Duckett, Robert G. Evans, Ullrich Heilemann, Terri Jackson, Marcus Kruse, Theodore J. Marmor, Annabelle May, Alan Maynard, Andreas Ryll, Markus Schneider, R. B. Scotton, and Clive Smee. He appreciates greatly the assistance of others who hosted conferences or research visits, including Earl Dick and the College of Commerce of the University of Saskatchewan; Ken Fyke and the Greater Victoria Hospital Society; the Goethe Institut of Boston; the Japan Society of New York; Monique Jérôme-Forget and the Institute for Research on Public Policy in Montreal; Alan Maynard and the University of York; Kate Moore and the Consumers Health Forum in Australia; and Aki Yoshikawa and the Comparative Health Policy Project at Stanford University.

White acknowledges an even greater debt to colleagues who read the first draft manuscript: Larry Brown, William A. Glaser, George D. Greenberg, Joseph Houska, Eric Peterson, Mark Peterson, and Thomas Rice. He learned much about health care policy from Mark Goldberg and other colleagues in the Health Care Study Group. At many points he was aided also by members of the Brookings community of scholars: Henry J. Aaron, John J. DiIulio, Jr., Christopher Foreman, Thomas Mann, Dahlia Remler, and, especially, Joshua Wiener. The author is thankful to Shannon Buchanan, Carole Plowfield, and Anthony J. Sheehan for research assistance, and to Cynthia Terrels for word processing support. Janet S. Mowery edited the manuscript; Eric Messick, Mary Anne Noyer, and Laurel Imig checked it for accuracy; Julia Petrakis prepared the index; and Ellen Garshick proofread the pages.

Most especially the author wishes to thank two scholars, William A. Glaser and Theodore R. Marmor, for advice, help, and criticism.

The views expressed here remain the author's alone and should not be ascribed to any of those whose assistance is gratefully acknowledged, nor to the trustees, officers, and other staff members of the Brookings Institution.

Bruce K. MacLaury
President

May 1995
Washington, D.C.

Contents

1

Introduction: Health Care Choices

*I*N 1993 and 1994, the U.S. government engaged in a massive conflict over reform of the nation's health care system. Unlike many other issues, the ills of American health care could be defined simply: health care costs too much and too many Americans go without needed care. Yet agreeing on a cure for those ills proved to be exceedingly difficult.

American observers of the two years of political struggle, in which a blizzard of charges and countercharges enveloped at least a dozen different plans and many dozens of issues, might conclude that guaranteeing access to and controlling the costs of health care is an extremely difficult and complex undertaking that is fraught with risk and uncertainties—a bold experiment in social engineering. From outside the United States, the issue looks a bit different.

The foreign perspective was nicely illustrated when I attended a conference about Canada's health care system in Saskatoon, Saskatchewan, in May 1993. Why, I was asked by Canadian health care scholars and practitioners, did Hillary Rodham Clinton think she could gather five hundred experts for three months and design the ideal health care system? After all, they pointed out, thousands of people in many countries had struggled for decades without finding the perfect system. But she doesn't have to design the perfect system, I replied. She just has to come up with something better than what the United States has now. In that case, they all asked, what was taking her so long?

Learning from Others

The reaction of my hosts on the Canadian prairie suggests an important conclusion about reforming American health care: No health

1

care system is perfect. Any proposal will have flaws. Therefore the right question is: Do measures exist that can improve conditions substantially within a reasonable amount of time?

If the goal is to do much better rather than to achieve perfection, the right answer is: The measures exist to achieve that goal.

Every other advanced industrial nation has virtually universal access to decent medical care, at much lower cost than in the United States. My Canadian hosts assumed we could select from among the measures used in their and other countries and design a program that improved our access and costs relatively easily. That is not to say that the United States could or should copy any country's institutions exactly. A history of any country's health care politics would show how inherited institutions and values constrained choices. Americans could not *adopt* Canada's, or Germany's, or any other country's structure. But they could *adapt* those approaches to America's inherited conditions.

Some Americans believe that the United States is unique and that it therefore cannot learn from other countries' experience. On its face, this theorem requires some unlikely corollaries. Australia, Canada, France, Germany, Japan, the United Kingdom, and all other advanced industrial countries guarantee health care to all their citizens. Their systems are very different from one another, but to say that the United States requires a system that is more different from all of theirs than they are from each other begs belief. Is America more different from Canada than Canada is from Japan? Are Australians more similar to Germans than to Americans? Do the British and French share systems of universal health coverage because of their cultural similarities? That would be news to both the British and the French.

Arguments that the United States cannot learn from other countries ignore the fact that, from popular culture to technology, modern life testifies to the ways ideas and practices flow across borders. People who face the same difficulties, for the same reasons, can count on some of the same responses to help. Thus Americans learned to employ Japanese methods of managing factories, and many of our current institutions of social protection, such as the social security system, were modeled on examples from overseas.

By the same token, health care is not a different phenomenon in the United States than in other countries. It is more expensive, yes.

But its basic dynamics are the same. They are grounded in technology and the sociology that follows from that technology.

In all industrialized nations there is an ever-increasing division of medical labor, caused by the increase in specialized knowledge. Hospitals evolved from institutions for mainly palliative care for poor people to temples of high technology. Although there are some differences in national norms about treatments—and variations within countries, too—research in one country is relevant in others, and innovations diffuse rapidly. Technology reshapes institutions and roles in roughly the same direction: for example, new forms of anesthesia have made surgery possible outside the hospital, challenging the hospitals' preeminence.

Physicians everywhere see themselves as professionals and resist regulation. They have developed similar ideologies and have even organized in response to similar "threats," such as the rise of medical clinics, in very different countries. Other participants in the health care system—economists, bureaucrats, nurses, allied medical professionals, and so on—everywhere believe physicians have too much influence.

The underlying economics of health care is as universal as all economics. The nature and incidence of health care costs is such that there is no advanced economy in which any but a distinct minority of medical services are purchased out-of-pocket, from personal or family cash flow or savings. Instead, each has versions of the approach that in chapter 2 I describe as shared savings.

In every country, unless the economy is growing very quickly, medical costs are likely to grow more quickly. Spiraling health care costs derive from the success of medical technology. New ways to treat conditions create longer life spans. The elderly consume more medical services than younger people and so have greater average medical expenses per person. Their longer life spans also mean that a larger share of the population is retired and not working, so the consumption of health care rises relative to the supply of productive workers. As populations age, therefore, the share of national product devoted to health care naturally rises, and policymakers in virtually every advanced country believe they face a health care cost crisis.

Because the challenges are common, responses around the world share many features. These features are one of the themes of this book, in which I explain what many countries do and how well their systems work. I call the range of strategies and institutions they have established the *international standard*. I believe that the United States can learn from other countries but understand that many Americans might not want to.

Whether the United States creates a system that guarantees health care to all Americans is a political choice, and anyone who infers that other countries made the choice because they had consensual political systems has not studied the politics. Australia's universal health insurance has existed only since 1984. Canada's was not fully implemented until 1971. France, Germany, and Japan were filling in gaps until the 1960s and 1970s. Many of the same forces that are most resistant in the United States, such as physicians worried about autonomy and small businesses objecting to any government taxes or mandates, had to be overcome everywhere. Was it less difficult elsewhere? Evidently so: they have done it, and the United States has not. But whenever national health care guarantees have been created, they have been strongly opposed by forces that claimed they were too radical a change.

Competing Solutions

An American political battle over health care that centered on understanding, interpreting, and slandering foreign experience and its relevance to the United States would have been a simpler debate, and this would have been a simpler book. Instead, the American reform struggle of 1993–94 involved both conflict over the international standard approaches and controversy over a supposedly uniquely American way to provide affordable health care to all Americans.

This second controversial approach was called *managed competition*. The push for managed competition was explicitly an attempt to avoid adapting other countries' methods, but the debate over these competing solutions barely deserved that name. This book fills in many of the gaps. I begin by describing and evaluating the international standard.

I have chosen six countries for comparison: Australia, Canada, France, Germany, Japan, and the United Kingdom. All except Australia are members of the "Group of Seven," the world's seven largest capitalist economies. Australia, Britain, and Canada, with which most Americans share a language and heritage, are the countries with which most Americans most easily identify. Japan and Germany are the countries most likely to be identified as "competitors," and are so cited in arguments that health care costs burden U.S. firms in international markets. Australia, Canada, and Germany are federal systems that provide examples of how authority can be allocated among levels of government. France and Australia have significant levels of supplementary private insurance in addition to national guarantees. France, Germany, and Japan all provide health insurance in a way that is neither directly part of the state nor part of for-profit competition.

Of these systems, the Canadian and German systems are used most often now as models for American proposals. Australia and France may be viewed as variations on, respectively, Canada and Germany. Japan and the United Kingdom are included both because their experience is sometimes made part of the policy argument and to further demonstrate that the core measures of the international standard are present even in those countries whose systems of health care finance and delivery have some aspects that Americans would be particularly unlikely to adopt.

International Standards

No two countries' systems are identical, yet certain similarities among the six other systems are prominent, particularly when compared with the U.S. system.

COVERAGE. All of these countries provide virtually universal coverage—a minimum of 99 percent—in a system of shared savings for health care. All achieve universal coverage by compelling individuals to participate in the system. Germany provides an alternative for 20 percent of the population, which is not required to join one of the "sickness funds." But that choice is limited to the people with the highest incomes, who, being well able to afford private insurance, are almost all insured in one manner or another.

Every country covers all "medically necessary" hospital and physician services and at a minimum provides pharmaceutical benefits for the poor and the elderly. In all cases the definition of medically necessary excludes "extras," such as private rooms and elective cosmetic surgery, but it never explicitly excludes treatment for painful or life-threatening conditions.

All six countries have some degree of inequality because the minority of the population with enough money can buy extra services. But that "tiering" of health care is exactly opposite the pattern in the United States, where most people have fairly decent coverage but a large segment has much less. In other countries, everybody is guaranteed decent standard coverage, and a few have more. One approach creates a (weak) "safety net" for the poor; the other creates an "escape valve" for the well-to-do.[1]

FINANCING. In the United States, discussions of how to finance health care tend to focus on whether insurers can charge different prices to different people (whether they can risk-rate or should community-rate) and on how to subsidize individuals who cannot afford the price. Ultimately this approach requires an assessment of each individual's income, and a separate, precise subsidy to each person or family that is helped. The international standard for financing health care is very different in both theory and practice.

In the other countries, the vast majority of health care costs are not paid by people "buying" insurance in the same way that they purchase other commodities. Instead, they contribute to a system. Their contribution is determined by rules designed to relate costs to ability to pay and to gather enough money to pay for the resulting health care. If everybody pays according to these rules, there should be little need for separate, specially calculated subsidies to individuals.

The contributions are related to ability to pay in one of two ways. The first is to charge not a flat price but a proportion of income—especially of wages. This could be a tax paid to the government or a premium paid to separate health insurance funds. Often the charge is paid by both employers and employees, much like the American taxes that pay for government social insurance programs such as social security and medicare. The second approach is to finance health care from the general revenues of government. Because these funds come from taxes that also tend to be proportional to income, the basic effect is the same. People who earn less pay less. People who earn more pay more.

In all six countries the cost of covering families is related only weakly, if at all, to family size. Single people and two-income families help pay for single-income families with children. The young and the old also contribute by the same rules. But because payments are related to income, a person who earns low wages at the beginning of a career does not pay as much as an older, more established worker. In all these cases the rules of contribution mean that, over the course of an average life, a person subsidizes others at some points and is subsidized at others. Health care costs remain a fairly steady proportion of income throughout one's life.

COST CONTROL. Each of these countries limits costs through systems of regulation. These involve standard fee schedules or budgeting—usually both. All have fee schedules for medical procedures. Even if the schedule is not binding, as in Australia, or has exceptions, as in France and Germany, it affects the large majority of prices.

All except Japan directly budget a large part of health care spending. Australia, France, Canada, and Britain budget the hospitals; Germany and to an extent Britain and Canada budget ambulatory care. Japan uses fees to control costs more stringently than do any of the other countries.

Each country also limits capital investment for the largest part of hospital care. Most do it through direct budgeting, but some limits are established by fee regulation in Japan and by a combination of licensing and criminal sanctions in France. All use their capital investment controls to prevent a medical technology "arms race" among hospitals.

National cultures and political happenstance affected how each country reached the international common ground of financial arrangements. Despite their similarities, many aspects of these countries' health care systems differ. After an introduction to the terms of health care debate and the American health care system, the first half of this book describes the similarities and differences within the international standard. It includes much detail, both as evidence of similarity and to show that choices can be made within the similar approaches.

Managed Competition

In the U.S. debate the theory of managed competition had many variants, but all diverged in some basic ways from the international standard.

COVERAGE. The major documents that put managed competition on the American policy map called for ensuring health care coverage for all Americans.[2] But there were many forms of managed competition proposed, and many did not provide for universal coverage. Some would have allowed the survival of medicaid as a distinctly inferior lower tier of medical care.

FINANCING. The basic logic of managed competition did not say what to do about inequalities in ability to pay for health insurance. Any such proposals would be tacked on to a managed competition structure.[3] But it did include two points that implied financing different from either the American status quo or the international standard. Unlike in the United States, the managed competition proposals would have banned (or in their diluted forms restricted) risk-rating, the practice by which American insurers charge higher prices to people who are more likely to be sick. Inequalities in health would not affect prices. Unlike the international standard, the managed competition theory required that people pay some portion of their health care out-of-pocket, as a purchase in the market. They would be buying a commodity, not contributing to a system.

COST CONTROL. As part of its theory of cost control, managed competition would require that people purchase insurance in a market. In the international standard, even if there are many separate insurance funds, costs are controlled through rules about payment and budgets that are applied to (almost) the entire system. Managed competition would divide health care financing into competing plans, each of which would try to reduce its own costs through *managed care*. Each payer would seek to negotiate lower prices with providers, or control the volume of services by its providers, separately. Those that provided better combinations of cost and services would be rewarded in the market with higher prices or more business. Because individuals would pay out-of-pocket, they would have an incentive to choose the more "efficient" plans.

Managed competition, unlike the international standard, has never been tried. Whether and with what consequences it could control health care costs would depend on the actual incentives from the competition and on whether competing plans successfully managed their health care. In the second half of this book I begin by analyzing experience with managed care and the logic of the proposed competition and then consider the possible implementation of managed competition by discussing two prototype plans that were part of the 1993–94 American debate. Both parts of my assessment reveal severe weaknesses in the case for managed competition. The Clinton administration sought to address many of these difficulties with its own plan, and this book discusses both why the Clinton approach was more likely to work and the major problems that remained.

Failures and a Synthesis

The obstacles to health care reform in America in 1993–94 were many, but one was the immense confusion generated by the presence of two competing models, neither of which was well understood. The Clinton plan attempted to merge managed competition with the international standard. That made some policy sense but proved virtually impossible to explain. The administration barely tried to explain some particularly complicated but significant aspects of the plan, such as its cost controls.

This failure to communicate occurred in part because Bill Clinton became trapped in his own rhetoric—not just his health care rhetoric, but his broader political rhetoric as well. It was not just the rhetoric of health care but of a broader political stance. He proposed government action to solve or ameliorate social ills but wanted the activity to occur outside of government bureaucracies. If that could work, it might appeal to the dichotomy within the American public: majorities want services but do not like the government.

Unfortunately for the president and perhaps the country, as explained in chapters 8 and 9, the strategy would not work. The evidence that managed competition could control costs was too weak to overcome obstacles that have been built into the legislative process in order to prevent increases in the federal deficit. Implementation of either a strong version of managed competition or the Clinton compromise required extensive mandates and regulations that were opposed by almost all of the social forces that objected to adapting the international standard.

Both politicians and other policy analysts wished to believe that, rather than choosing among versions of the international standard and managed competition, they could do enough with halfway measures. In this book's conclusion I explain why most versions of that approach would accomplish little. Yet there was one partial measure, freeing the states to set up their own systems of universal coverage and cost control, that could represent real progress.

While the national battle raged, similar conflicts were occurring in many states. A range of federal regulations and programs made state reform even more difficult than it had to be, by foreclosing many of the measures of the international standard. The conclusion therefore explains the measures that the federal government could take to help states choose their own approaches.

Ending there, however, would beg the question of what approach makes the most sense for the United States. The evidence clearly favors adapting the international standard over managed competition. But there are good reasons to try to build the best features of the managed competition approach into an American reform. The conclusion suggests how that might be done. The result would be different from any other system in the world—but similar enough to guarantee lower costs and universal access without sacrificing quality of care. Whether it will ever be enacted by any level of American government remains to be seen.

Plan of the Book

The complexities of health care policy, of doing justice to seven countries, and of explaining two approaches require a long book. Much of the argument includes detail that some readers may choose to skim, just to see that the generalizations are based on evidence. Other readers may find that this detail is the book's most useful part, either as an introduction to other nations' approaches or as a critique of American proposals. I have tried to allow readers to choose, by providing a structure that allows people to find both the basic points and the full argument.

Part one, American Health Care and the International Standard, consists of chapters 2 through 6. Chapter 2 begins the analysis by providing basic data comparing American performance with the international norm and summarizing the major issues in health care policy. Chapter 3 describes the current American health care system. By identifying the major aspects of this most complex system in the world, I highlight the features that will seem, after comparison, most questionable. But I also identify those features that, because they are not easy to change, set limits on the measures that the United States can adapt from other countries.

Chapters 4, 5, and 6 provide descriptions and analysis of the six comparison countries. Chapter 4 focuses on the two main models, Canada and Germany. Chapter 5 provides less thorough descriptions of health care in Australia, France, Japan, and the United Kingdom. It documents the ubiquity of the methods of coverage, financing, and cost control summarized above. It also shows that many modifications of the Canadian and German models are possible. In Chapter 6 I evaluate the international experience. I discuss the extent to which differences in quality or other factors might justify American costs and conclude that they do not. I consider the range of choice offered by international experience, identify areas where there may be more choice than some reformers think, and highlight subjects that have not received enough attention.

Part two, Competing Solutions, begins with a discussion of the theory of managed competition. Chapter 7 relates managed competition to a broader theme of international health care reform, the "internal market." It explains the theory and its presumptions, in order to show both its attractions and its weaknesses. That requires some further discussion of how some of the measures on which the theory relies, forms of managed care, have performed in the United States. The chapter concludes by analyzing the internal market reforms of the British National Health Service. I argue that these measures do not provide any support for managed competition within the United States but have some merit within the British context.

Chapter 8 provides a form of thought experiment about how managed competition would work in the United States. I look at two prototype bills, the Chafee and Cooper-Grandy proposals (introduced, respectively, by Senator John Chafee (R-R.I.) and Representatives Jim Cooper (D-Tenn.) and Fred Grandy (R-Iowa). In addition to the theoretical problems, managed competition would face two other broad difficulties. First, in order to win political support, the legislative proposals compromised important parts of the original theory. Second, measures that theorists consider fundamental would be exceedingly difficult to implement.

Chapter 9 reviews the Clinton compromise. The administration found solutions to the most severe implementation difficulties, but only by dropping one major aspect of the theory and moving toward the international standard for financing. It improved on managed competition's theory of cost control also by moving toward the international standard, with "backup" fee regulation and budgeting. The Clinton proposal still had two sets of problems. On the one hand, synthesizing competition and budgets would have been difficult to implement. On the other, it lost the support of managed competition's true believers and so had no political advantage over a plan that would have more directly adapted the international standard.

Chapter 10 then relates the substance of health care reform in America to its politics. The approach presented relies more on the international standard than on managed competition for reasons of both substance and politics. The evidence does not support claims that managed competition will work better, and managed competition in the end was a distinctly minority position. It was attractive rhetoric because of what it was not: neither the international standard nor the status quo. Yet managed competition, done right, is a system of extensive regulation that would restrict all parties: insurers and providers and patients. It was attractive to each group only without the restrictions. In the conclusion I suggest an approach that would be both substantively and politically superior.

Part One
American Health Care and the
International Standard

2

Challenges and Choices for American Health Care

*H*EALTH care reform became an issue in America because of questions of cost and access. The basic differences between arrangements in other countries and in the United States are associated with one huge difference in results: American health care costs far more.

Tables 2-1 and 2-2 and figures 2-1 and 2-2 display the data. As table 2-1 shows, American health care costs in 1991 totaled 13.4 percent of the U.S. gross domestic product (GDP). Canada was second, on this table and in the world, at 10.0 percent. Put differently, Canadian costs, as a share of the economy, were three-quarters those of the United States. France, at 9.1 percent, was third.

Yet as the table also shows, the differences were not always so great. Only since the early 1980s have American health care costs as a share of the economy risen much more quickly than those in other countries, as figure 2-1 makes clear. And that suggests an important point: *Other countries' health care arrangements do not guarantee better cost control. Instead, other countries give governments and insurers the capacity to control costs if they choose to do so.* During the 1960s and 1970s, other countries frequently increased medical costs even more than the United States, because their citizens were willing to pay that price. During the 1980s health care costs aroused considerable anxiety in all the countries discussed in this volume. In the United States the efforts of government, employers, and insurers to control costs were continual and extensive. Managed care proliferated; employers frequently changed the policies available to their employees; employees paid larger shares of premiums; providers reorganized themselves in response to new demands; and costs spiraled upward. Policymakers in other countries

15

TABLE 2-1. *Total Health Care Spending as a Percent of GDP*

Years	USA	Australia	Canada	France	Germany	Japan	UK
1961	5.5	5.3	5.8	4.5	4.8	3.4	4.0
1966	5.9	4.7	6.0	5.4	5.5	4.6	4.2
1971	7.5	5.9	7.4	6.0	6.3	4.7	4.6
1976	8.6	7.5	7.2	7.0	8.1	5.6	5.5
1981	9.6	7.5	7.5	7.9	8.7	6.6	6.1
1986	10.8	8.0	8.8	8.5	8.6	6.6	6.1
1991	13.4	8.6	10.0	9.1	8.5	6.6	6.6
Average annual growth rate (in percent)							
1961–71	3.24	1.07	2.34	2.99	2.64	3.10	1.40
1971–81	2.46	2.41	0.22	2.69	3.35	3.58	2.84
1981–91	3.43	1.46	2.88	1.42	−0.24	−0.03	0.87

Source: OECD Health Data, CREDES.

were more successful at controlling costs because their arrangements gave them stronger tools.

Some analysts argue that measuring health care expenses as a portion of GDP is the wrong test, because the ratio depends on the denominator, economic growth, as much as on the numerator, health care cost growth. Therefore a country that does a good job of controlling health care costs might seem to have done poorly because its economy grew only slightly. But the criticism begs a question: if your income is growing more slowly than your health care costs, shouldn't you be trying harder to control costs? Still, the data could be deceptive, so table 2-2 and figure 2-2 display the trends in terms of spending per capita. Because currency values change, and exchange rates often have more to do with international trade flows than with the ability to purchase goods in a given country, spending is expressed here in terms of purchasing power parities. This method compares health care expenses in terms of ability to purchase a market basket of goods, translated into U.S. dollars.

Because GDP per capita is higher in the United States, the purchasing power comparison shows the United States spending even more, relative to other countries, than the GDP comparison. In 1991 what the United States spent would have bought twice as much in comparable goods in Australia or Japan, more than 70 percent more in Germany, and almost 50 percent more in Canada. Because GDP grew more quickly in most countries, the comparison does dampen

TABLE 2-2. *Health Care Spending per Capita in Current Prices, PPP$*

Years	USA	Australia	Canada	France	Germany	Japan	UK
1961	150	106	118	84	102	34	83
1966	222	128	169	140	154	75	110
1971	379	236	289	231	248	142	157
1976	672	471	483	429	510	280	297
1981	1,222	760	854	805	925	587	525
1986	1,822	1,072	1,364	1,135	1,215	839	741
1991	2,867	1,407	1,915	1,650	1,659	1,267	1,035
Average annual growth rate (in percent)							
1961–71	9.69	8.30	9.36	10.68	9.24	15.24	6.62
1971–81	12.41	12.42	11.44	13.28	14.08	15.24	12.82
1981–91	8.91	6.35	8.41	7.44	6.01	8.00	7.01

Source: See table 2-1.

PPP $ = purchasing power parities

the difference in trends. But figure 2-2 still shows that in the 1980s other countries gained much greater control of their costs.

One may choose to spend more for better access to and quality of health care, and defenders of the American status quo claim that the United States does. But this book's analysis of other countries' systems and comparative data should cast great doubt on arguments that greater choice, sicker patients, or higher quality of care justifies the American level of spending. Instead, America spends more because of how it has chosen to organize its health care system. The organization of health care can be divided into three topics.

The first issue is what we mean by health care, its *definition*. Where does the health care system stop and the rest of the world begin? For example, are school lunches a health care program? What about drug interdiction? These issues determine the objects of reform.

The second issue is how health care is *financed*. How is money collected, from whom, on what terms? To whom is the money paid, in what amounts, on what basis? These issues most directly affect the economic stakes in the system and are therefore of greatest interest to many policy players (particularly employers and government budgeters).

Last is how health care is provided, the system of *delivery*. What kinds of providers exist, how do they relate to each other, and how do patients choose providers (or vice versa)? These issues have most to do with the effectiveness of treatment and how people experience care.

FIGURE 2-1. *National Health Spending as Share of Gross Domestic Product, 1961 through 1991, Seven Countries*

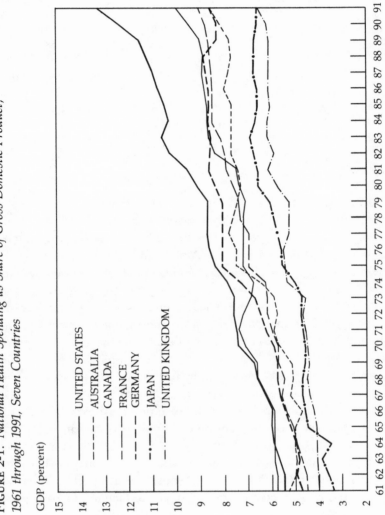

Source: OECD Health Data, CREDES.

FIGURE 2-2. *Total Health Spending per Capita at Current Prices, PPP$*

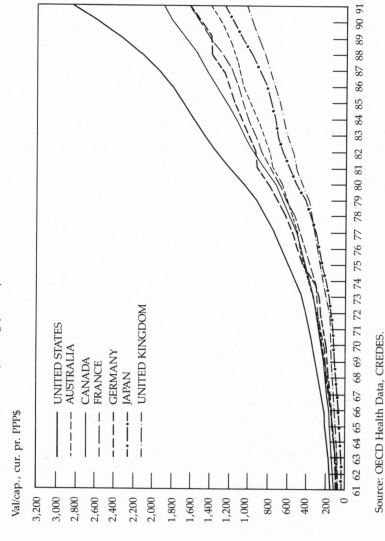

Val/cap., cur. pr. PPP$

Source: OECD Health Data, CREDES.

Broadly conceived, American reform that adapted the international standard would focus on financing; in contrast, managed competition would emphasize changing the delivery system. The former would seek savings by paying less per unit of care; the latter would change the pattern of care. Adapting the international standard would require the most change in (and in some reforms the elimination of) financial institutions, the private insurers. Managed competition would require the most change for health care providers (possibly driving some of them out of the market).

Neither approach would change the definition of care. Arguments about the boundaries of health care attract many analysts and many political factions. Yet proposals based on a revised definition of health care have not been a major theme of the American reform debate, for good reason.[1]

Defining Health Care

Food and shelter, dietary habits, whether and how much people smoke or consume alcohol, whether they live somewhere with much crime or dangerous traffic, and a raft of other matters determine levels of illness and injury in a population. These illnesses and injuries can be considered the input to a health care system; its efforts to fix the problems are its output, and the overall results are health outcomes. From this perspective it should be evident that two different health care systems could be equally proficient at treating disease and injury, but the health of the population in one could be worse than in the other simply because its problems were worse to begin with.

A broad definition of health issues therefore could focus on "wellness" rather than curing disease. Health policy could be conceived as including nutrition programs, the fifty-five-mile-per-hour speed limit, large taxes on tobacco, or any number of other things that promote health but are unrelated to delivery of medical services per se.

Difficulties with the "Wellness" Model

On the political left, emphasizing the health effects of income inequalities strengthens arguments for income redistribution. A focus on diet and other "holistic" concerns, on the grounds that these would give people more control of their own lives, fits the left's mistrust of the medical establishment, which some believe serves corporate capitalism and makes people dependent.

On the right, the argument that differences in health outcomes are caused by behaviors, such as smoking and drinking and shooting each other, makes the payoff from finance and delivery reform seem less certain and therefore becomes a reason not to change the status quo.[2]

In the center, budgeters worried most about cost control can claim that greater spending on programs such as nutrition aid would allow lower spending on medical care. Such arguments can be used to justify doing less about medical care and sometimes making budget cuts.

Attractiveness across political factions is not, unfortunately, a good criterion for reform. President Clinton was criticized for the scope and complexity of his proposal. Yet a broader definition of health policy would require even more sweeping proposals. If the "real problems" are the pathologies of poverty, environmental degradation, and crime, then reform requires new nutrition, housing, and general poverty policy, sweeping new environmental regulations, and massive reforms of the police and criminal justice systems. Any such proposals raise complicated issues of justice and efficiency, not to mention political support, that make reforming the rest of health care policy look relatively tractable.

If health care policy includes everything, then it means nothing. The "medical model" includes a discrete something: delivery and financing arrangements that can be identified, related to each other, and governed. The institutions that carry out those arrangements cannot be expected to meet all social needs, any more than the schools can replace parents. Conservatives who imply that government should address issues of behavior rather than health care financing are, in effect, saying that government should define its task as the most thorough imaginable regulation of daily life.

Some basic aspects of wellness promotion, such as immunizations, prenatal care, and screening for breast cancer, can and should be part of the medical care system. But it is the medical model, not the wellness model, that responds to the core concern of average citizens. They worry not about the average health of the population but about their own health once they are sick. Nobody ever died of short life expectancy. There is no "right" to be healthy, because that is not in society's power to provide. But there are arguments for equity in access to treatment once sick. National health care guarantees are ways to protect individuals against the fear, pain, and expense of illness. Subsidies are based on empathy for individual people. Insurance is based on personal fear. For all these reasons liberals who emphasize the importance of wellness are putting second things first.

By the same token, prevention is not always better than cure. It certainly is not cheaper.[3] Even when it saves money in the long run, prevention probably requires more spending in the short run. Spending on child nutrition, for example, can reduce later illnesses related to malnutrition, but it will do little or nothing to reduce the incidence of disease in the first year the money is spent. Therefore spending on such prevention cannot replace spending on care, and it should not help with budget deficits. There is no good budgetary argument for prevention as a replacement for cure.

Public health measures should be funded well because they are good policy. Education campaigns, financial incentives (such as tobacco taxes), and other efforts to change behavior are desirable for their own sake. But policymakers should resist seductive arguments that they can avoid reform of health care finance and delivery by focusing on subjects for which policy instruments are even less reliable, and social disruption could be even greater, for less immediate return.

Practical Issues of Definition

Deciding what to include in the medical model is difficult enough. There are three broad issues: what constitutes effective care, what is necessary care, and the consequences of insurance.

EFFECTIVENESS. If people think some form of care does not work, they are unlikely to accept national policies to pay for it. But effectiveness is not so easy to measure. The French and Germans pay for some spa treatments. Should they? Mental health benefits vary widely. Pharmaceutical treatment for some conditions is so obviously effective that it is normally covered. But what about psychiatric therapy? To some people, paying into a fund that pays for other people's therapy is like being forced to pay someone else's church dues.

NECESSITY. New information can add or subtract treatments from the definition of effective care. Definitions of necessary care also change with transformations of society. Once upon a time, long-term care could be left to families—partly because families were geographically closer and partly because few people lived long enough to be much of a burden.[4] When there were fewer very old people, physical therapy to improve their independence did not seem so pressing; now it is a major medicare expense. Although social trends are similar from country to country, populations may value different care differently. Insurance coverage for spa treatments, dental care, long-term care, and mental health care differs from nation to nation and from plan to plan within the United States.

INSURABILITY. Each form of care also raises peculiar problems of insurability.[5] Insurance cannot work if it creates the need against which it is supposed to protect people. That is, the ability to pay with someone else's money should not raise consumption of all medical goods. No one gets a cardiac bypass for the heck of it; neither does anyone purposely contract the flu or get in a car accident because insurance will pay the medical bills. But mental health spending some-times involves dependency relationships between professionals and patients, in which the need is defined by a transaction between the two more than by anything others could measure. Dentistry has strong cosmetic elements, and the boundaries of necessary and unnecessary cosmetic treatment are hard to define. Long-term care often involves support services, such as cooking and cleaning, that could be provided by family—unlike most medical services.

In each of these cases, there is reason to fear that the act of insuring will increase demand and cost. Thus though agreeing on a definition of care may not solve America's health care problem, it is a major issue. What should be guaranteed to all citizens? In the absence of a clear objective standard, Americans might look at what other countries have decided.

But insurance may have similar effects for other types of treatment as well. The question is not just whether a condition will be treated, but in what ways and with how much intensity. That brings us to questions of financing and delivery, and especially the role of insur-ance itself.

Financing Health Care

Is health care a commodity like any other, or a public good, such as police services, that fits poorly in a market? Many countries have

decided it is not a normal commodity but also not something government should provide directly.

Why Health Care Is Not a Normal Market Commodity

In an ideal market, suppliers do not have the authority to tell consumers what they need to buy. Consumers have the information and
flexibility necessary to shop around for the best deal. There are many
buyers and sellers, enabling "relatively free and easy entry into the
market by new buyers or sellers," "no one of whom is so big as to
have a significant influence on the market price."[6]

Health care markets cannot be ideal. Patients cannot know enough
about medical care; they often are too sick to shop; the job of the
doctor is to tell her customer what he needs; hospitals frequently have
local monopoly power, and creating new hospitals is very difficult.

Many markets are not ideal. That is an argument for regulation but
not for dramatically altering the market mechanism. In a normal market, the volume and variety of goods and services still is determined
by individual choices. Because purchasers have only limited incomes,
when they consider buying some good they have to think about the
other goods on which they will not be able to spend that money—
what is known as the "opportunity cost." Total spending on a particular set of goods and services—food, movies, housing, or whatever—
reflects the sum of these constraints on individuals.

Mismatches between individual desires to consume and ability to
pay are not a problem in the market but one of the points of the market.
In a market there is no such thing as a "need"; there are only "wants."
Market prices force people to prioritize what they want. Neither the
United States nor any other modern country distributes health care
services through normal market mechanisms because consumers and
voters, in the face of pain and fear of death, object to price constraints
on the purchase of health care. Individuals wish to avoid constraints
on themselves and find them hard to accept (though many of us do)
as a consequence for others. Within limits, other commodities, such
as food and shelter, might also be considered needs rather than wants,
and societies can choose to guarantee some minimum of each.[7] Health
care is especially subject to modifications of the market mechanism
because that is in the self-interest of many nonaltruistic persons, and
the direct incidence of pain and fear in the face of illness provides the
most direct tug on human sympathies.

INDIVIDUAL SELF-INTEREST. In most circumstances, people get around the constraint of limited incomes by delaying a purchase, anticipating the need and saving for it, or borrowing and paying later, with interest. These safety valves work poorly for health care. Delay is usually unattractive, and often, such as for setting a broken limb or treating pneumonia, a very bad idea. Saving is not practical for serious illnesses, which can be very expensive and may require treatment before enough money is in the bank. Seriously ill people are very poor credit risks.

To protect themselves, individuals join systems of *shared savings*. They pool their money, contributing at regular intervals. When another member needs to spend, the pool pays, and when you need to spend, it pays. But only a fraction of members have large expenses in any one year, so no single person needs to contribute as much as if everyone saved separately, and an adequate amount can be collected fairly quickly.[8]

Private insurance, public insurance, and national health services all are forms of shared savings that protect against an unpredictable risk of health care expense. People with private insurance pay premiums and then collect benefits as payment for services. In public insurance systems, people pay taxes and collect as they would for private insurance. In countries with national health services people pay taxes and collect benefits directly, in kind.

Because all of these systems pool and use shared savings, a person does not use her own money when she consumes medical services. People who are not spending their own money are more willing to spend than those who pay out-of-pocket. Many analysts conclude that insurance is the reason for spiraling health care costs, because it eliminates price constraints at the point of service. But that is the whole purpose of health insurance. And that is why insurance requires nonmarket methods of cost control.

The real choice is among health insurance with regulation, insurance without cost control, or no insurance at all.

SUBSIDY ISSUES. Only people who are very wealthy or both very healthy and confident are likely to object to the idea of health insurance. But many could object to helping pay for other people's insurance.

What does "helping to pay" mean? That depends first on whether you believe health insurance should charge more to people who are more likely to get sick: whether health insurance is a form of *casualty insurance* or *social insurance*.[9]

Providers of casualty insurance normally charge people according to a risk factor. People with wood houses thus may pay more for fire insurance than people with brick or stucco houses. Calculation of risk, called *risk-rating*, and writing policies to fit, or *underwriting*, is the companies' job.

But there are reasons to think health insurance is different. A person may choose a brick or a wood house as part of a series of trade-offs; but he does not choose his genes or age or gender or many other factors that affect health risk. Further, the best indicator of health risk is an existing illness, or *preexisting condition*. A health insurer that raises a sick person's rates or refuses him coverage is doing something more akin to canceling fire insurance during a fire than to assessing risk in advance.

Private health insurance first developed, in the United States and elsewhere, by charging a basic rate to all members of a community, or *community-rating*. Over time in the United States that principle has been destroyed by the private market's competition. Still, the beneficiaries of risk-rating—young and healthy persons in safe jobs—might consider community-rating a subsidy from themselves to others.

One issue then is whether insurers should risk-rate or community-rate. The other is whether payments should be related to ability to pay. Whether you support income-based subsidies for any purpose is a matter of your personal values, but in all societies support for subsidies depends on the good or service involved. No modern country, for example, expects people to compete in a market to buy elementary and secondary education.[10] None objects to competition to buy televisions.

All seven countries in this study, the United States included, have substantial income-based subsidies for the costs of health care. They may be justified by high-sounding values such as "rights" and "solidarity," but self-interest is also a factor. Financial circumstances may not be as likely to change as health status, yet few incomes are secure; even people with good jobs cannot count on keeping them in an unstable economy. Even a person who can protect herself might not be sure of protecting her children and parents.

Subsidies based on income therefore allow people to protect themselves and their families against risks throughout the life cycle. People pay more for the elderly and the poor as part of a compact, in which they expect others to pay when they are older or if they become poor. In the United States, medicare is a system of shared savings against the risk of high medical expenses in old age, just as social security is shared savings for pensions.

Neither individual interest nor community sympathy extends to everything that might be defined as medical care. If something is relatively cheap, such as over-the-counter medication, there is no reason not to allocate it in the market. If the efficacy of a form of treatment is not accepted by a clear majority of the community—a good working definition of "alternative medicine"—then people will not agree on saving for it. But these examples support the basic point: the size and unpredictability of medical expenses, and agreement that services are necessary and should not be forgone on account of cost, cause societies to find nonmarket ways to guarantee that some types of care are paid for.

Financing Issues

In creating a system of shared savings, normally in the form of social insurance, each nation must first decide who should be included. Second, it must decide what care to include. More coverage may mean more costs. But it is not quite that simple, because if expensive forms of delivery are covered and less expensive forms are not, people might forgo the latter and end up needing more of the former.

The third choice is the form of savings. This book describes four major options: general revenue taxation, premiums or payroll taxes paid to government, premiums paid to nonprofit funds that are governed differently from either government bureaus or private firms, and premiums paid to private firms.

The fourth decision is who will subsidize whom and how large the subsidies will be. Within governments, subsidy issues often involve not only individuals but also regional interests. In federal systems, for instance, there are arguments that richer states should assist poorer states. But even in Britain and France, geographic representation in the legislature makes regional disparities an issue.

These choices are sometimes contested with weapons of political symbolism. They nevertheless can have real substantive consequences, especially for cost and complexity.

Payment Issues

Health care financing includes not just who pays for what, but to whom the money is paid, how it is paid, and how much is paid. Some analysts distinguish the allocation of payments from financing, but here we will consider them together.[11]

Hospitals, doctors, and other providers may be paid by charges per service: this is called *fee-for-service medicine*. In America hospitals charge for individual aspirins if they can get away with it. Most other countries pay physicians per service, and even more pay per prescription for pharmaceuticals. Another method of allocation calls for an agreed-upon sum to be paid to a provider for all services provided during a year. For a physician this would be a salary; for a hospital, a budget. In between lies a range of payment mechanisms. Physicians may be paid a part-time salary, called a *sessional fee*. Sessions normally are defined as half a work day, and a hospital, for example, might pay a subspecialist, whose services are not needed full time, for five sessions per week. Hospitals may be paid a lump sum for each day of care, except for a limited set of extra services: a *day rate*. Hospitals may also be paid a lump sum for treatment of a patient who has received a given diagnosis; in America's medicare system this is called the *prospective payment system (PPS) for diagnosis-related groups (DRGs)*. At a higher level of aggregation is the payment of one fee for all treatment for a person for a year, whatever he or she may need; this per capita payment is known as a *capitation*. In Great Britain, for example, a general practitioner receives a capitation payment to cover all care within certain bounds for each patient on her list. An American health maintenance organization (HMO) receives a capitation to cover all possible care for each of its patients.

In general, the more aggregated the level of payment, the less the payers know about what they are buying. That makes overseers nervous, especially when they are bureaucrats, who believe their job is to keep records. But it is also much harder for providers to manipulate and increase charges in a highly aggregated system. It is easier to invent extra tests on a cancer patient than extra cancers.

Another issue is whether the same fee is paid for all services of a certain type, according to a *fee schedule*. All fee schedules have two elements. One is the ratio between two fees. For example, the charge for an initial office visit might be twice that of a return visit, and the fee for a breast biopsy might be two-fifths of the fee for a liver biopsy. These *relative values* can be expressed as a series of points per service. Then the actual fees depend on how much is paid for each point, the *conversion factor*.

Relative values determine the relative incomes of providers, so are very controversial within the medical profession. They are of interest to policymakers because they provide incentives to supply more of some forms of care than of others. For any set of relative values the conversion factor determines both actual incomes of providers and total costs to payers. Within some limits, therefore, payers care more about the conversion factor and may be willing to let physicians work out the relative values among themselves.

Another question is whether fee schedules determine what the provider can charge or only what the insurer will pay. Physicians everywhere want the right to charge more, and systems provide a variety of options, ranging from practice outside the context of the national guarantees to direct extra charges. In the latter case, the physician bills the patient directly for the portion of the charge that exceeds the amount on the fee schedule. This is called extra billing.[12]

In many cases, policymakers have decided that patients should pay some amount out-of-pocket in order to discourage frivolous use of services. This cost sharing takes three basic forms: a copayment, a deductible, and coinsurance. A copayment is a flat fee per service— for example, $10 for an office visit to a dermatologist. A deductible is an amount that a beneficiary must pay before the insurance begins to contribute—for example, $250 in expenses before the insurance begins to contribute. Coinsurance requires that the beneficiary pay a proportion of the bill—for instance, 20 percent of hospitalization costs. Cost sharing, in contrast to extra billing, does not increase provider incomes. Normally a physician can choose to accept only the insurer's share; this is called *accepting assignment*.

The form of payment can affect the health care system in many ways. Highly aggregated payments are less easily manipulated by providers who seek to multiply charges but can provide a contrary incentive to do less than is necessary. Whether cost sharing reduces total costs is controversial, but it surely transfers some from the insurance fund to the consumers of services. Fee schedules can be used to influence both costs and the kinds of care that are delivered. Extra billing and cost sharing can affect access to services. Greater and more appropriate regulation of payments is a major reason why the other countries in this study are able to provide more equal access to care and lower costs than the United States.

Delivering Health Care

The quality, cost, and accessibility of medical care are also affected by how care is delivered. These issues include the types of doctors and hospitals available, how individuals choose their providers, and links between physicians and between physicians and hospitals.

Physicians and Hospitals

A central relationship in the provision of health care is the relationship between the physician and the hospital. To begin with, what kind of care is provided in the hospital, and what care is provided outside? Inpatient care is provided to patients who stay in the hospital overnight; ambulatory care is provided by physicians (or other professionals) in offices outside the hospital; and outpatient care is ambulatory care provided by a hospital through a clinic.[13]

The modern hospital developed its prominence by being the doctor's workshop, the place where she could find all the tools for modern medicine. While more and more high-technology services can be provided outside the hospital walls, the hospital remains the center for critical care, and hospital care is the largest category of medical expense. Physicians practicing in hospitals provide care as part of exceedingly complex organizations that limit their autonomy. But the physician remains the crucial operator within these systems, and the contractual relationship between the hospital and the doctor is a key component of any health care system.

In all countries the house staff, physicians who receive salaries from hospitals, includes interns who have just graduated from medical school and residents who are training in specialties. All systems have some complement of salaried professors, who are paid for teaching and research and provide clinical services as well. In the United States and Canada, however, most of the physicians supervising the treatment of patients are not house staff but physicians who have both office-based practices and admitting privileges at a hospital. In France, Germany, Japan, and the United Kingdom, the house staff largely includes these more senior physicians. There is a greater distinction, especially in Germany, between physicians who provide ambulatory care and those based in hospitals.

The differences between hospitals that rely on salaried house staff and those that rely on office-based physicians with admitting privileges are myriad. Salaried staff have less incentive to generate business (though they still may overtreat out of professional pride or curiosity). Salaried staff are part of a hierarchy under the authority of the chief of each clinical service. Their activities can be coordinated and they can be rewarded and punished far more easily than can doctors in a system that uses the admitting-privilege model. Whether having salaried staff is good or bad, however, depends on the quality of the chief of service. The hierarchical model may discourage innovation and criticism of the chief.

It is easier to coordinate treatment within a hospital if the physician in charge of each patient is in the hospital full time, but sometimes the coordination of inpatient and ambulatory care can be difficult. In a system that grants doctors admitting privileges, doctors have financial incentives to hospitalize patients who visit their offices; if the two spheres are separate, office-based physicians have reason to avoid hospitalization, because at that point they lose both control of care and access to fees.

The relationship between hospitals and doctors matters in other ways as well. If doctors can use expensive capital equipment only by using the hospital as their workshop, then controlling hospital investment is an effective way to control costs. If a doctor refers a patient for elective surgery to the hospital as an institution, there is less chance that the patient will have to wait than if the referral is to a specific consultants (specialist) within the hospital (as in the United Kingdom), or if an admitting physician seeks a bed from his own quota.[14] But the patient will have less choice about who provides the surgery.

Many health care policy analysts seek a third model for the relationship between doctors and hospitals, in which the hospital and doctors are part of the same health maintenance organization. The physicians have admitting privileges to the hospital but do not have financial incentives to overtreat because they are not paid separately for each service. They may practice as a group rather than as independent practitioners or salaried subordinates to the chief of service. From the standpoint of the issues raised above, such an integrated health maintenance organization sounds like a superior form of delivery.

Managed competition has attracted many analysts because it promised to create a world of such HMOs. But as chapter 7 argues, there must be serious doubt that it could do so, for two reasons. Patients and physicians tend not to prefer this form of delivery in spite of its theoretical advantages. And building these organizations properly is very difficult.

Hospitals and Other Institutions

In addition to the relationships between hospitals and doctors, the delivery of health care involves relationships among hospitals themselves and between hospitals and other organizations. Many people who need simple nursing and monitoring do not need the expensive physical and human infrastructure of a hospital. Instead they need an extended-care facility, such as a nursing home. Yet frequently either financial incentives or a lack of nursing home capacity forces many such patients into an acute-care hospital. Treatment of more difficult cases requires specialized staff (nurses and technicians as well as doctors) and special equipment and also depends on having physicians on duty twenty-four hours a day, in case a crisis arises.[15] In all health care systems, then, there are tiers of hospitals, ranging from small, often suburban institutions that specialize in obstetrics or simple elective surgery, to the giant academic medical centers. Treatment of some chronic disorders, such as mental or physical disabilities, may also require specialized facilities. Yet separating these patients from the rest might reduce their access to the best facilities, depending on whether the separation is for reasons of medicine, class, or stigma.[16]

Health care systems must also decide how to allocate resources among institutions of the same type. The most controversial decision involves capital investment: on what basis will the capacity to provide the most expensive forms of care be distributed? In an unregulated system such as the United States has, hospitals might compete for physician affiliations, and thus for business, by overinvesting. Three hospitals in an area might each buy an expensive piece of equipment, such as a lithotripter (which uses sonic waves to dissolve kidney stones) when there is only enough legitimate business in the area to justify one machine. In a regulated system, decisions to make large capital investments must be made by a central authority. Then overinvestment is less likely, but gathering the necessary information and designing and enforcing a facilities plan is never easy.

The link between educational and treatment institutions may be the most complex of all. It involves the priorities of three different activities: teaching, research, and treatment. It usually involves budgets for each task and therefore difficulties in allocating overhead costs among them. It creates complex social and economic incentives: the prestige of and funding for research, for instance, might create a medical staff oriented to providing care that is more "cutting edge" than appropriate.

Any health care reform must include choices about medical education and the physical capacity of the system. A nation may choose to have no policy at all, but it must then accept the consequences.

The Medical Profession

How physicians are trained determines what treatments patients receive. Most of the issues about doctors can be subsumed in the conflict between two goals: specialized treatment and coordinated care. On the one hand, each of us wants to be treated by someone who is an expert on our particular problem. On the other, if we have several problems, we want a doctor who understands their relationships and who can diagnose a hidden problem.[17]

Therefore the key delivery issue involving doctors is the role of the primary care physician (PCP), the doctor you see when you have not been diagnosed as needing a particular specialist. One issue is how much the primary care physicians can do themselves. In other countries the general or family practitioner is more likely than in America to provide pediatric, obstetric, and gynecological services. A second issue is whether primary care physicians must function as "gatekeepers" by approving access to specialists. Routing specialist care through a primary physician helps coordinate care and can serve as a screening device to reduce spending on specialists. It also may delay access to specialist treatment and be seen by patients as an inconvenience.

Should a patient be able to choose among all primary care physicians, as they can in Canada or Germany? Or should choice be constrained, as it is in the United Kingdom and in the United States under some insurance plans? Should primary care physicians be able to refer patients to any physician they wish, or should they be restricted to a limited set of the physicians by the terms of an insurance contract, as they are in many forms of American managed care? Even if choice does not influence quality—a questionable assumption—the degree of choice is clearly important to the public and to providers. It would be a major issue in the American controversy over managed competition.

Beyond Hospitals and Doctors

Although hospitals and doctors are vital, they are only part of any medical system. Other professionals, especially nurses, both make the system run and have political interests that often differ from those of doctors and hospital administrators. And huge businesses, such as pharmaceutical manufacturers, are an integral part of the health care economy.

Who should decide what to pay for outside of hospitals and doctors' offices? Should patients be able to go to a chiropractor or physical therapist or nurse practitioner and have the services paid for by insurance, without a doctor's referral? Advocates of those services claim they are more efficient and comparable in quality to those provided by doctors, so should be funded directly. Physicians argue that those providers generate extra services of lower quality.

Advocates of HMOs argue that they can coordinate care to ensure that it is received from the most appropriate provider. In theory the capitation payment provides incentives for efficiency; whether the HMO managers *are* efficient, and whether their choices for patients can be more satisfactory than the choices patients make for themselves, is less clear.

Conclusion

Inevitably, arguments about the roles of physicians, hospitals, and other providers are almost inseparable from arguments about the definition of health care itself. Financing arrangements influence behaviors and roles, while the roles shape costs and incomes. The conceptual distinctions among finance, delivery, and definition should not blind anyone to the links between them.

Yet the differences are fundamental to debate about health care policy. Particular interests emphasize reform of specific aspects of the system: public health professionals and alternative providers emphasize definition; insurers emphasize delivery; and employers care more about financing. Cost control that emphasizes reform of delivery will have advantages and disadvantages that are different from those that come with cost control that focuses on regulating payments. In short, the losers and the winners and the institutional barriers to success vary according to whether reform emphasizes the financing, delivery, or definition of health care.

Except to define the benefit package, this book now dispenses with arguments about the definition of health care. If health care is everything, then it cannot be analyzed or reformed. The balance of this book focuses on financing and delivery in the United States and six other countries in the early 1990s, and possibly in a future America.

3

The American Health Care System

*T*HE most obvious difference between the American and all other health care systems is that the American system does not guarantee care to all Americans. A large number of Americans are without health insurance at any given time, and an even larger number have a period without it at some point during each year.[1]

How Americans Are Insured

In 1992 the most authoritative estimates reported that 56.7 percent of Americans obtained their primary health insurance coverage from a group policy through their employer or the employer of a family member—including the federal government and the military. By the same estimates 7.3 percent were covered mainly by insurance they purchased individually, 12.4 percent relied on medicare, and 8.2 percent on medicaid. That left 15.4 percent uninsured.[2]

The percentage of Americans without insurance rose from 14.1 percent in 1988 to 15.4 percent in 1992 because increases in coverage through medicare and medicaid offset only part of a decline in the proportion with primary coverage through group plans from 59.7 percent to 55.6 percent. These figures reflect an average of 38.9 million persons uninsured at any given time.[3] An estimated 58 million were uninsured at some point during the year, and at least 21 million were uninsured for the entire year.[4] In no other country in this study is as much as 1 percent of the population uninsured.

Public Programs

Medicare covers health care for the elderly and persons with end-stage renal failure. Employees and employers pay equal percentages

36

of payroll to finance medicare hospital coverage, Part A of the program. Beneficiaries then pay a community-rated premium set at about 25 percent of the costs for medical services, Part B; the balance is paid from general revenues.

Medicaid is a program for the poor, jointly funded by federal and state general revenues. The covered population is determined by a combination of federal mandates and state options. Its general revenue funding means that costs are paid proportionally to incomes.

Federal, state, and local governments also fund a wide variety of special programs from general revenues, including community health clinics, medical research, city and county public hospitals, care for the military and their families, and veterans' programs.[5] Through this assortment of government health care programs, the United States provides income-based subsidies for a large part of the health care received by Americans. Within medicare, the United States already provides the most significant subsidy that has to be established to create any national health care system: support by current workers for the expenses of the elderly.

MEDICARE COVERAGE. Medicare is available to any older American who has worked, or had a spouse work, long enough to be vested in the social security system.[6] Therefore 99 percent of the elderly are insured, 96 percent of them through medicare.[7] But medicare benefits are not comprehensive, so almost 70 percent of the elderly supplement medicare with private "medigap" insurance.

Medicare cost sharing includes a deductible ($696 in 1994) for each year's first sixty days of hospitalization, and a copayment ($174 in 1994) for each of the next thirty days. After that, a person can dip into a lifetime "reserve" account of sixty days, but with double the copayment. After the 150th day there is no coverage.

Medicare pays 80 percent of the amount on its fee schedule for medical services. Doctors are encouraged to bill only the 80 percent (to "accept assignment"), but patients are liable for the full 20 percent coinsurance if the physician demands it. Legal extra billing is rare; restrictions implemented in 1990 reduced its volume from 7.0 percent of total charges in 1990 to 1.4 percent in 1993.[8]

Medicare's coverage for care other than that provided by hospitals and physicians includes six months in a hospice for the terminally ill and limited provisions for skilled nursing care, but no general nursing home benefit or prescription drug benefit.

As a result of these exclusions, cost sharing, and the fact that the elderly are particularly likely to need care, in 1987 they paid over 37 percent of their medical costs from private funds. The large majority of these costs were paid out-of-pocket, not from supplemental insurance such as medigap. In 1991 elderly households spent an average of 11.3 percent of their gross income on health care.[9]

MEDICAID COVERAGE. Medicaid spends only 29 percent of its total on children and adults in families, though they are 72 percent of the beneficiaries. Medicaid has become the default insurance for long-term care, available only if a potential beneficiary has spent (or otherwise made invisible to the government) almost all assets other than a house. Medicaid spends 38 percent of its funds on the nonelderly disabled, who are 15 percent of its beneficiaries. It spends a third of its funds on the elderly, either for nursing homes or other aspects of medigap coverage, though they are only 13 percent of its beneficiaries.[10]

The federal government sets a mix of medicaid eligibility requirements and options, provides over half of any state's costs, making somewhat larger payments to poorer states, but leaves many decisions to the states. For some categories of persons, eligibility for medicaid is linked to eligibility for the aid to families with dependent children (AFDC) program, and state regulations vary greatly as to how low a family's income must be to qualify for AFDC. As a result, in 1992 only half the people in families with income below the poverty line received medicaid benefits; another 18.4 percent had some private insurance.[11]

Medicaid benefits sound more generous than almost any other package available. All or almost all states offer pharmaceuticals, prosthetic devices, dental and optometry services, and even eyeglasses. But states seem to discourage application for the program by requiring potential beneficiaries to complete complex application forms, and access to care for medicaid beneficiaries is limited by several factors. One is a shortage of providers in areas where the poor live, because few physicians choose to practice in those neighborhoods. Another is the fact that states have normally paid much lower fees for medicaid services than providers receive from private insurance or medicare. In 1993, on average medicaid physician fees were 73 percent of medicare levels. "A large body of research," as one report puts it, "indicates that low Medicaid fees result in low physician participation in the program and affect the number of Medicaid patients physicians are willing to treat."[12] Some of the care that might have been provided on an ambulatory basis is replaced by outpatient care in hospitals, often through the emergency room.

BUDGETARY IMPACTS OF PUBLIC PROGRAMS. During the 1980s, medicare and medicaid costs burgeoned as medical inflation combined with growth in the beneficiary populations. Congress took numerous steps to reduce the pace of medicare cost growth, but it still grew rapidly relative to the rest of the budget. Congress also enacted "several major mandatory expansions of Medicaid eligibility," courts began to enforce provisions requiring that medicaid fees be closer to other payers', and states responded to these higher costs with "innovative" financing strategies to pass the buck to (or collect more bucks from) the federal government.[13] Federal medicaid spending grew 29 percent between fiscal years 1991 and 1992.[14]

Health care reform became a budget issue because of this experience. While the federal government did a better job of controlling its costs than most private payers did, demographics and the need to keep public payments somewhat in line with private payments produced estimates of continued cost growth into the next century. The Congressional Budget Office reported in 1993 that all of its current estimates of future growth in federal spending as a share of GDP were due to medicare and medicaid estimates.[15] If health care costs did not increase, the budget deficit would fade away.

Private Insurance

Most Americans, as they contribute to care for the elderly and the poor through government, obtain insurance for themselves through their employment contracts. Employers offer coverage through one or a small number of insurers;[16] the employer normally pays most of the premium, and the employee contributes a portion. Many employers self-insure: they establish the rules for their own programs and pay claims directly. Often these self-insured companies hire an insurance company to administer the claims process.

The federal government encourages employers to provide group insurance by treating employer payments as a business expense. Employee compensation in the form of health care benefits is not subject to income tax, whereas if the employer paid the same amounts in salary and employees had to then buy insurance, the income would be taxed first. The Congressional Budget Office estimated the revenue forgone at $75 billion in fiscal year 1994.[17]

LIMITED AVAILABILITY. Employer coverage is strongly related to an employee's income and the size of the employer.[18] At the highest income levels and in the largest firms, approximately 90 percent of employees have coverage through their employers—and many who do not have chosen to be covered by a spouse's employer instead. Smaller firms and those that pay lower wages are much less likely to provide (meaning pay a large part of the premium for) insurance. Firm size affects the employer's decision about providing insurance because the cost of marketing and administering insurance per employee goes down as the number of employees rises; so insurance companies charge much higher overhead costs per beneficiary to small firms than to large ones. Wage level is an even bigger factor: for small firms that pay low wages, the cost of health insurance is a much larger proportional cost than for large firms. Coverage that costs an employer $4,000 per employee is a much larger portion of total expenses for an employer whose employees earn an average of $12,000 than for one whose average employee earns $40,000.

Many employees of small firms obtain insurance through a family member's coverage or by buying it themselves. As table 3-1 shows, that is a good thing.

In 1992 only 12.6 percent of workers earning less than $20,000 per year in a firm with fewer than ten employees received health insurance through their jobs, while 91.3 percent of workers earning more than $50,000 with a firm of over 1,000 employees were insured through their jobs.[19]

American workers might also have no insurance because insurers have decided people in their line of work are too risky. Insurers might exclude businesses whose employees are prone to risky behaviors (restaurants and bars because of proximity to alcohol; flower shops because insurers think employees are more likely to be gay and therefore at greater risk for AIDS), businesses where the work itself has health risks (logging, dry cleaning), and those whose employees might be unusually oriented toward pursuing treatment of health problems (hospitals, clinics).[20]

TABLE 3-1. *Workers Aged 18-64: Private Health Insurance Coverage by Employee Earnings and Firm Size, 1992*
Percent unless otherwise specified

Firm size	Under $20,000	$20,000– $49,999	$50,000 or more
Fewer than 10			
Direct from firm	12.6	34.8	43.6
Any private	58.0	79.0	90.3
10–99			
Direct from firm	29.9	69.6	76.5
Any private	61.9	88.0	95.5
100–999			
Direct from firm	43.0	83.1	88.5
Any private	71.7	94.6	97.2
1,000 or more			
Direct from firm	42.9	86.6	91.3
Any private	73.6	95.6	97.7

Source: Employee Benefit Research Institute, "Sources of Health Insurance and Characteristics of the Uninsured," *Special Report and Issue Brief* 145 (January 1994), table 34, p. 62.

Individual purchase of insurance is not a solution in many of these cases because it is very expensive, and employers who do not pay for insurance are not likely to be providing higher wages instead. On average, the cost for coverage for a family of four in 1992 was around $5,000. That is a lot of money for the average family, whose *pretax* income is around $37,000.[21] Eighty-eight percent of the uninsured in 1992 were in families with estimated adjusted gross incomes of less than $20,000 per year. Fifty-two percent lived in families headed by full-time, full-year workers; 8 percent in families headed by full-year, part-time workers; and 17 percent in families headed by full-time workers who experienced some unemployment.[22]

A small proportion of uncovered workers are uncovered by choice. The typical example is a young single person whose health risks are low but who works in an "unsafe" and officially low-wage job, say, as a waiter, who decides to forgo paying the high cost of an individual policy until his risks are greater. Most of the uninsured simply do not have the money to be insured.[23]

All people who are neither elderly nor part of a large group are at risk of being denied insurance in the market. A person who has insurance may not be able to keep it because a contract expires and is not renewed, or is renewed at a prohibitive rate. One example is particularly salient. When Lee Atwater, then chairman of the Republican National Committee, was stricken with a brain tumor, the committee's insurer, when the contract was up for renewal, proposed a 52 percent rate increase. The insurer was doing its job: protecting the firm's profitability. The RNC was just another unlucky, smallish firm. It shopped around and found alternative coverage for only 26 percent more than it had been paying. Some employees decided they could no longer afford family coverage at those rates.[24]

COVERAGE AND EXPENSES. Employers who provide coverage usually require employees to contribute to the premium. About half of employees contribute to individual coverage and two-thirds to family coverage. Survey data suggest that employee contributions to individual coverage in 1993 were about 18 percent of plan costs, while their payments for family coverage were about 29 percent of costs. These figures had risen from 10 percent for individuals and 25 percent for families in 1988. The proportion of the total paid by employees is higher if we include the taxes paid for medicare and other public programs.[25]

When employers self-insure instead of paying premiums, they keep the money and disburse it to pay medical bills. Self-insurance is essentially unregulated, being protected from state insurance premium taxes, benefits standards, and reserve requirements by provisions of the Employee Retirement Income Security Act (ERISA). Because of these advantages, the number of self-insured companies grew extremely quickly in the 1980s; they now cover well over a third of all full-time employees and a large majority of those in large companies.[26] American self-insurance is different from the "company funds" in Germany and Japan in that the American approach is unregulated. There are no standards for benefits, no guarantees that they will continue, no process of redress if a claim is denied, and rarely an official employee voice in governing the plan. Many companies drop coverage if an employee is no longer able to work, and unless challenged by a strong union, employers may unilaterally change the terms of their plans, eliminating a beneficiary's protection.[27]

Because insurance is a contract between each employer and each insurer, or simply part of employment in the case of self-insurance, it is not portable. Private plans have vesting periods before a new employee is covered and normally lapse when a person changes jobs, and many exclude pre-existing conditions. All of these aspects help explain why some people are without insurance for parts of a year. Other countries use employment as a convenient and distributively just device for collecting money; only in the United States does the extent or even existence of coverage vary greatly from workplace to workplace.

The profusion of types of American private insurance makes summarizing their benefits impossible.[28] Aside from the tens of thousands of self-insured firms, the United States has more than a thousand private insurance companies, which offer an even larger number of packages.[29] Yet some patterns stand out. Unlike in other countries, many plans cap total spending on a patient, so people can exceed the limits of their coverage for catastrophic illness or injury, for example.[30] Virtually all private plans cover hospitals, physician services, laboratory work, and pharmaceuticals. But there are large differences among plans as to whether they cover benefits in full or require some form of cost sharing. Except in HMOs, the vast majority of benefits have limiting conditions.[31]

Surveys that estimate the proportion of Americans' medical expenses that are paid out-of-pocket nevertheless find that, in spite of the increase in the proportion of Americans without insurance, out-of-pocket payments for care have declined as a share of expenses. Their estimated level in 1991, 19.2 percent of medical spending, was the lowest ever recorded.[32] How could this be, given all the talk about a health insurance crisis? Out-of-pocket costs fell relative to total costs, but grew relative to incomes, because health care costs grew much faster than incomes.[33]

The growth of costs made health care less affordable to employers as well as employees. Employers kept reducing the value of coverage, from the employees' perspective, by implementing cost-saving measures such as restricting the choice of doctor. Employers also passed some cost increases on to employees by increasing the employee contributions to premiums. In one set of surveys, employee payments for family coverage doubled from 1984 to 1989, at a time when median family incomes rose by about 30 percent.[34] In spite of all these measures, health insurance costs rose so quickly that employers still increased their own spending even more quickly than they raised direct employee costs, so the employee share of costs fell even as employee payments rose. Both employers and employees felt like losers in the process.

The lower out-of-pocket spending might also mean that access to health care for the uninsured is declining. As insurance coverage is reduced, more costs would be paid out-of-pocket only if people without insurance could afford to pay. Because the level of insurance is related to income, and insurance coverage has been declining because of high costs, people who lose insurance might well be consuming only the health care they can get for free.

However it is paid for, American health care is becoming less and less affordable for individuals, their employers, and the government.

Paying Providers

American health care providers are paid different amounts and in different ways by different payers.

HOSPITAL PAYMENT. A hospital that is owned by or has a contract with an HMO may be subject to a budget or paid a capitated amount per enrollee in the HMO. Otherwise the hospital is paid by fees, calculated per service per day, or per diagnosis. The form of payment varies with the payer and often involves a mix of means.

Each hospital makes up a list of charges and tries to collect as much from payers as possible. But what it collects from each payer varies greatly, from medicaid on the bottom to some unlucky corporation or insurer that pays the posted price. Payment varies according to the power of the payer.

Hospitals cannot bargain with medicare at all. The federal government determines both the charge structure and the payments, and such bargaining as occurs is power politics in Congress. The federal share of the budget is too large for hospitals to act as if they had a choice about accepting the rates, and hospitals mainly fight over the formulas by which the Health Care Financing Administration (HCFA) pays them.

Medicare sets its payments to hospitals according to diagnosis-related groups (DRGs); that is, it pays a set amount for treatment of a patient according to the major diagnosis. Teaching hospitals claim that they need bonus payments because their patients are sicker than the average for each given diagnosis and that they have extra expenses associated with teaching. Medicare therefore adjusts the prospective payment system of fees per DRG to pay teaching hospitals more and for other factors such as proportions of impoverished patients in a hospital and geographic differences in average costs.

Hospitals cannot bargain much with medicaid because the payers, state governments, are almost always in well-publicized fiscal crisis. State governments also license hospitals. Because they cannot charge medicaid patients enough to recoup their costs (or so they claim), some hospitals try to discourage medicaid patients from visiting them for treatment. Hospitals are in a better position to deal with Blue Cross/ Blue Shield, the largest private insurer, than with either medicare or medicaid. But the local version of Blue Cross is also usually a very large payer and often knows more than other payers about the hospital because Blue Cross is frequently the agent for paying medicare claims. So the hospital cannot charge Blue Cross as much as it would like either.

All of these differences help explain why hospitals' posted charges have hardly any relationship to their receipts. "The most remarkable item in Stanford Hospital's balance sheet," one set of observers concluded, "is that it actually received only $312 million of the $603 million it billed its patients. The rest is accounted for by bad debts it will never collect, and the discounts it is forced to give large payers like Medicare, Medicaid, and managed care organizations."[35] What is truly remarkable is that Stanford stays in business yet persists in claiming that its charges are related to its costs.

The academic medical centers (AMCs), like Stanford, because they are unlikely to turn away medicaid patients, may be more likely than other hospitals to have such bizarre-looking charge structures—but other hospitals have them too.[36] Hospital "costs" as reflected in "charges" are list prices much like those for furniture or stereo equipment. Hardly anyone pays the posted price for any of these items— which means "discounts," also, are largely fictional. From the standpoint of the higher payers, the whole process is simply cost-shifting: the hospitals ask less powerful payers to pay some of the costs for the more powerful.

One might argue that cost-shifting is only fair; after all, the less powerful payers self-insured to get the advantages of nonregulation, so should be willing to pay the costs of having less market power. Fair or not, a system of different prices for different payers creates large social costs. Because each payer is continually trying to negotiate separate discounts, challenging bills, and trying to establish a favorable charge structure, hospitals must keep the books on a wide variety of payment rates and in a wide variety of categories. The Johns Hopkins Hospital, for example, has eighteen thousand charge categories for payment by five hundred different insurance plans.[37] As anyone who has ever tried to decipher a hospital bill knows, from a patient's standpoint the results are very hard to comprehend.

Paying hospitals with budgets rather than charges per service would involve much less overhead. Many hospitals do receive some budgeted funds. Academic medical centers that are part of the state university receive large state appropriations. They also generate income from the federal government in the form of support for research. Yet because they also must collect for patient care, their accounting can be even more complicated than that of other hospitals.

Hospital payment in the United States is therefore exceedingly complex. It also includes less of the cost of care provided in the hospital than is covered by payments to the hospital in many other countries. Admitting physicians, and sometimes specialists within hospitals, are paid separately, a situation that not only requires more separate bills but also creates conflicts over payment and incentives to provide more services.

PHYSICIAN PAYMENT. Salaried doctors have little reason to compete with each other for the right to perform a given service. In America, however, specialists wage war over the right to perform services such as transluminal coronary angioplasties (radiologists vs. cardiologists) or surgery on hands (orthopedic vs. plastic surgeons). Conflict is exacerbated by the large number of specialists competing for income. In an extreme case, a hospital purchased extra equipment so both groups of competing physicians could provide the same service—raising the hospital's costs. There are fewer such turf battles at AMCs, where clinical professors tend to be on salary.[38]

Physician fees, wherever incurred, are subject to the same dynamic of bargaining power, prices, discounts, and cost-shifting as hospital charges. Of course, American payers have not been trying so hard to constrain physicians for quite as long as they have sought to limit hospital payments. And physicians are more politically powerful than hospitals, so medicare is just less than a decade behind in using its bargaining power on doctors, with private payers (tentatively but eagerly) following.

In the late 1980s the Health Care Financing Administration created a standard set of categories and fees for physician payment under medicare, which is being expanded in the 1990s to include all physician services. This structure is called a resource-based relative value scale (RBRVS) because it purports to relate fees to each other based on the relative value of the resources used in providing a service.

RBRVS raises many issues, including how to judge relative values. It is seen by virtually everyone as a tool to transfer income from procedurally based specialists, such as surgeons, to those who spend more time on diagnosis.[39] But the real importance of RBRVS is that it can be the basis for fee schedules. A medicare schedule cannot be adopted directly by other payers (it is not much help on obstetrics, for example). But any form of fee schedule would make cost-shifting harder to hide and would also enable better comparisons among providers and arguments about what costs *should* be.[40]

Because the market for insured health care is not a normal one, some of the savings from lower fees can be countered by providers who increase their volume of billings. They can do so because it is more common for a physician to tell a patient what she needs than the reverse. This ability to increase billings has its limits. Some providers need prescriptions from others to create demand. But the "behavioral offset"—physicians behaving differently to maintain their incomes—remains significant.[41] In order to counter this effect, Congress created the medicare volume performance standard (MVPS) system of fee adjustments. This structure, "sets an annual volume target through congressional action or, if Congress does not act, through a default formula. The difference between this target and actual volume partly determines future physician payment rate updates, with low volume growth rewarded by higher updates."[42] And vice versa. In essence this approach sets a prospective budget for medicare physician targets, which can be calculated as the product of fees and projected volume. If costs exceed the budget, they may be recovered through lower fees in subsequent years.

In the early years of their implementation, volume performance standards have been a rousing success. The Physician Payment Review Commission (PPRC), an independent organization created by Congress to monitor the system's performance, reports that "Medicare spending for physicians' services rose at an average annual rate of 4.8 percent between 1989 and 1993, compared with 12.1 percent between 1980 and 1989." If anything, MVPS has been more successful than analysts hoped. It works because very few physicians could refuse the medicare business even though the fees are substantially lower than the average private fee. The decline of medicare fees relative to private reimbursements has not reduced beneficiaries' access to physician services. But by 1994 the PPRC commissioners by 1994 were concerned that further restraint within medicare, if not matched in the private market, could cause some doctors to begin refusing to accept medicare patients.[43]

Other payers did not achieve anything like the MVPS for two reasons. First, they have not had the market power to enforce the fees. Second, they cannot do it fairly. HCFA can honestly claim to know virtually the entire volume of services to an entire class of beneficiaries, and to adjust on that basis. Every other payer has a mixed bag of beneficiaries, so cannot claim an objective basis for setting targets. Instead, other insurers are left to control costs without overall volume adjustments. Because they cannot adjust fees to volume, they try to directly limit the volume of care.

VOLUME AND MANAGED CARE. Limiting volume directly is known as managing care. The advocates of managed care can cite reams of evidence that the medical profession has no coherent standard as to when many procedures should be used. The best evidence is a huge variation in rates of specific procedures, not just from state to state but among small communities within the same general area.

There are many ways to manage care. Some, such as providing a special manager to coordinate the many forms of treatment for complex and extremely expensive cases, are not controversial. Others, such as requiring preapproval of hospital admissions, were once controversial but are now ubiquitous. Still others, such as getting large group practices to provide all care for a person for a single capitation fee (the logic of a group- or staff-model HMO) are beloved by health policy analysts and are more common in the United States than elsewhere, but are not so popular with patients and physicians.

From both patients' and physicians' perspectives, the most evident form of managed care is detailed review, by insurers, of treatment decisions. A payer may require preapproval of a procedure, or may establish rules and disallow cases that it says do not fit. But in either case, physicians feel they are harried by clerks (or nurses) who make decisions over the telephone without knowing much about the patient. Patients face uncertainty about whether their costs will be reimbursed. The confusion and anxiety are magnified by having to deal with multiple payers with different personnel and different rules. Some patients find that when their insurance changes, so do the rules of coverage and reimbursement. Providers must keep track of the different rules of dozens of plans, most of which change frequently. The result is a regime of distrust and continual change.[44]

The United States has lower rates of visits to physicians than any other country in this study—though that may be due less to review than to high cost sharing, high prices, and lack of universal insurance. It also has lower rates of hospitalization and shorter lengths of stay in the hospital.[45] Visits have not been increasing, and hospitalization has been decreasing. For all these reasons, one might expect American arrangements to have controlled the volume of care well enough to control costs at least as well as other nations.

But American health care costs still skyrocketed through the 1980s and into the 1990s. Patients spent less time in the hospital, but the intensity of service, and the expense to deliver it, rose dramatically. In 1980 the average community hospital had 394 employees per 100 daily patients; in 1990 it had 563. The number of in-hospital operations declined, but the number of outpatient surgeries tripled. So did the number of inpatient diagnostic tests.[46]

In short, outside of medicare, American methods of paying for health care services were better at creating confusion than at controlling costs.[47] American methods of paying for health insurance therefore became less and less able to cover the costs. Levels of insurance slowly declined, and individuals' out-of-pocket costs rose.

Delivering American Health Care

Like its system of financing health care, America's systems for delivering and paying for medical care are notably more complex than those of most other countries. Many doctors work in more than one hospital, making governance of medical staffs difficult; specialists are harder to coordinate because there are more of them; and the proliferation of forms of managed care means rapid change in patterns of gatekeeping and referral.

Physicians

American doctors go through extensive training to work long hours for high pay.

NUMBERS AND TRAINING. The typical medical school program requires, after four years of college, four more years of "undergraduate" medical education. During the final two years, students receive some clinical training. Virtually all graduates then must complete some graduate medical education in order to be licensed to practice medicine. This education is obtained in residency programs, mainly in hospitals affiliated with medical schools.[48] Normally only one year of residency (as an intern) is needed for licensure, but up to eight years (for neurosurgeons) may be required for certification as a specialist.

The United States has over 230 physicians in active practice per 100,000 persons—about the same as Canada, more than Japan or Britain, but fewer than Germany or France. On average, physicians work about sixty hours per week, forty-seven on patient-care matters, but have more weeks off (five) than most Americans. Interns and residents work extremely long hours for pay that is low relative to their level of training and effort. Many also graduate from medical school with substantial debt: about 79 percent of 1990 graduates had some debt (the average was $46,224); and about an eighth had debt of over $75,000. Given the length of their training and the size of their debts, it is understandable that most physicians feel entitled to incomes that are much higher than those of most other Americans.[49]

Graduates of foreign medical schools (international medical graduates, or IMGs) fill gaps in American supply, for instance as residents in less popular fields such as institutional psychology, radiology, and pathology. Many are Americans who could not gain entrance to U.S. medical schools so attended offshore. Often they fill a need for primary care physicians that U.S.-trained medical students do not wish to meet. IMGs constitute about one-fifth of American physicians, but concerns have been periodically raised about their training. Their admission to residency programs was restricted after studies in the 1970s and 1980s suggested that the quality of their medical knowledge was lower than desired, and international graduates still perform much worse on licensing tests than the American norm. The presence of these international graduates is important, though, both because they fill in some gaps in the American delivery system and because any efforts to structure physician supply would be conflated with attitudes toward immigrants.[50]

DISTRIBUTION AND SPECIALIZATION. It is much easier to find a doctor in urban than in rural areas. In 1988 one study found three times as many primary care physicians per person in the most urban than in the most rural counties, and fourteen times as many specialists.[51] As a result, physicians in less populated areas see substantially more patients and spend more hours seeing them than do physicians in large cities.[52] It is also easier to find a physician in the suburbs and wealthy parts of a city than in impoverished neighborhoods. "In vast stretches of inner city New York," the *New York Times* reports, "there are only a handful of doctors, and virtually none who offer patients a reasonable standard of primary care."[53]

An unusually high proportion of American doctors are trained to specialize. Barely 10 percent of American doctors in 1987 called themselves general practitioners (GPs), the standard term for primary care physicians. But because a specialist such as a family practitioner (FP), internist, pediatrician, or obstetrician-gynecologist may be a person's regular physician, between 33 and 40 percent of physicians (depending on who is counting) are mainly primary care providers. However counted, that is fewer primary care physicians, and more specialists, than in other countries.[54]

Two-thirds of physicians practice in offices, the vast majority with admitting privileges to a hospital.[55] Many practice in more (for example, a nice suburban hospital for simple cases, and a high-tech academic medical center for difficult ones). Hospitals therefore must compete for admissions by making those physicians happy, such as by having the fanciest equipment. Hospitals have large house staffs (25 percent of all physicians), but most of those are residents and interns.[56]

The emphasis on specialization feeds on itself. If you can see a specialist for a problem, why see the "nonexpert" GP? If fewer people go to the GP for a common condition, such as pregnancy, the GP will become less expert. America's system of malpractice insurance then further inhibits GPs from doing the work, by charging doctors who do fewer procedures higher malpractice insurance relative to their income from those procedures (a particular problem in obstetrics).

Historically, doctors in all seven countries have preferred to practice alone, as self-employed professionals. Group practice by specialists of the same type offers less independence but the ability to share the costs of equipment and administration (both of which are growing rapidly). A multispecialty group can offer a wide range of medical services and can also increase consultation among providers with different expertise. Groups also may offer less personal care and have their own coordination problems. Groups may be organized as corporations paying salaries, or as partnerships with each physician as a partner. In either case, physicians trade some independence for the opportunity to share risk and expenses. Among physicians outside hospitals, group practice is more common in America than in any of the other countries described in this book.[57]

Institutional Care

Long-term or chronic care, especially for the aged, is a complicated system on its own, and the potential expenses of long-term care are so great that it is highly unlikely that any reform will do much about it. I have chosen not to address it carefully in this book because it is so complex, the financing seems so intractable, and the subject is covered thoroughly in another recent book.[58] This work focuses instead on the costs of the current American health care system, of which one major component is hospital services for acute care.

The American supply of hospitals is dominated by private nonprofit hospitals—many owned by religious organizations. In 1991, 66 percent of hospital beds were provided by the nonprofits, 10 percent by the for-profit sector. The rest, just over a quarter of the beds, were in federal, state, or local facilities. It is hard to identify much difference between the behavior and efficiency of the for-profit and private nonprofits.[59] If private institutions are more efficient, the savings go largely or entirely to investors.

Americans spend a great deal of money on hospitals: $288.6 billion in 1991, or 43 percent of all spending on patient care. But hospital expenditures did not rise as quickly in the 1980s as other forms of spending, and "the hospital is not as dominant a provider as it once was or still is in other countries."[60] Hospitals and doctors tried to avoid regulation by moving care to ostensibly freestanding ambulatory care facilities. Examples include kidney dialysis units, and radiology group practices with close relations with hospitals. Some payers encouraged the shift, believing those facilities would be cheaper.

The growth of various freestanding centers increased controversy over self-referral: physicians sending patients for tests to laboratories in which they have a financial interest. The American Medical Association (AMA) is engaged in internal struggles over whether to ban or how to limit the practice. Congress and the Department of Justice have also shown an interest, on antitrust and kickback grounds. But there is such a proliferation of such labs, under so many different arrangements, that it is hard to tell what is going on, with what consequences.

Back in the traditional hospitals, the nature of care depends greatly on hospitals' relationships with doctors and medical schools, and on hospitals' catchment areas—the areas from which they get most of their patients. Care is different in a suburban community hospital and an urban academic medical center, because staffing, hierarchies, schedules and patients differ.

A suburban hospital can generally provide sophisticated care, such as cardiac bypass surgery, but it is not as likely to have clinical professors who are able to provide extremely specialized care for "interesting" cases. All hospitals want the most advanced equipment, but the academic medical centers must have it for research and training. These centers rely heavily on residents and interns for delivery of care and, most important, are likely to have a much lower-class population of patients.

Many of the AMCs are in inner cities. They are likely to have large outpatient departments to train the students (residents) and serve the local population, which feeds into the inpatient wards; the emergency room not only gets emergencies but also serves as an outpatient clinic for some of the population.[61] All of this is the good news: if a major teaching hospital is in the inner city, then either a large and endowed institution or a state government pays for some care for the inner-city poor.

When local hospitals receive little funding for education, poor populations must frequently rely on a hospital financed by a strapped city or county budget. Such hospitals—for example, Cook County in Chicago, Boston City, and Charity in New Orleans—have interns and residents to do the work because of their relationships with a training program, but nowhere near the resources of a freestanding university hospital. All hospitals in the inner city try to convince medicare that they deserve an extra subsidy for treating a poorer, less-insured, and often sicker population. The federal government calls these dispro-portionate share payments. One of the huge issues for American health care reform is what will happen to the academic medical centers and the remaining urban public hospitals if payment systems allow competing insurers to favor hospitals that are less expensive because they have lesser teaching and subsidy burdens.

Another major issue is how a bias toward specialized, high-tech-nology medicine, created in part by how medical education is financed and how physicians are paid, is reinforced by arrangements for capital investment in American medicine. There are hardly any measures in place to prevent a "medical arms race" among hospitals that seek the most advanced technology in order to attract physicians and generate revenue. Measures to restrain capital investment, if backed by political and financial power and will, can restrain costs and maintain high-quality care in the United States, as shown by the dramatic success of Rochester, New York. But that experience was based on highly excep-tional circumstances, especially the leadership of two giant corpora-tions with a history of public service that dominated the local market and could cooperate with a Blue Cross plan that insured more than 70 percent of area residents.[62]

Doctors and Hospitals

Outside of Rochester, the American health care delivery system is more expensive than other countries' in part because expensive equip-ment is spread more widely, with less attention to need, and in part because it relies more heavily on specialists. Because for years insurers would pay whatever physicians and hospitals billed, and hospitals relied on physicians to provide patients, hospitals competed for pa-tients by having the best equipment, and insurers ended up paying for excess treatments and higher charges per treatment. At one time also physicians could refer patients to any specialist they wished, and patients could go directly to a specialist without referral.

The rise of managed care and of more aggressive bargaining by insurers has begun to change this basic pattern. Insurers have become more likely to refuse to approve a given service or to insist on a lower price. Hospitals still need to attract physicians by offering the best equipment, however, so they are caught between the demands of doctors and payers. Meanwhile insurers are limiting choice of and access to specialists by building closed panels, in which a person covered by a plan either cannot use or must pay a surcharge to use any provider who is not on special contract to the plan. A patient might find that her doctor of twenty years' standing is no longer part of her insurance plan; a physician might find that many of his patients can afford referral only to three nephrologists whom he does not know. One of the key issues in reform is whether these new restrictions on choice of physician are necessary. Advocates of the international standard say no; advocates of managed competition say yes.

Ensuring High-Quality Care

The American system of health care financing reduces the quality of care for at least one group of people: those without insurance. Estimating these effects is difficult, because people who go without treatment by definition are not seen by anyone who could estimate how they should have been treated. Yet careful analysis suggests that over the course of a year the uninsured "have about 60 percent as many ambulatory health services contacts and about 70 percent of the inpatient hospital days in the year as they would have had if they had health care coverage."[63] The uninsured are twice as likely to be hospitalized for conditions that are treatable through appropriate ambulatory care and are more likely than the insured both to delay needed care and to say they did without care that they felt they needed.[64] "As others have documented," Katherine Swartz writes, "being hospitalized while being without health insurance frequently means receiving fewer services than insured patients and running a higher risk of dying when hospitalized." Further, persons who get sick while uninsured then have a pre-existing condition that may prevent future coverage; "Thus even a short uninsured spell does not have the benign implication many would ascribe to it on the basis of a short duration."[65]

Chapter 6 discusses the trade-offs between these health care losses and the putative advantages of American methods of financing and delivery; here we must note only that a system that fails to guarantee insurance has overlooked an obvious step for guaranteeing quality health care.

Other measures could focus on regulating the quality of providers. The most direct approach is licensing. These powers are lodged almost entirely in state governments. States cede most of their powers of quality control to professional bodies—the state medical associations, the Joint Commission on Accreditation of Healthcare Organizations, the Accreditation Council for Graduate Medical Education, to name only a few. Revoking a physician's license to practice is rare. Withdrawal of medical staff privileges at hospitals is also an effective sanction but is also rare.[66]

MALPRACTICE LITIGATION. The other major form of quality regulation is through the court system. The filing of malpractice suits is a very emotional issue, rife with dubious conventional arguments.

Physicians argue that an out-of-control tort system subjects them to persecution by sharp lawyers looking to make money, greedy or misguided claimants, and juries prejudiced against doctors or interested in gouging their "deep pocket" insurers. All of this may be true, but it is also evident that physicians are not eager to regulate themselves and that the incidence of mistakes due to negligence is much greater than the number of internal disciplinary actions or malpractice suits. A 1984 Harvard University study of over thirty thousand hospital records in New York found adverse events caused by negligence in about 1 percent of cases. A 1974 California study of over twenty thousand cases found similar levels of negligent error. Both studies were performed by physicians, and the latter was cosponsored by the California Medical Association. Comparisons show that the amount of negligent error was eight to ten times the number of malpractice suits, sixteen to twenty-five times the number of successful suits, and a much larger multiple of the amount of disciplinary actions by medical boards.[67]

There is little objective reason to believe that jury determinations, or settlements, are shaped by bias. "It appears," Peter Budetti and Stephanie Spernak conclude, "that a substantial majority of the compensation awarded does go to parties who have meritorious claims under current negligence principles."[68] Many physicians would argue that those principles favor plaintiffs and that the standard of evidence should be higher, but the chairman of an AMA task force on professional liability noted that malpractice defendants are "winning 60% to 80% of cases that go to trial. Perhaps," he suggested, "we could get that number up to 95 percent by going to a tougher evidence standard, but . . . the whole idea appears self-serving."[69]

Thus it is hard to support arguments that physicians are being persecuted for nonexistent malpractice. But some court decisions do not appear to make much sense, and the system is often unfair and illogical.[70] Further, all people make mistakes in their work at some time, even "negligent" ones, and physician reviewers of decisions by others have the benefits of leisure and hindsight. There is no reason to believe that every incident of alleged malpractice constitutes "negligence."

What, exactly, should the malpractice system do? It should have two purposes: to provide remedy or at least redress for a tort, by compensating an injured individual; and to benefit society as a whole by making physicians and hospitals more likely to practice high-quality medicine. The system does not do a very good job of the former: a large part of costs are absorbed by lawyers and insurers, building a case against medical providers is difficult (they do not want to provide incriminating data), and redress can be delayed for years; but in the end the malpractice system does provide some redress. No policy analyst can suggest what amount of opportunity for redress is appropriate.

There is little reason to believe, however, that the system does anything to improve the quality of medical care. Guilty physicians who settle suits before trial undergo no professional sanction and can keep the details secret. The system thus does not reduce threats to subsequent patients. Studies show virtually no link between adverse malpractice experience and changes in patterns of practice, and behaviors that physicians ascribe to fears of malpractice do not appear to be related statistically to levels of suits or premiums.[71] If the goal were to encourage high-quality medicine, measures to improve professional self-regulation would be much more logical.

So physicians are right to criticize the malpractice tort system. Yet their usual argument, that it is a major cause of high U.S. health care costs, is almost certainly wrong. The cost of malpractice insurance is about 1 percent of total system costs.[72] Therefore the effects must be indirect: essentially, that fear of suits causes physicians to practice "defensive medicine," doing more to avoid being sued for errors of omission.

It is impossible to measure "defensive medicine," but there are strong reasons to doubt its importance. Most evidently, the argument is self-serving: physicians and hospitals that earn more money by doing more claim they are doing so out of fear, so they (and insurers) can blame lawyers for doctors' incomes! The argument also ignores the fact that American medical practice has always been far more invasive and aggressive than any other to which it has been compared. Historian Martin S. Pernick wrote that Dr. Benjamin Rush, a signer of the Declaration of Independence, tried to convince practitioners and patients that "to cure Americans would require uniquely powerful doses administered by heroic American physicians." Oliver Wendell Holmes asked, "How could a people . . . which insists on sending out yachts and horses and boys to outsail, outrun, outfight and checkmate all the rest of creation; how could such a people be content with any but 'heroic' practice?"[73] Since American medical practice was notably aggressive long before malpractice suits became an issue, one might infer that aggressive practice causes the suits, not vice versa.

The primacy of practice norms, rather than the legal system, is made evident if we ask: why do physicians expect to be sued for doing too little rather than too much? Usually in life, errors of commission are easier to identify than errors of omission. The system could only be biased in favor of punishing errors of omission if physicians, patients, and juries all are part of a culture that expects heroic action.

Do doctors believe they would do less unnecessary work if the malpractice system were weakened? Yes. Warnings about malpractice suits permeate medical education, and fear is part of physicians' culture. But individual doctors also express pride at being more thorough and careful than other practitioners.[74] In countries where the fear of lawsuits is low, such as Germany, doctors explain "excess" procedures by blaming patients for expecting services (especially prescriptions) whether they are necessary or not. These physicians argue that they have to provide the extra test in order to keep the patient's business. The same pressures operate, and the same arguments can be made, in the United States. And when studies estimate the cost of defensive medicine, careful analysis "reveals that many practices ascribed to defensive medicine, such as maintaining more detailed patient records and referring more cases to other physicians, might be needed to provide adequate medical care."[75]

For all these reasons, there is little reason to believe that restrictions on malpractice litigation would have much effect on American health care costs, and one should hesitate to greatly reduce patients' opportunities for redress on those grounds. But the system also is doing little to improve the quality of medical care, and limiting redress in return for stronger quality controls makes sense, as long as redress in egregious cases remains possible. If that saves money, all the better. A trade-off of this sort would reduce the level of anxiety among physicians (or focus it in a productive direction: meeting peer standards). And holding physicians responsible for doing "too little" makes no sense within systems of cost control dedicated to punishing them financially for doing "too much."

Conclusion

The American health care system has many virtues. It is also designed, or nondesigned, to create confusion and extra costs.

The structure of insurance creates administrative expense in insurance offices, which pay to sell policies and assess risk and design special policies because customers cannot afford the standard ones. The fragmentation of insurance into thousands of plans, many of which try to regulate volume and set their own prices, requires extremely complex billing and accounting operations in hospitals and doctors' offices.

The U.S. insurance system not only does not guarantee access to care, but some aspects of it, such as risk-rating, are designed to discourage access. The status quo creates great uncertainty and confusion about what is covered, and that uncertainty affects not only patients but physicians, who must deal with ever-changing regulations even within large plans such as medicare and Blue Cross/Blue Shield.

The delivery system ensures a large supply of specialists and research-oriented hospitals to supply the latest, most-advanced care to people who can pay for it, and even to some who cannot. It provides relatively easy access to specialists for the well insured. It is not as good at coordinating care or ensuring primary care. The high level of specialization creates incentives for a higher volume of specialized care than in other countries, regardless of need. So does the competition among hospitals for business from admitting physicians. Regulation of hospital investment barely exists.

Because of differences among insurers, a given physician may be in many different "delivery systems," defined as a set of rules about the care they can deliver. The variety of basic relationships—of forms of group practice, of ways to capitate group practice, and of referral structures as insurers try to limit the networks they offer to patients, makes the system's topography harder to map for the United States than for any other country.

We have just scanned the surface in this chapter, but should have seen enough to recognize differences as we move north of the border and across the seas.

4

Canada and Germany: The Two Most Common Models

CANADA and Germany are the prototypes for two of the three basic approaches to health care coverage within the international standard. In Canada insurance is provided by the government; in Germany by nonprofit sickness funds within a framework of regulation. (A third approach, a national health service such as the United Kingdom and some other nations have, has not been a major contender in American reform proposals for the past few decades.)

The German approach is the more common internationally. Only Australia has adapted the Canadian methods. But Canada remains the most obvious model for American reform because of the proximity of the two countries. Canada, which shares a 4,000-mile border with the United States, has teams in the National Basketball Association, the National Hockey League, and both major and minor league baseball, and whose citizens drive on the right and winter in Arizona and Florida, is as unforeign as another country could be. It shares with the United States a basic pattern of medical care delivery, office-based physicians with admitting privileges to hospitals, and a system of medical education. Americans may not choose to add health care financing to the list of similarities, but it is surely within the bounds of cultural possibility.[1]

Canada

Canadian health insurance is operated by the ten provinces.[2] The federal government's role has been to offer money to the provinces that meet certain conditions.[3] Each province runs a system in which patients face no restriction on choice of physician, with very little managed care.

Development

The American and Canadian health care systems developed in the same manner, for the same reasons, for much of the twentieth century. Canadian hospitals were accredited by the U.S. Joint Commission on Hospital Accreditation until well after World War II; after the United States created a grant program to finance the building of hospitals in 1948, Canada created one in 1949; and Blue Cross was created in Canada as well as in the United States. The two countries' health care costs followed nearly identical trends until Canada's national health insurance was entirely implemented in 1971.[4]

The two systems began to diverge when the province of Saskatchewan created a hospital insurance program in 1947, followed to varying degrees by British Columbia, Alberta, and Newfoundland. In 1957 the federal government passed the Hospital and Diagnostic Services Act, partly in response to pressure from other provinces that sought to do the same but wanted federal support. In return for federal payment of half of hospital costs nationwide (by a formula that favored poorer provinces), the act required that provinces make all insured services available on uniform terms (which eliminated any means-tested approach) and that provinces approve both hospital budgets and purchases of capital equipment.[5]

Once it received help on hospital payments, Saskatchewan moved on to medical services insurance, enacted in 1961. Medical insurance everywhere is far more controversial than hospital coverage, because doctors are more prickly and powerful than the people who run hospitals. Saskatchewan doctors went on strike. The final compromise allowed doctors to maintain their own "physician-controlled plans as agencies for the transmitting of doctors' accounts and doctors' payments" and therefore, it is argued, prevented any government effort to restructure health care delivery. But the government's achievement was far more important: it created the first universal medical insurance system in North America.[6]

In 1964 a Royal Commission, appointed three years earlier to get the hot potato off a conservative federal government's lap, surprised observers by issuing a sweeping call for federal cooperation with the provinces to help them fund public medical insurance.[7] At the end of 1966, Parliament passed the National Medical Care Insurance Act. It set four conditions (or principles) for federal contributions to provincial insurance expenses. The provincial plans had to be:

—*Comprehensive*: covering all medically necessary services provided by physicians;

—*Universal*: providing coverage to all legal residents of a province (with a three-month waiting period, as it developed);

—*Publicly administered*: either directly by the provincial government or by an authority directly responsible to it, so the federal government would not be subsidizing a private power;[8]

—*Portable*: so beneficiaries would also have coverage when away from their home province or, if they moved, until they became vested in their new province's plan.

Provinces that met these standards could, after 1968, receive a payment of half the national average per capita cost—a formula that increased the subsidy to the less wealthy provinces.[9]

It took until 1971 to bring all provinces and territories into the system. In Quebec implementation became embroiled in conflict over the province's place within Canada itself. Quebec made more of an effort to create an integrated network of hospitals, community health clinics, and other social services, while during the 1970s establishing more stringent cost controls than the other provinces. Still, the Quebecois version of Canadian health insurance remains identifiably Canadian.[10]

In terms of both cost control and access, the Canadian system after 1971 was far more successful than its neighbor's south of the border. Since 1971, all Canadians have had extensive health insurance. As table 2-1 showed, American and Canadian costs as shares of GDP were roughly equal (about 7.5 percent) in 1971; by 1982 Canada's had risen only to 8.4 percent, while the United States was spending 10.3 percent of GDP on health care.[11]

Nevertheless, two pressures for change developed. Many provincial plans allowed some form of extra billing, and some included cost sharing, for small daily room and board charges in hospitals, for example. Even though the large majority of procedures were billed at the set fees, physicians claimed the right to extra bill as a matter of professional dignity. A president of the Saskatchewan Medical Association proclaimed that extra billing was "the single factor that separates the medical profession from being legislated into a civil-service, union-like position."[12] But critics argued the extra charges created inequalities between those who could afford to pay them and those who could not.

The critics won the political argument, and in 1984 the Canada Health Act, passed unanimously on the eve of an election, established a fifth core principle, "accessibility." It sought to force provinces to forbid extra billing and cost sharing by calling for the federal government to deduct the amount of such charges from its payments to any province. Faced with fierce opposition from medical associations and wishing to retain the revenue from cost sharing, the governments of a number of provinces did not comply until they had forfeited some federal money. The conflict reached its height in Ontario, where physicians opposed the province's implementing legislation with a twenty-five-day strike. But there was little popular support for higher medical costs, the major Toronto news media took the government's side, and the strike failed.[13]

In the end, provincial compromises with doctors tended to include higher fees and more acceptable procedures for setting them. Over time these procedures evolved to include more formal roles for physicians in negotiations and, normally, some system of arbitration. In essence, eliminating the "safety valve" of extra billing forced both doctors and governments to work out ways to ensure acceptable settlements.[14]

The second pressure for change was budgetary. Doing better than the United States was not good enough. In 1977 the federal government, trying to stabilize its costs, negotiated with the provinces a new system of grants called Established Programs Financing (EPF). The formula in essence paid half of provincial health care costs through 1986.[15] But the federal government soon began to cut other transfers and since 1986 has increased its funding less than the rate of inflation.[16] The consequences of this federal budgetary squeeze have yet to work themselves out. The federal government's ability to enforce the five principles of the Canada Health Act could be threatened as the federal contribution falls—though the principles are popular in the provinces, too. The most likely result, though still a number of years away, would be provincial adoption of some cost sharing.[17]

Already, however, the provinces have had to confront fiscal strains from both lower federal contributions and the Canadian recession of the 1990s. The crunch hit in 1992, and provinces responded by drastically restraining spending. After fourteen years of uninterrupted growth, real public sector health care spending per capita fell in 1992 and again in 1993. Spending as a share of GDP did not grow from 1992 to 1993, while U.S. health care spending rose by half a percent of GDP. The difference in costs between the two countries leaped from 33 percent to 42 percent.[18]

The experience since 1991 makes even clearer than before the superiority of the Canadian approach for cost control and universality. Yet while some analysts of the Canadian system think it can easily make these savings without endangering quality, others are uneasy. It is too early to tell. So in order to reduce the chance of misrepresenting the consequences of a less expensive system, this book focuses on the differences in 1991, instead of later. The goal of the analysis in chapter 6 is to establish a cautious baseline estimate of possible savings from reform; if more is possible, all the better.

Finance and Benefits

Provincial funds are gathered from a mix of federal transfers that favor poorer provinces, general provincial revenues, employer payroll taxes in four cases (Quebec, Ontario, Manitoba, and Newfoundland), and premiums in two others (Alberta and British Columbia). Neither form of dedicated fund exceeds a quarter of any province's costs.[19]

Where premiums exist, there are special provisions for assistance to people with low incomes. For instance, in British Columbia subsidies ensure that no single person with an income below $11,000 (in Canadian dollars) pays any premium, and a family with two children does not pay unless its income exceeds $20,000. The application form is as simple as the American 1040EZ income tax form—unlike the thirty-page medicaid applications common in American states.[20]

Residents of each province receive insurance cards, which they present when they go to the doctor or hospital. In British Columbia the application form is two pages long. It requests no information about risk, because there is no risk-rating. Because there is no cost sharing or balance billing, patients need only present their cards in order to take care of their bills. Physicians have no economic reason to discriminate against certain types of patients, and they have very low billing expenses.

Canadian health insurance therefore is about as simple as such a thing could be. The benefits vary slightly among provinces and do not include some items that are covered in other countries or in high-end

American private insurance. There is no general dental coverage, but most provinces provide some assistance for pediatric dentistry, and all cover in-hospital oral surgery as part of hospital care. Many provide limited optometric and chiropractic coverage, and a few cover some physical therapy.

Financial support for pharmaceutical expenses is included in separate programs, generally for seniors and other categories of the needy. In British Columbia, for example, "Pharmacare" support is available to seniors, recipients of social assistance (our "welfare"), and disabled persons. Above a deductible amount, the provincial plan reimburses 80 percent of costs, and all costs are paid once any family's pharmaceutical expenses reach $2,000 in a year.[21]

Every provincial plan insures all medically necessary physician and hospital care. This includes anything a hospital can do unless it is specifically excluded, and any physician service on the fee schedule. Because there is virtually no cost sharing, no extra billing, and no cap on total insurance payout, hospital and medical benefits are better than the vast majority of private American insurance plans. Provincial coverage is far better than American medicare's.

Private insurance is allowed for anything not covered by the public plans. An estimated 80 percent of the population has supplementary coverage for items such as private rooms and dental care. It is financed primarily through employers, and as in the United States is treated as a business expense for tax purposes.[22]

In theory the Canadian form of financing could underfund a system for two reasons. First, each government can claim the other should have primary responsibility for raising the money. The federal government especially is able to cut its contributions and blame the provinces for any consequences. Second, without a dedicated payment for health care, it is easier for the public to believe that more could be spent without raising taxes, by cutting other programs. But these attributes could also be seen as advantages. Partial federal financing allows equalization among richer and poorer parts of the country. And forcing each government to choose how to spend its money may be viewed as desirable.

Paying the Hospitals and the Physicians

Canadian hospitals receive prospective, lump-sum budgets from each province's Ministry of Health.[23] Whether the amount is "negotiated" or "imposed" is a matter of opinion—but there is little doubt that the ministries have the upper hand. As fiscal conditions have tightened, governments have relied more on their own internally developed allocation formulas and less on submissions from the hospitals in deciding budgets. The job of the hospital administrator is to allocate that budget.

Requiring hospitals to adhere to budgets controls their costs. Budgeters are less likely to reallocate funds among recipients to increase efficiency, creating "winners" and "losers," than policy analysts would like.[24] But as the decline in number of hospital beds suggests, ministries have made some difficult choices, including closing hospitals. Most of the operational choices are left to the hospital administrators themselves, who have to decide, for example, how many cardiac care beds to maintain and what to do if demand for some service outstrips the budgeted resources. Somebody in the hospital has to allocate scarce beds among admitting physicians.

Unlike that of an American administrator, the Canadian hospital manager's job definitely is not to increase market share.[25] One could infer that hospitals might try to restrict their activities, doing as little as possible for their total payment. Yet the provincial budgeters are in a position to reward hospitals that do more and to punish those that seem guilty of slacking. In addition, admitting physicians, who are paid per service, have strong incentives to pressure the hospital to be as efficient as possible, because their incomes are at stake. "Historically," economist Robert G. Evans reports, "this has been successful; the throughput of Canadian hospitals has been going steadily up while bed supply has been going steadily down."[26]

Hospital administrators' tasks are made more difficult in Canada by one factor that would not be as significant in the United States. Unions are much stronger, and bargaining with hospital employee groups takes place at the provincial level. Provincial officials tend to allow wage increases that are greater than budget increases, leaving the administrators to account for the difference.

Physicians, meanwhile, are paid according to a fee schedule. Unless they "opt out"—choose not to participate in the insurance system at all—they must charge the set fee.

In all provinces, fee schedules were originally derived from the schedules created by provincial medical associations as part of preexisting physician-organized prepayment (in essence, Blue Shield) plans. The inherited relative values represented custom and internal medical politics rather than any comprehensive analysis. They have to be modified at short intervals to include new procedures. They are modified less frequently in response to traditional criticisms (primary care providers being underpaid relative to specialists) and evolutionary developments (as some procedures become easier, such as retina operations, more are provided at lower cost, so receiving the same fee as before is a windfall for those providers).

Provinces have tended to stay out of fights over relative values because the disputes are essentially about relative incomes within the medical profession, and it is better to have doctors blame each other than the government for the results. Physicians also prefer to settle this among themselves. "Indeed," Jonathan Lomas and colleagues write, "the relative value of fee items has been, in most provinces, a jealously guarded determination of the medical associations."[27] If a province decides to redo the entire schedule, it will rely on the provincial medical association to do most of the work, as British Columbia was doing at this writing.[28]

Provinces care much more about the conversion factors that translate relative values into payments. In setting these updates, Canadian provinces have constrained fees more effectively than the United States. Some restraint was accidental, because both sides underestimated inflation in the 1970s; some was part of broader national policies of wage and price control; and some, especially in Quebec, was aimed specifically at doctors.[29] Over two decades, Canadian physician fees per service fell to 59 percent of fees for American medicare and to less than half the fees charged to American private insurers.[30]

Physicians' relative incomes did not change as much because practice expenses for malpractice insurance and billing are much lower in Canada and volume of services per physician increased more quickly in Canada. Fee controls also appear to have affected higher-paid specialists more than generalists, so the income difference between typical Canadian and American physicians is not as great as the difference between averages.[31] The increased volume per physician and growth in the number of physicians meant that costs, while controlled more effectively than in America, still rose. Although paying lower prices for more services probably seems desirable to the average consumer, the provinces sought greater cost control.

Governments desired "to move the focus of negotiations from medical prices (fees) to average incomes (the product of fees and the quantity of services), and finally to total medical expenditures on physicians' services (the product of average incomes and the number of physicians)."[32] Until the mid-1980s only Quebec had adopted significant measures beyond fee schedules. By 1993 provinces were using several different methods. One method is to adjust fees for levels of utilization. In New Brunswick, for instance, excess spending in one quarter is paid back by discounting fees for the following quarter. By 1991 only a couple of provinces did not have some sort of method of adjusting fees to utilization.[33] A number had also adopted measures to reduce fees to physicians once their incomes exceeded a threshold. In 1993, for example, Ontario would pay the full bill until a physician's gross billings reached $C402,000; two-thirds of the fee for billings that raised the gross toward $C452,250; and one-third of any billings above that total.[34]

Each province's policies and politics differ from the others. But there is a clear trend toward more extensive negotiation between the province on one side and the doctors on the other. The government has a larger voice in total spending and the physicians more say on distribution. Having good data about existing costs and trends is very important; otherwise negotiations can bog down in arguments about facts. Over two decades, provinces have found that a pure adversarial approach does not work as well as mutual accommodation. Thus when British Columbia tried to impose new cost controls by legislation, it was defeated by the British Columbia Medical Association and in 1993 had to accept a new master agreement in which the BCMA has extensive rights.[35]

Following diverse paths, almost all the provinces have now reached a point where the province and physicians negotiate according to formal processes that include, for some issues, arbitration. William A. Glaser rightly emphasizes "the extraordinary significance of arbitration between an association of providers and a government."[36] Kicking and screaming in many cases, both sides have been dragged into recognizing that they have to live together, that rules are necessary, and that neither side should be able to impose its will. The government may have the upper hand because ultimately it raises the money, but both sides are better off cooperating. Some current proposals, such as setting guidelines for particular treatments, or agreeing to "delist" some procedures that officials feel are frills but doctors figure people will pay for willingly, require that the provincial ministries and physician organizations support each other against any protests.[37]

Delivery of Services

There is little reason to expect any differences in the outputs of Canadian and American medicine due to the organization of medical care.

PHYSICIAN SUPPLY AND TRAINING. Canadian and American undergraduate medical education are interchangeable: both countries' residency programs recognize each other's medical school training. As in the United States, international medical graduates work in some geographic areas that Canadian-trained doctors prefer to avoid (usually very cold and empty ones).[38] The major educational difference is financial: Canadian students pay only nominal tuition, so Canadian doctors graduate with less debt and less reason to argue that they need specialist incomes to pay it off.

Canada has similar numbers of physicians per person and proportions of residents and interns as the United States, but at least 50 percent of Canadian physicians function as general practitioners.[39] GPs commonly assist in surgeries and are frequently in charge of the delivery of babies—one hospital medical director estimated that, even in his urban hospital, obstetricians were involved in only about 30 percent of cases.

Because of the large number of GPs who provide a wide variety of services, provincial health care systems assume a person will go to a GP first and to a specialist once referred. Canada has no formal gatekeeping system, capitations, or risk-bearing arrangements. But if a patient goes to a specialist without a referral, the specialist may not be paid as much for the initial consultation as when a referral is made. The system might produce delays if GPs were not plentiful and going through them were mandatory, but access is easy. Specialists might object if, as in the United States, there were so many of them that they were in desperate competition for business. But that is rare in Canada. The system would seem overly bureaucratic if a person needed approval for every specialist visit. Instead, referrals are for a period of time such as six months, and if the GP and specialist have a good relationship, renewal is frequently done by phone.

HOSPITAL STRUCTURES AND CAPITAL SPENDING. Most Canadian hospitals are nonprofit societies governed by a board of trustees with bylaws approved by the provincial minister of health. There are hardly any for-profit hospitals in Canada. In 1990 Canadians spent more time than Americans in the hospital: very roughly, hospitals had about 10 percent more acute-care beds per person, about a day longer average length of stay, 10 percent more admissions per person, and about 10 percent higher occupancy rates.[40]

Canada has and uses more beds but has and uses less equipment. Every Canadian province strictly regulates the purchase of new equipment. Controls are more specific for larger items, and hospitals receive funds that they may choose to allocate among smaller items (the definitions of large and small vary by province). A province might pay for only a portion of capital costs, and hospitals raise money privately for the rest. But approval is needed if any government money is involved, and if a hospital pays for a purchase entirely with private funds, the provincial Ministry of Health may refuse to increase the operating budget to pay for running the equipment.[41]

Capital allocations do not produce an entirely planned or "rational" allocation of resources, because different hospitals have different levels of prestige and ability to raise the private funds needed to add to public funding and buy some items. But the budgeting process does give special attention to high-tech equipment, and items such as lithotripters and magnetic resonance imaging (MRI) machines tend to be concentrated mainly in the academic medical centers. As a result, equipment is used more intensively in Canada, and both the costs of the machines and the salaries of the technicians who use them can be spread over a larger number of uses.[42]

The capacity of the Canadian health care system contributes to Canada's lower expenses. Most evidently, lesser capacity for more expensive treatments means that those treatments are not as likely to be overused and that each use costs less. A somewhat broader role for general practitioners may reduce the need for referrals, while the lower number of specialists enables them individually to maintain the volume necessary to create high incomes while collecting much lower fees.

The delivery arrangements also provide wide choice of doctors. There are no gatekeepers with incentives to refuse referrals, and there is no need to wait three weeks for an appointment at one's HMO. Still, the Canadian system has not created total and equal access to care. As they are everywhere, rural areas are underserved relative to urban; that is one reason the Canadians bring in international medical graduates. And free access to medical care does not eliminate inequalities in health that are based on differences in shelter or nutrition or other factors. It does mean that every sick Canadian can go to a doctor without worrying about the cost.

Americans who wish to scare their fellows away from universal coverage argue that, in order to achieve that coverage, Canadians (and all other peoples) have to accept inferior medical care. Chapter 6 analyzes that charge in greater detail. In the end, the fact that quality is so hard to measure will allow some people to conclude what they wish. But the preponderance of evidence suggests that, after all possible adjustments, American health care quality could at best be very marginally better than Canada's. Canada has better choice, much better access, and much lower costs.

Germany

In the standard terms of American policy debate, Canada might seem to offer the only alternative to the American way of saving for health care. Canadians save through government insurance, Americans (mostly) through private. One is "the state," the other "the market," and people can take sides depending on what they think of those labels. The German form of shared savings is not a compromise between these two models. It is the original to which all others should be compared.

Sickness Funds and the Financing of German Health Care

During the Middle Ages, European societies developed webs of obligation and help for medical expenses. Guilds of working men— bakers, smiths, and the like—created funds to help members with the costs of hospital care, to pay for funeral expenses, to help disabled fellows, or to aid bereaved families. Journeymen who did not have guild status formed fraternities for similar purposes, and miners also formed associations. In short, members of a nonhierarchical community saved together on the basis of that membership.[43]

Such community-based insurance had no more to do with the market than with the state. It was not sold on an open market, purchase was compulsory rather than voluntary, and prices were not set in relation to risk but as a flat rate or a share of income. As the modern economy was invented, the organization of work and workers changed. But the needs remained, and therefore, as William A. Glaser summarizes:

> Similar arrangements were created among the industrial workers of the nineteenth century. They too needed invalidity payments; their widows and children also needed funeral expenses and death benefits if the worker died. Mutual aid societies within individual plants and towns were created by trade unions, political parties, employers and churches. To make benefits more reliable, money had to be collected more systematically; every member paid a predictable subscription fee, and some employers contributed administrative help and cash . . . all workers in the plan were expected to join and pay; all members were eligible for standard benefits regardless of variations in contribution due to length of membership and income level; retired members might receive pensions even when they no longer contributed. Nonmembers were not covered.

"The national health insurance laws beginning in the 1880s in Germany," Glaser explains, "made social solidarity official policy and eventually spread it to entire populations."[44] Universal coverage took a while, and the results tend to look more like patchwork quilts than like the seamless garment of the Canadian design. Over time the state came to regulate the sickness funds substantially, just as it regulated the market. But the fundamental aspects of sickness funds remained— membership according to location or occupation rather than choice, contributions based on income (with single persons subsidizing families) rather than risk, and fund management obligated to the members rather than to any investors.

In the mid-1870s, Germany had about 10,000 relief funds with 2 million members. In 1883 Chancellor Otto von Bismarck of Germany expanded and systematized this structure. The law provided for employees to contribute two-thirds, and employers one-third, of the costs, and for governance of each fund by a board similarly constituted by representatives of employees and employers. The government set the minimum benefit level by statute, and it included sick pay, medical expenses, and hospital treatment.[45] The law's key provision was that it made membership compulsory for employees with incomes below a certain level, about three times the average wage, in specific types of industry. By 1885, 4.3 million workers were members of the funds.

Bismarck's system of sickness and other insurance was expanded as the economy and society evolved toward its modern form. Separate funds for salaried employees (white-collar rather than blue) had existed since the early nineteenth century and were included in the regulatory framework in 1913. A 1927 law creating unemployment insurance also provided for continuation of membership in the sickness funds for persons who lost their jobs.

Even the Nazis did not threaten the basic benefits, though they did take control of the funds' administration, purging socialists and Jews. After the Third Reich was destroyed, the victorious Allies found little reason to reform the social insurance schemes. In 1951 the contribution rates and representation on the boards of the primary funds was changed to an even split. Otherwise, change was incremental. In December 1970 the income threshold for mandatory membership in the sickness funds was indexed, and voluntary membership in those funds was made possible for all employees. In 1972 membership was expanded for farmers and their families; in 1973 time limits on hospital treatment were abolished; and in 1975 all students were included in the statutory scheme.[46]

Since the early 1970s, the health care policy agenda in Germany, as elsewhere, has come to emphasize cost control rather than expansion of coverage. Controlling costs is never easy, and the payers had to learn how to do it. But by the late 1980s West Germany had created fairly effective institutions to control costs. As the figures in chapter 1 show, they were quite successful by international standards. But a combination of the demographic pressures for higher spending, the costs of reunification, and the recession of the 1990s worsened fiscal conditions in the early 1990s. The Germans, who sometimes perceive fiscal crisis in anything other than perfect stability, adopted new cost control measures at the end of 1992.

In order to win support for those measures from the opposition Social Democratic party, which controlled the upper house of Germany's parliament, the government of Chancellor Helmut Kohl had to endorse significant changes in the rules for membership in and contributions to the sickness funds. As is the case with Canada, we do not know how those new policies will work, so the description that follows focuses on German institutions as they existed in 1991. The concluding part of this section then describes the 1992 reforms.

Financing and Benefits

In 1989 Germans were insured by more than 1,100 different funds. The primary funds, serving 57 percent of the population, could be formed by a single employer or workplace, a craft, a trade group, or an occupation (agricultural workers, miners, seamen). At least seven hundred of these were for single employers, but they enrolled only 11 percent of the population; 37 percent enrolled in the 268 community-based funds that pooled all employees not in one of the other funds.

Blue-collar workers with earnings less than the threshold (DM 58,500 per year in 1991) had no choice of fund.[47] All white-collar workers, and those blue-collar workers with earnings above the threshold, could join a substitute fund. The eight blue-collar and seven white-collar substitute funds enrolled 31 percent of the population. Six of the latter were nationally available, and among them they enrolled by far the largest part of the 31 percent of Germans who were covered by substitute funds.[48]

Above the income threshold, Germans are not required to join a sickness fund.[49] Self-employed persons may be members only if they have previously been in a fund (for instance, in an earlier job). Higher civil servants (which in Germany includes teachers) are directly reimbursed by the state for at least half of their expenses and buy private insurance for the rest. Most Germans who have a choice nevertheless choose to join a sickness fund. As a result, about 10 percent of the population has private insurance, and about 2 percent (such as members of the military and the police) has direct government coverage. Perhaps 100,000 persons do without insurance.[50]

Germans pay much less than Americans out-of-pocket for health care—approximately 7.5 percent of the total in 1987.[51] They pay a larger visible contribution, on average, for their insurance: half. Whether that makes any economic difference is a matter for economic theologians. It likely makes the public more enthusiastic about cost control.

FINANCING SICKNESS FUNDS. Each sickness fund requires that employers and employees contribute a fixed percentage of wages up

to the same cap above which persons have a right to refuse membership in the fund. The employer pays half and the employee pays half.
The financing principles are therefore virtually identical to American
social security and (until the cap was removed in 1993) medicare part
A. People with lower incomes pay less but get the same benefits.
Unlike in America, payments are made to a nongovernmental entity.
The maximum contribution is set by law, but the board of any fund
can choose to exceed that limit. In 1992 the average was slightly higher
than 13 percent of the covered payroll.[52] Because each fund represented a different pool of persons, with different incomes from which
to draw contributions and different morbidity profiles, premium rates
varied substantially.[53] Because most companies and employees would
not maintain separate funds if doing so were more expensive, company
funds, with an average contribution rate of 11.5 percent, had lower
rates than either community funds, averaging about 13.5 percent, or
substitute funds, which averaged 13 percent with slightly more generous benefits. The range of premiums, about 10 to 15 percent for all
but rare cases, still represented large disparities relative to income,
which the Social Democratic party wanted to eliminate.[54]

Contributions to health insurance for the unemployed are made by
the unemployment insurance system, which contributes an amount
equal to the average contribution for all workers.[55] Retirees pay a proportion of pension incomes, in keeping with the principle that people
should contribute according to their means. Because the elderly do not
have employers, they pay the full share (13 percent) out of private
pensions. Payments out of public pensions are more complicated.
Though ostensibly they are moving in the same direction, the actual
figure is closer to the usual employee percentage.[56]

The rest of the cost for the elderly is covered by employee and
employer contributions. Roughly 3 percent of the 13 percent employment-related contribution is dedicated to the cost of pensioners. It is
treated as a separate pool of money, and a system of interfund transfers moves money from funds with fewer elderly than the norm to
those funds with more. This dedicated payment is thus similar in both
amount and source to America's 2.8 percent medicare payroll tax.

SICKNESS FUND BENEFITS. Sickness fund benefits vary slightly, but
the minimum, mandated by government, is quite extensive. In 1991 it
included all physician care for illness, without copayments; some am-

bulatory preventive care (for example, cancer checkups for women over thirty, and vaccinations but not annual comprehensive physicals for adults); substantial dental benefits (80 percent of materials and 100 percent of labor for dentures); and hospital benefits with only very small copayments (10 DM ($6–7) per day for the first fourteen days).

German coverage for pharmaceuticals is universal and among the most extensive in the world, requiring small copayments. A small number of mainly over-the-counter medications, about 18 percent of the spending on pharmaceuticals, is not covered. Since 1989 Germany has had a system of "reference prices" for comparable drugs, so the funds pay more than the generic price but less than the price of some brand name medications.[57]

The system also includes extensive income benefits (sick pay) and much more generous benefits than most other systems for aids such as glasses, hearing aids, and prostheses. It even pays a substantial portion of expenses once every three years for "the cure" at a spa— often prescribed for recuperation from serious illness. Mental health benefits are covered but not talked about much, perhaps because Germans believe in them less than Americans do. Until the 1990s long-term care was covered only by a means-tested public program. Legislation to create a new long-term care program was passed in 1994.[58]

PRIVATE INSURANCE. People who purchase private insurance receive coverage that generally pays providers more, may provide some extra benefits, often has cost sharing, and because of the higher payments buys better service. Purchasers who go a long enough time without claims occasionally even receive rebates. Some purchasers consider private insurance to be more prestigious than public; in a sense they pay more for the prestige of paying more. Private insurance may also be believed to have higher status.

The financing of German private health insurance differs from American in two important ways. First, no risk-rating is allowed. Unlike in America, less healthy people do not pay more. Second, German insurers charge a level premium. Actuaries estimate a person's expenses over a lifetime and then establish a base premium that, paid annually, is expected to cover lifetime costs. Level premiums are a device for limiting adverse selection in a nonmandatory system. A person who buys insurance at a young age will pay more than the actuarial cost for likely services at that age. But, having paid those costs, he receives in essence a discount in later years. A fifty-year-old who has been in a plan for ten years is charged more than one who has been a member for twenty. Level premiums thus provide some incentive to buy insurance and a very strong incentive to stay with the same insurer; a person who switches plans enters the new one at the higher rate charged to people her age.[59]

Private insurance could create adverse selection in another way: eligible individuals might go private while young and without a family, then join a sickness fund when the private charges for family insurance exceed the sickness fund contribution. Germany has therefore banned persons with private insurance from (re)joining the sickness fund system unless their eligibility status changes.[60]

Paying the Bills

West Germany was divided into eighteen regions, some equal to a state (Land) and some essentially cities. In each region, physicians in order to bill the sickness funds had to be a member of the Association of Sickness Fund Physicians (Kassenärztliche Vereinigung, or KV).[61] Each type of sickness fund formed its own regional associations.

In 1977 legislation created an organization called Concerted Action, consisting of about seventy representatives of various interests who meet twice a year to set guidelines for cost trends in each sector of health care (hospitals, pharmaceuticals, ambulatory and dental care, and the like). Its deliberations have been strongly influenced by staff and a standing council of expert advisers. Although it has no formal authority to set prices, Concerted Action has established a standard of "reasonableness" to which both negotiators and an arbitrator might refer.

With those standards as a guide, the sickness funds in all regions negotiated to hold down the costs of both hospital and physician services.

HOSPITAL PAYMENT. In 1991 and earlier, when sickness fund associations negotiated with hospitals, they agreed on budget targets on the basis of past experience, possible new needs, staffing levels, and other common subjects of budgeting. These were converted into day rates by dividing the budget by the number of expected days of care. Each fund then paid for the days that its members spent in the hospital. To limit incentives for excess stays, the funds paid hospitals only

25 percent of the rate once the number of days exceeded the targets, but 75 percent of the rate for each day under the target that was *not* billed![62]

Unfortunately, the hospitals preferred to receive extra payments, even if they were only 25 percent, the rationale being that if hospitals lost money, payers might choose to reimburse them in the next year's negotiations. Hospital cost controls in Germany were less successful than physician cost controls—a reverse of the normal pattern.[63] Germany, virtually alone among the nations of the world, has budgeted ambulatory care more strictly than inpatient care. That difference was narrowed in 1992.

PHYSICIAN PAYMENT. The National Association of Sickness Fund Physicians (Kassenärztliche Bundesvereinigung, or KBV) and the national associations of each type of sickness funds negotiate, periodically, a relative value scale. This establishes, for the entire country, a point schedule with about 1,700 items. A home visit, for example, is worth 360 points, and a telephone consultation with a patient 80.[64] Given this relative value scale, regional physician associations at one time negotiated the conversion factor, and thus a unique regional fee schedule, with the regional associations of each type of sickness fund. The substitute funds always paid a bit more (around 10 percent) as evidence of their socially superior status (and suggesting that their members would receive better service). As had been true for decades, physicians billed not individual funds but the regional physician association (KV). The KV collected the vouchers each quarter, totaled them up, billed each fund for its members, and then passed the payments back to the physicians (who had received monthly estimated payments based on previous billings).

This administratively simple system (from a physician's point of view) did not thoroughly control costs, because the volume of services rose more than expected. In 1986, therefore, the sickness funds won a system in which, instead of negotiating the conversion factors, they negotiated the total regional payment by the primary funds to the physicians. There is no longer a negotiated conversion factor. Instead, the KV receives each quarter's vouchers, adds up the number of points, and divides that into the payment total to determine the payment per point. Therefore, if physicians do more than expected, payment per point is reduced automatically and immediately.

Some services are exempt from the cap, largely preventive services believed to both improve the quality of care and, by reducing illness, perhaps even save money.[65] To protect against proliferation of billings in ways that would give some physicians an advantage over others, the funds and doctors in 1987 agreed to separate caps for physician consultations, laboratory tests, and other services.

If a physician finds innovative and perhaps illicit ways to increase his volume of billings, he is not exploiting the sickness funds—he is exploiting other physicians. That fact gave extra impetus to the KVs (physician associations) to regulate outliers among their members. In each region, a committee consisting of four representatives of the funds, four representatives of the physicians, and an annually rotating chair, conducts a retrospective review of physician practice data. Using the centralized billing data, they are able to construct profiles of each physician's practice, compare physicians of similar training, patient mix, office staff and so on, and identify those who provide or prescribe much more services of particular types. The reviewers also can flag particularly expensive cases. Then physicians from the physician association consult with the individual doctor to identify reasons for the deviations (such as that a physician was placed in the wrong peer group). If the committee wishes, it can deduct identified excesses from a physician's future reimbursements.[66]

A physician who objects to the committee's decision may appeal to a review board. The process is oriented more toward counseling than sanctions. There is usually very little disagreement within the committee between fund and physician representatives, because the physicians have more incentive than the funds to discipline other physicians.

This system reduces the average volume of services, to which each physician is being compared, only by limiting some high volumes that raise the average. But it has that marginal effect, while the review makes fraud and abuse somewhat less likely. More important, in this system physicians, rather than outside regulators, govern physicians, which reduces their ability to complain about insurers or the government and makes them more likely to address their own behavior.[67]

How, an American might ask, could the sickness funds get away with imposing such a system? They "get away with it" because they did not impose it: it was created through negotiations. But, then, why did the doctors accept it? At one level the funds exploited, perhaps unintentionally, divisions within the physicians' groups. The funds had resisted paying for new services on the grounds that relative values should be revised, but any revision of relative values was likely to start a fight between GPs and specialists. So there had been a deadlock, pressure for change built up, and the physicians agreed that in the context of a major revision, with unpredictable effects on volume and incomes, *temporary* measures were justified to provide system stability. Once they were created, these measures became the status quo.

But the flexible conversion factor seemed much less revolutionary than it might have, because of a history that has ironic overtones for the current U.S. debate. The sickness funds were simply returning to an approach made possible by legislation more than fifty years earlier, one that appealed to physicians at the time because it abolished closed panels, the equivalent of American HMOs.

At one time, sickness funds contracted with limited groups of doctors, often setting up clinics. German physicians first organized, in the early twentieth century, to fight against this system. In 1931 and 1932 the government banned the negotiations between sickness funds and individual physicians that created exclusive contracts, and required funds to negotiate with all physicians through the newly created KVs. In return it allowed payments to the KVs by capitation (essentially creating a global budget). During the fat years of the 1950s and 1960s physicians convinced the funds to abandon this system, but this was a matter of negotiation, and the funds needed no extra authority to recreate the system in 1985.[68]

By 1991, therefore, Germany was in the highly anomalous position of having controlled ambulatory care payments better than hospital or pharmaceutical costs, at least as compared with expectations. German physician incomes were already falling because of the rapid increase in the number of physicians before 1986, even though only fee regulation was in effect. The hard cap on total billings locked in the trend, and by 1989 the average earnings of office-based physicians had fallen to about four times the average private sector wage, from about 5.5 times in 1975.[69] These trends shaped the cost control measures in the reforms adopted in 1992 and implemented beginning in 1993.

German methods of cost control, combined with a robust economy, stabilized health care costs in the 1980s as a percentage of GDP. They rose from 8.1 percent of GDP in 1977 to 8.7 percent in 1981, but were only 8.5 percent in 1991. During this same period, American costs rose from 8.7 to 13.4 percent of GDP.[70]

By 1991, however, ordinary citizens' incomes were stagnating in the poor economy throughout Europe, and German reunification added huge costs to the federal budget, which were financed by higher taxes and higher interest rates. Sickness fund premiums escalated substantially from 1991 to 1993.[71] Further increases in the health insurance contribution rate seemed too great a burden for individuals and corporations.

Delivery of Health Care

German health care delivery differs from America's and Canada's in significant ways.

PHYSICIAN SUPPLY AND TRAINING. Education in Germany is funded by state governments, as a right of citizenship, and therefore medical students are able to attend medical school and graduate debt-free. As a result, Germany has 20 percent more physicians per person than either the United States or Canada, and the supply is rising rapidly. State (Land) governments have clearly trained too many physicians.

German medical education combines the eight years of American college and medical school into one six-year period. But eighteen months of further training is needed for full licensure; a total of four years is needed for certification as a sickness fund GP, and further clinical training is required to become a specialist; so the education is functionally equivalent to that in the United States. As is true in most countries, procedurally oriented specialists earn higher incomes than generalists.[72]

In a near-perfect illustration of Wildavsky's law—"even Stalin and Beria couldn't get doctors to move to the countryside"—as many as ten or fifteen thousand German physicians may be unemployed, yet there are still shortages in rural areas.[73]

In addition to having more doctors, Germany has a stronger wall between hospital-based and office-based practice. About 12 percent of acute-care hospital beds are allocated to office-based physicians, primarily in a few specialties—otolaryngology, pediatrics, and gynecology. There are also some part-timers in hospitals. But the norm is for an office-based physician not to have admitting privileges and for hospital physicians to be permanent, salaried staff. Office-based physicians instead work in private "clinics," which may be well supplied with expensive diagnostic tools but in the absence of residents and a permanent salaried staff cannot handle complex cases.[74] Thus once your regular physician refers you to the hospital, he is out of the loop. A German colleague of the author, asked about this, recalled that her mother's doctor did visit her when she was hospitalized, even in another city—*during visiting hours*!

Among ambulatory care physicians, there is no formal distinction between primary gatekeepers and referral specialists. Members receive voucher booklets (one for medical and one for dental care). The norm is to use one voucher per quarter and present it to the first physician visited. This physician then provides a transfer voucher for seeing a second physician, or the patient may also just use another voucher from the booklet. None of the sources consulted for this book reported obstacles to seeing more than one physician in a quarter.

Most office-based physicians are in solo practices, although perhaps because of rising expenses for equipment, the number of group practices is growing.[75] At least as many doctors work in German hospitals as in office practice. The chief of service is the boss. He has formal authority within the hospital, but can also allocate to other doctors a share of the fees he receives for special attention to privately insured patients.[76] Otherwise referrals are by transfer voucher to the hospital itself, not to an individual physician.[77]

This referral structure may explain why there is not much talk in Germany about waiting lists. One's ambulatory care physician has little financial incentive to recommend a hospital procedure. And, if one is to enter the hospital, the wait is for the hospital itself, not for a particular specialist. When people are divided into groups, each waiting for a specific service provider, the likelihood of a conflict is greater than if they all wait together for anyone from the pool of providers. That is why banks now have people wait in one line for all tellers rather than in specific lines for each teller, and why getting in the "wrong" check-out line at the supermarket is so irritating.[78] Therefore the odds of having to wait are lower if one goes directly to the hospital rather than to a specific physician.

The huge supply of doctors ensures that, though physicians are eager to have private patients, they compete to deliver services to everyone. Germans visit physicians at nearly twice the rate per year that Americans do, are hospitalized more often, and stay longer in the hospital.[79] The longer lengths of stay are commonly ascribed to the financial incentive for longer stays in a system that pays hospitals by the day and to a shortage of nursing-home beds. Be that as it may, there is no doubt that the supply of hospital beds and physicians, along with universal coverage, allows easy access to beds and to physicians.

HOSPITALS AND CAPITAL EQUIPMENT. Public hospitals, owned by federal, state, or local governments, account for just over half of all beds; private voluntary (mainly religious) hospitals account for 35 percent, and private proprietary hospitals, normally owned by doctors, for 14 percent. Even private hospitals receive most of their capital budgets from state governments. Hospitals are allowed more than a thousand dollars per bed for annual routine maintenance, but major investments require separate funding.

There is little reason to believe that German planning is particularly coherent; but, as in Canada, the individual states' efforts to put high-tech equipment in the academic medical centers and to limit funding for most other capital purposes during the 1980s did reduce the growth of high-tech capacity.[80] In both countries these methods inherently put the most demanding programs in the most advanced centers with the most expert staff and thereby concentrate experience with new procedures in the hands of physicians who can be fully employed and thus expert in their work.

Office-based physicians are said to have bought large amounts of equipment, in part to compete with hospitals.[81] But the system of fee regulation for physician expenses was so strong that this was the doctors' problem, not the payers'.

The 1992 Reforms

The Structural Health Reform Act of 1992 created new payment regulations in response to the financial problems associated with unification. It did not, unlike American reform proposals, contemplate significant change in the delivery of medical care. But as part of a political deal, it included what should be substantial change in how Germans pool their funds for health insurance.

COST CONTROLS. The 1992 act preempted the Concerted Action process for 1993–95 by freezing the sickness fund contribution rates.

To enforce that target, the Act subjected each sector of health care "to a separate, strict, and airtight budget cap the growth of which is directly linked to the payroll base."[82] Although the 1992 reform includes constraints on doctors, its main purpose is to restrain cost growth in other sectors, on the assumption that physicians have borne enough of the burden so far.

The law mandates multiyear budget targets for the hospital sector. If a hospital exceeds its target for a given year, it must pay back the individual funds for that excess at the end of the year.[83] Thus budgets have become more binding. Although a fund might, as previously, allow a hospital to earn the money back in the following year, the funds were forbidden to negotiate overall hospital spending increases that were larger than the funds' growth in income; so in order to compensate a particular hospital for losses, they would have to take the money from others.

These hospital spending limits have raised a few questions. First, what is the effect of wage settlements? The bill allows the cap to be adjusted upward to pay higher wages, so it is not as tight as it may seem at first glance. Second, how can funds ensure that hospitals do not simply reduce services to meet the targets? In the German system admitting physicians do not lobby for greater productivity, but the funds have some ability to monitor amounts of services directly—for example, by requesting access to patient files. If patients begin having trouble getting admitted for procedures, there will be an increase in complaints, or the records will show a sudden increase in services provided by private clinics. If a hospital claims to be providing extra services, the payers may demand precise documentation. Americans should remember that the regulators, in this case, are local associations in regions averaging about 3 million persons, rather than a distant federal government. Thus while the methods used to monitor hospital performance are hardly perfect, they should be sufficient to prevent egregious slacking.[84]

A second set of measures targets the costs of dental care. Per capita, dentists are better paid than physicians, partly because their number has grown more slowly. As a result, the number of patients (or customers) has not fallen as quickly for dentists as for doctors. The 1992 law applied budget targets to the dental sector, reduced fees for dentures and orthodontic treatment by 10 percent, cut dental technician fees by 5 percent, delisted some dentures considered not medically necessary, and created mechanisms to reduce fees further if volume exceeded targets.

The most dramatic measures in the 1992 reforms addressed pharmaceutical costs. Save for creating a few copayments, West Germany had made little effort to constrain pharmaceutical costs before 1989. Because the government regulated markups by pharmacists but not the wholesale prices set by manufacturers, West Germany had among the highest pharmaceutical prices in the world. Joined with a medical style that favored use of a great many drugs, and more generous insurance, German policies supported higher spending on pharmaceuticals than in the United States, in spite of the much lower spending on health care as a whole.[85]

The 1992 law froze total pharmaceutical spending at the 1991 level through 1994. Small increases in copayments were a minor means to that end. Price cuts and incentives for doctors to reduce their prescribing are far more significant.

The reference-price system had already begun to reduce the disparity between German and other countries' pharmaceutical prices. The act mandated a 5 percent cut in prices of all prescription drugs not covered by the reference-price system, cut over-the-counter prices by 2 percent, and froze those prices through 1994. The rules for application of reference prices were simplified so they could be applied to more products. Then the act made physicians responsible for total prescription costs.

If in 1993 costs were up to 2 percent higher than the target, the sickness fund physicians and the drug companies would both somehow be assessed for half of the excess. Much more significant, the same review procedure that had been applied to physician fees can now be applied to prescription costs, with lower thresholds (if the physician's prescribing exceeds the pharmaceutical cost target by 25 percent or more, the burden of proof is on him to justify his costs; if his costs are between 15 and 25 percent above the target, the control doctors will investigate, but they must show why the prescribing is not justified). If a physician's prescribing costs are too high, the funds may deduct excess costs from the physician's own fees.

Overreacting, German physicians reduced their prescriptions so much that total charges for prescription drugs sold in February 1993 were 30 percent less than in February 1992. Physicians prescribed more generics and issued prescriptions for smaller packages. They also became much more hesitant to satisfy patient expectations that the doctor "do something" by prescribing harmless but not particularly useful medications. By midyear the physicians may have been less panicked, so drug spending per sickness fund member was only 20.6 percent less than in the first six months of 1992.[86] But the incentives for individual physicians, and the price cuts, ensured that the sickness funds would more than meet their savings target.

The new cutoffs for profiling review and creation of the pharmaceutical spending category are the 1992 act's major change in physician reimbursement. The legislation was designed to impose costs on the pharmaceutial manufacturers and on those physicians who provided excessive services, rather than on physicians as a whole. The act therefore allowed ambulatory surgery and preventive care to rise faster than the funds' income. The short-term price limits, more stringent budgets, and requirement that physicians bear risk for exceeding some targets were described as emergency measures, to respond to an economic crisis for which everyone must share the burden. In theory, long-term measures in the act would reduce the need for its drastic temporary controls later.[87]

These long-term proposals of the 1992 act are based on standard critiques of health care systems in general and the German system in particular. They include the establishment of diagnosis-related groups so hospitals can be paid according to the amount and type of services provided, not according to how much they were paid the year before; encouragement of outpatient treatment by hospitals; disincentives to specialize; reduced training of new physicians and measures to force them to practice in underserved areas; development of a formulary of approved drugs (rather than a list of those disapproved); even moves toward gatekeeper models for primary care and cost-per-case payments.

Two things should be noted about this long-run agenda. Some of the measures had to come sometime. Most countries have drug formularies, and there was no way established physicians could live with the projected increase in their numbers, given any plausible level of cost control. But a number of the measures are more statements of intent according to common international notions of what-would-be-nice, than settled proposals that can be expected to work. Some are nowhere near implementation. Others, such as the DRGs, are closer— but whether they will save money is an open question. DRGs give hospitals better arguments for more funding, and ambulatory surgery may cost less per case but can also increase volume.

THE PRICE OF REFORM. One last set of provisions was not about total health care costs but about the equity of premiums. In 1994 a new process of risk adjustment was to be introduced, setting up interfund transfers based on numbers of insured dependents, age and sex distribution of the insured, and incomes. In 1995 this process will supersede the current set of transfers that pay for pensioners.

How much equalization these changes produce will depend on the formula, but a second provision of the law could be quite effective. Beginning in 1997 substitute funds will be required to open membership to everyone. If people are in fact paying attention—which cannot be taken for granted—members of funds with higher rates will switch to the substitute funds. But as they acquire less healthy or less wealthy members, the substitute funds' rates will likely rise. Free choice of funds therefore could nearly equalize rates (if the transfers have not already done so) and consolidate the number of funds.[88]

These equalization measures were the price of Social Democratic party support for the cost controls. The main exception seems also to fit that party's base: company funds can refuse to accept nonemployees of the company. Therefore large industries with good risk profiles or high wages should be able to pay a smaller contribution rate—a benefit to both big labor and big business.

The system that results will likely include some large national funds, some company funds, some local funds (in fairly low-cost regions), and much more expensive private insurance for a small proportion of the population. That distribution of options sounds somewhat like the Clinton administration proposals.

Summary: Germany and Canada

As with the Canadian case, it is wiser to evaluate German methods of financing and delivering health care as of 1991 than to guess how new initiatives will work. Also as in Canada, budget problems caused by forces larger than the health care system itself have caused governments to define as a "crisis" levels of spending and access that would seem wildly successful in the United States.

Germany controlled costs more effectively, with even more generous benefits, than Canada did. Some aspects of Germany's greater success must be related to the salaried status of hospital doctors and the small number of admitting physicians. The former directly lowers payments, while both eliminate most incentives for doctors to prescribe expensive inpatient treatments (unless a patient has private insurance). Other advantages and disadvantages may cancel each other out. Germany has many more physicians and more hospital beds than Canada. Occasional reports suggest Germany has greater capacity to provide high-technology care, but that may be false.[89] Administration also must be more expensive in Germany than in Canada (comparative data on this subject are hard to find, and hard to judge if found). But Germany has a less invasive culture of medical practice. Living next to the United States affects both Canadian patients and doctors.

Canada's much less fragmented insurance system gives its citizens the advantage of, at least until 1997, more equal contribution rates as a portion of income. With Germany moving in Canada's direction rather than the reverse, American inequalities are harder to defend. But because Germany finances health care directly rather than through general revenue, and contributions are deducted from unemployment checks and pensions as well as wages, the principle that everyone must contribute in rough proportion to income is illustrated more clearly in Germany. And the German method of financing has other advantages. It shows that health insurance can be separated from the government accounts. Because funding is separate, it is not caught up in the intergovernmental transfer politics endemic in Canada and the United States (with medicaid).

The German example shows that successes like those of Canada can be achieved with a different financing structure. A country can even have separate insurance for a small portion of the population—as long as it is the wealthy, not the poor or the middle class. For cost control what matters is not how many payers there are but whether they work together or separately.

The German example also reinforces the importance of physicians' role in governing a successful health care system. In both Canada and Germany the payers and the doctors must find a way to get along; and the payers have learned that contentious intraprofession issues, such as relative values, should be left mainly to the physicians to settle.

Both countries' systems also therefore require that physicians be organized into more representative bodies than exist in the United States, and that those bodies be granted some authority by the state.

Physicians in neither country can impose their will by going on strike. Yet neither can either government, or German sickness funds, simply impose terms on physicians. In both countries, the trend is toward finding ways to get physicians to control volume within each payment area (a province in Canada, a region in Germany), though the process is far more advanced in Germany.

There are many other similarities that were mentioned in the introduction, such as the importance of fee schedules and of budgeting. The reviews of Australia, France, Japan, and the United Kingdom will help establish how fundamental these features are: they work everywhere, not just in Canada and Germany. Those two countries have shown that there are different paths to some of the same ends. The other cases provide further options within the international standard.

5

Alternatives: Australia, France, Japan, and the United Kingdom

*T*HE health systems of Australia, France, Japan, and the United Kingdom are less commonly suggested as models for American reform than those of Canada and Germany. Each country, however, can teach us something about our health care alternatives.

Australian and French arrangements provide illuminating variations on, respectively, the Canadian and German models. They can help us judge the effects of adjustments that Americans might choose to make in adapting either a system of government insurance or of regulated sickness funds. Great Britain and Japan represent more distant models than the other four. Yet both provide tests of some commonly overstated claims about health care systems and further illustrate the basic elements of the international standard. The following descriptions, therefore, emphasize what seems most useful to the American debate.

Australia

Australia, like Canada and the United States, is a nation of continental expanse, federal structure, and British heritage. Unlike in Canada, its advocates of full-fledged national health insurance have not fully triumphed. Arguments over "public" and "private" medicine have separated the parties, with Labor on the former side and the Liberal and Country Party coalition (hereafter, the coalition) on the latter.

Development and Tensions

The current Australian health care system, established seemingly permanently when Labor regained power in 1984, includes a public

91

guarantee of care but gives private insurance a role that is larger than anywhere else in this study but the United States. Unlike in Canada, private insurance legally can provide many of the same benefits as the public system and in some cases offers greater convenience and choice. It does so by paying for "private" status in a public hospital or for a large part of the charges of a private hospital. Public coverage does not include private hospital stays. But the private hospitals do not as a system offer the same services as public, especially in terms of emergency or intensive care. The care received in private hospitals is of a more elective nature.

These differences have created a dynamic in which people who are more certain of needing care are more likely to choose to buy private insurance. Because higher-cost people are more likely to choose private coverage, rates should rise, lower-cost people should drop out, rates should rise further, and the private system should eventually collapse. As one of the designers of the dual Australian system explained it, the market could drive Australia to "Canada by stealth." But the federal (or Commonwealth) government has tightened its funding to the public system, especially the transfers to the states that largely fund hospital care. As a result, more people have reason to use the private insurance "safety valve" to guarantee convenient access to care. These countervailing pressures to drop and maintain private coverage has been a complex set of cross pressures that in the early 1990s roughly stabilized the proportion of Australians with private insurance, but at rising costs for that coverage.

Australia's systems of physician and hospital payment differ from both Canada's and America's for historic reasons. In order to pass a constitutional amendment allowing Commonwealth financing of health care in 1946, advocates had to include language forbidding "any form of civil conscription." This certainly banned any version of the British National Health Service (which was the point), but a 1947 Supreme Court ruling has been interpreted as banning compulsory fee schedules as well.[1]

The Australian states set up extensive systems of public hospitals long before the Commonwealth became involved in health care. Normally physicians and surgeons treated the poor for free in return for the right to use some hospital beds for paying patients. Public hospitals normally also had outpatient clinics. Private hospitals arose mainly so that middle-class patients could avoid association with the lower-class nonpaying types.

The medical staffing arrangements, and the growth of a private alternative, are similar to developments in the United States. But in Australia, public hospitals had a more secure financial base than in the United States. And because their role in medical education was not seriously challenged by private institutions, many of the scientific advances of medicine after World War I were concentrated in the public hospitals. Although a few large private nonprofit institutions did develop, they never became dominant, as they did in both Canada and the United States.

Therefore state governments had more direct influence on the provision of health care than in the United States. Hospitals' reliance on admitting physicians foreclosed the German-style separation of ambulatory and inpatient sectors. Physicians who wanted to provide the most advanced care had to practice in the public hospitals, even if they could do lucrative work in private institutions. Physicians' joint practice in public and private hospitals shapes the interaction between public and private insurance, as well as the controversy about waiting lists in the public hospitals.

Public Sector Financing

In 1984 Australia adopted what it calls medicare. All permanent residents of the country, and some visitors, may join, and all pay for the system whether they join or not.

Australian medicare pays directly only for ambulatory services. A tax of 1.4 percent of personal income, the "Medicare levy," raises some of the costs of that program; most are paid from general revenues. The states provide hospital care, but the federal government provides grants to states for their public hospital systems on the condition that they provide free hospital services to all medicare members.

Australian states have weak taxing powers, so a large part of their general revenues is in the form of Commonwealth Financial Assistance Grants. Thus in addition to the 40 percent or so of hospital costs paid for by dedicated Hospital Funding Grants, much of the rest of states' hospital expenditures are derived from federal transfers that have been shrinking (relatively) as a consequence of policies to limit federal budget deficits.[2] State leaders argue that the Commonwealth government now has power without responsibility: it can restrain spending and leave the states to figure out what services to reduce.

The Commonwealth actors, meanwhile, have to worry that the states will reduce the wrong services: for example, outpatient services, on the theory that those could be duplicated within the physician service program of medicare. The Commonwealth budget is charged directly for general practice and specialist medical and diagnostic services outside hospitals, but the states pay for medical care by general practitioners (GPs) in hospital casualty (emergency) departments and for specialist services in hospital outpatient clinics; the Commonwealth pays directly for pharmaceuticals provided in the community, but the states pay for drugs provided by the hospital services. These overlaps guarantee that one of the most contentious parts of the governance of Australian health care is the periodic negotiation of medicare agreements between the Commonwealth and the state governments. The Commonwealth can unilaterally determine its own payments but not the terms of state participation. State participation is settled by contract, not mandate. The Commonwealth therefore searches for terms to ensure that the states do not reduce existing services that might be provided outside of the hospital, while states of course seek freedom to do so.[3]

A separate federal program, the Pharmaceutical Benefits Scheme (PBS), "subsidises the cost of a wide range of drugs and medicinal preparations." PBS covers 57 percent of prescription costs (this figure does not include additional government payments for drugs provided through hospitals). The various provisions in the Pharmaceutical Benefits Scheme are designed to mostly help those with greater financial or medical need, much like most provincial supplementary programs in Canada. There is separate government funding for allied health and preventive care such as vaccinations, community nursing, and other related activities.[4]

Because medicare is a national program run by Australia's Health Insurance Commission and pays at least a part of virtually every doctor bill, Australia reaps most of the administrative advantages of a single-payer system for ambulatory care.[5] Public hospitals are funded by a combination of public budgets and payments from private insurance. Private insurers pay public hospitals according to standard fees, so in public hospitals also Australia realizes the administrative savings of a simplified payment system.

PRIVATE INSURANCE. Private insurance pays mainly for care in private hospitals or "private" status in public hospitals (described below). Choice, less risk of waiting, and perhaps status are reasons for persons to purchase private insurance, and roughly 40 percent of Australians do. People with more money are more likely to buy private coverage, but so do over 20 percent of "contributor units" with gross weekly income under $A160.[6] This has been possible because private insurance has been relatively cheap: the average weekly family basic contribution in June 1991 was $A14.20.[7]

Australia bans the most destabilizing aspects of the American private market. Insurers must set rates for communities as a whole and accept all applicants. Although subtle discouragement is possible, its effect is limited by the fact that the government, as a vestige of the coalition's efforts to avoid a tax-based system, runs the largest market-based insurer, Medibank Private.

Insurers do not cover benefits in kind but instead make exact payments—for example, $A388–$A408 per day, for up to fourteen days, for advanced surgical care in a shared room in a private hospital.[8] And the private insurers are at risk for only 25 percent of the medicare schedule of physicians' fees for inpatient services. Their patients may need to worry about extra billing, but the insurers do not. Paying by large categories, such as a day rate, protects Australian insurers against the American hospitals' tactic of proliferating detailed charges.

Nevertheless insurance is more likely to be bought by persons who have kept their pre-1984 coverage than by younger persons who have less need and are not in the habit. The pool therefore becomes more risky. The persons who are most likely to buy or keep private coverage are those who expect to use it. The government has given this dynamic of adverse selection a push in two ways. First, to the extent that services in the public sector are harder to obtain, people may create more costs for the private insurance that they already have (for example, by going to a private hospital rather than as a private patient to a public hospital). Second, since 1984 the government has eliminated subsidies for private insurers, required them to pay some higher charges, mandated some extra benefits, and increased the risk of adverse selection by reducing pre-existing condition exclusions from two years to one.[9]

"What we find difficult to understand," a private fund administrator plaintively told me, "is why the government wants to prevent the extra coverage." The national director of the Australian Hospital Association has described private insurance as increasingly a "user pays" system, with "only the sick carrying insurance . . . counter to any stable insurance pooling of good and bad risk."[10]

Whatever the Labor governments may have thought about private insurance, they behaved precisely like any other budgeter by seeking savings that would make some other organization most directly responsible for the consequences (in this case, private insurers, who would have to raise private premiums). For a while, purchasers of private insurance were willing to pay, and the natural decline in rates of private insurance after the establishment of medicare slowed dramatically in the late 1980s. Survey data showed few of its purchasers were very price-sensitive. But for how long would they absorb premium increases of about 14.5 percent per year? In 1992 the proportion of Australians with "supplemental hospital cover," which pays for care in private hospitals, began to decline. It fell from 38.7 percent in mid-1991 to 34.4 percent on June 30, 1994.[11]

Paying for Public Care

Unlike Canada and Germany, Australia allows significant cost sharing for ambulatory care. Medicare has a fee schedule and will pay 85 percent of the amounts on that schedule. Doctors may accept assignment and bill medicare directly for the fee schedule amount ("bulk-bill"). If the physician does not bulk-bill, the patient pays the doctor the difference and claims the 85 percent from medicare.[12]

Because the fee schedule is not binding, a doctor may charge more, and the patient is responsible for that as well as the 15 percent coinsurance. Doctors' individual prices then depend largely on market factors. Nearly two-thirds of Australian physicians are GPs, and competition, especially in the large cities such as Sydney and Melbourne, is fierce. Many specialists, however, are in short supply. Therefore in 1990–91 70 percent of GP services, but only 26 percent of specialist services, were bulk-billed. The two balanced each other out, so total fees came to only 0.3 percent above the schedule![13]

One lesson, also learned in America, is that a loose labor market can help enforce a fee schedule even if it is not compulsory. But remaining fee differences can create restricted or unequal access to specialist care for persons with low incomes. Two policies mitigate the effects of unequal fees.

First, *private insurance is not allowed to pay fees above the medicare schedule*. A patient who wants to may pay more than the schedule fee out-of-pocket, but there is a real price constraint on such behavior. As Stuart Altman and Terri Jackson explain:

> The prohibition on insurance for extra-billing has been an effective means of limiting physicians' ability to break out of fee constraints by passing fee increases on to private patients and in turn to health insurance premiums. This has also prevented a bidding war between the public and private sectors in terms of which sector is able to provide better-quality (or at least higher-paid) medical care.[14]

Second, some specialists choose to accept the schedule fee for certain patients—for example, those who are eligible for various other subsidies such as for pharmaceuticals. Most important, however, the hospital outpatient clinics provide a safety valve for specialist care. My interview sources reported that they and other doctors send patients who they believe cannot afford outside specialist care to the outpatient unit. I could not find figures on the proportions of specialist services for the poor that are provided by the outpatient units, but less direct measurements suggest the figure must be very high.[15] According to a survey performed for the National Health Strategy review of Australian health care, 43.6 percent of the respondents receiving outpatient care had incomes below $A12,000 per year; only 6.2 percent of the general population had similar incomes. The former cannot be getting much specialist care elsewhere.[16]

At an outpatient clinic a person is more likely to be treated by a resident, by a less senior physician. But outside specialists may also work in the clinic, and the hospital it is part of may be better equipped than a specialist's office. So the poor do have access to care, even if it is not equal in all ways.

A similar story obtains for hospital care. Any person covered by medicare can be treated as a "public" patient at any public hospital. As a government brochure explains, "The hospital will choose a doctor to treat you. You won't need to pay for the doctor or the accommodation."[17] Public hospitals receive budgets directly from the state governments, much like all the hospitals in Canada. But unlike in Canada there is a separate class of patients, "private" patients with private insurance. Private insurance pays for hospital charges incurred at private hospitals and for "private" status in a public hospital. A patient with private status may select her own physician. In either a public or a private hospital, medicare pays 75 percent of the schedule fee for physician services, and insurance pays the other 25 percent—but never more.

Public hospitals also receive a fee for each private patient.[18] These fees give public hospital administrators important financial incentives to admit private patients.[19]

The fees to doctors, apart from their regular payment from the hospitals, give them too reason to serve private patients first.[20] Hospital physicians with admitting privileges, called visiting medical officers (VMOs) are normally paid by the session (for example, an amount per half day). Some public hospital doctors are salaried. But in either case, the physician may receive and earn more in the public hospital from direct payment. And in the private hospital, the physician may collect not just the schedule fee but somewhat more out of the patient's pocket.

Delivery and the Public/Private Hospital Division

Whether these different payment systems create serious inequalities is a matter of political debate. Doctors and hospitals play up stories about long waiting lists in order to extract higher payments from the governments. Private hospital operators do the same in order to build support for government action that favors private insurance as a safety valve or alternative.

PRIVATE VERSUS PUBLIC HOSPITALS. Australia's private hospitals, funded largely by private insurance, may be either for profit or not for profit. The latter tend to be owned by religious bodies, much like many hospitals in the United States. Australia's private hospitals have substantial capacity for nonurgent care, but the two sectors have different capacities for urgent care. Private hospitals are less likely to have residents, so physicians hesitate to admit patients who may need a doctor round-the-clock. Teaching hospitals, which are public, tend to have more high-tech equipment and definitely have more prestige. Few specialists feel they can eschew affiliation with a public hospital, and they therefore must care for public patients.

Private hospitals have more than a quarter of the beds and a somewhat larger share of admissions; but they have a somewhat smaller proportion of the bed days because they treat less serious cases, on average. An open question is whether, as capital funds for public hospitals are squeezed by the states, some private institutions will become serious challengers to the public ones for high-tech services. At present that is rare—but it is becoming more common. The much higher relative level of investment in the private sector is not justified in the market, but the capacity, nevertheless, is being created.[21]

The advantages of private care may be fewer than the formal arrangements suggest. Public hospitals try to encourage care by an attending specialist who already knows the patient. And having private status creates a perverse incentive for the attending physician to try to monopolize treatments, thereby denying the patient the full range of services from the hospital staff.[22] Nevertheless there are clear differences in convenience, and what an observer calls convenient the ill person may consider vital. Australians buy private insurance in part to avoid waiting for elective surgery and in part so they are able to choose their physician. Thus, for example, a couple may decide to buy private insurance a year before they begin trying to conceive a child so the woman can be assured that the same doctor cares for her from pregnancy through labor.

Chapter 6 discusses waiting-list problems and the reasons to believe they are usually exaggerated. Yet the use of admitting physicians does make waits more likely in Australia than in a different delivery system. As in Canada but not Germany, physicians are allocated a specific number of beds within a hospital, so there are many separate queues.[23] There is no doubt that the public budget squeeze and private alternative create unequal choice and access to elective surgery. Whether these constitute unacceptable differences in quality of care is a matter for personal decision. Yet no Australian goes completely without insurance or even has inadequate (by U.S. standards) coverage; there is no comparison in Australia with the unavailability of physicians to some medicaid patients in the United States, and even the cost of supplementary private insurance is less than that of many medigap policies for the U.S. elderly. Australian pharmaceutical benefits are extensive, and cost control has been effective.

AN INNOVATIVE RESPONSE TO MALPRACTICE. The institutions described so far exist throughout Australia. Australia, however, is a federal country in which states have substantial autonomy and some different policies. Queensland provided free admission for all to public hospitals when the rest of the country did not. Policies in New South Wales suggest an approach to dealing with malpractice.

As discussed in chapter 3, the U.S. system of redress in the event of malpractice does little for society as a whole or to prevent future occurrences. Punishing a doctor by making his insurance company pay a large judgment hardly seems much of a deterrent. Enduring the legal process itself may be more trying, but the doctors who win their cases are not supposed to have been punished. Monitoring physician performance and subjecting them to professional sanctions, such as the loss of hospital privileges or even their medical license, would be more appropriate. Some American states and medical facilities do impose such sanctions, but not without difficulties. Doctors do not like to confront other doctors, and of course an accused doctor may dispute the charges.

New South Wales has not found a way to solve all possible problems. It emphasizes quality control and protecting future victims rather than redress. But its approach merits consideration by American legislators, especially to improve patient protections, if reform also sought to satisfy physicians by restricting malpractice suits.

The Complaints Unit is a division of the New South Wales Health Department. It presents itself as an investigative and informative organization. People may complain directly to the unit, or complaints may be referred by "their representatives, service providers, the coroner's court, Registration Boards, Members of Parliament, the Ombudsman, consumer organizations, health professionals, state government authorities, and the Commonwealth Department of Health, Housing, and Community Services." The Complaints Unit has a toll-free telephone number and provides foreign-language interpreters.[24]

The unit's staff first tries to resolve a matter by asking the provider to explain the circumstances that have upset the complainant. Often, staff explained, all the complainant really wants is an explanation. The unit will dismiss (or so they say) obviously "vexatious, trivial or frivolous" complaints and will suggest alternative dispute resolution if that seems appropriate and is available.[25] If preliminary discussions do not suffice, the complainant is advised to make a written statement that provides the unit with authority to investigate.

Although the unit began without subpoena power, it could still gather sufficient information to substantiate the complaint and to determine whether to refer it to a higher authority. The unit does not recommend disciplinary action without first consulting "other independent practitioners of the same profession."[26] In the case of physicians the unit may recommend counseling by other physicians. Or, if it believes stronger sanctions are called for, it may present the case before either the Professional Standards Committee or the Medical Tribunal. Each is set up by the state medical board, which is controlled by physicians. In either case, the unit itself, not the patient, is the complainant. The Complaints Unit is the plaintiff in the public interest (like a district attorney), and its leaders are well aware that their interpretation of the problem may not always be the same as the patient's. The unit is more concerned about preventing further damage than about satisfying desires for revenge. Thus its concerns may be closer to those of physicians than of all victims or their relatives. I was told that in one case of a "boy who died it wasn't the intern's fault; it was a system problem. The family is very upset with us because we didn't have the intern, who had been in practice for two weeks, struck off the register" of practitioners.

The Professional Standards Committee includes two doctors and one layperson. No lawyers are present, and the committee can recommend fines up to $25,000, retraining, restrictions on practice, and some other sanctions. Only the Medical Tribunal can remove a physician's license to practice. It includes a judge as well as the two doctors and the layperson, and both sides have lawyers.

Physicians were suspicious of the Complaints Unit when it was created, but their organizations became more supportive over time. The unit's leadership was sensitive to the need for support from doctors, and its procedures have solved problems for physicians who want to provide high-quality care and avoid a malpractice crapshoot. First, the unit pays for the investigations. Second, the act of investigation does not pit one physician against another. Third, because physicians rather than juries make the final judgments, physicians can be reasonably sure that professional standards, rather than public resentments, determine decisions. Fourth, doctors who have served on the panels have seen cases that were real and shocking—and in some cases decided that removing physicians from the profession was appropriate. In less serious cases—a physician with a drinking problem, for example—they could tailor the punishment (perhaps suspend his license, require treatment for alcoholism, and then allow him to return with supervision). Fifth, the unit screens cases, so comparatively few reach the level of severe discipline. In 1991, out of 1,037 complaints closed, 128 were substantiated without disciplinary hearings, 32 conciliated, 36 substantiated in disciplinary hearings, and only one brought to a hearing and not substantiated.[27] Sixth, the unit does not provide evidence for subsequent civil suits that might be filed. Last, there is no due process problem because this is a statutory process: a physician whose license is revoked may appeal the decision to the state courts.

This system is not perfect. No system is likely to maximize the values of both quality control and redress. Put differently, its "near exclusive focus on the public interest . . . has occurred at the expense of protecting and defending individual consumers' rights."[28] But it is a very intriguing model for improving regulation of individual providers.

Conclusion

While the public and private insurance mix in Australia is not logically neat, once could argue that it is quite equitable. Everyone pays taxes that guarantee a basic level of care. People who want more or better care may buy it. If voters wanted more convenience in the public system they could vote for politicians who would raise their taxes to pay for it.

Australia therefore poses a number of questions for American reform. First, what inequalities are acceptable? Does Australia represent a viable compromise between Canada, with no cost sharing and no private provision of services covered by public insurance, and America, in which large portions of the population are guaranteed nothing at all and differences in payment depend more on luck than on choice?

Second, are binding fees really necessary? Germany shows that some variation by coverage type may be acceptable. Is the Australian trick of forbidding extra insurance enough, given favorable market conditions (such as many specialists) to provide ample physician supply to all at a reasonable price?

Third, if Americans wanted to move in the Australian direction on the first two questions, could they do that without much more direct control of the hospitals? American hospitals, unlike German, often do have large outpatient clinics. Is there some way to make sure enough top-rank specialists are tied to the right hospitals, and the right clinics, to cover the entire nation and to ensure that inequalities do not get out of hand? If so, the effect of reform on the academic medical centers would be crucial.

France

The French system of social insurance looks similar in many ways to that of Germany. The French model developed later but with many of the same tensions: physicians seeking autonomy and higher income; employees being easier to cover than the self-employed or workers in agriculture; competition among unions, employers, and the state for influence over the sickness funds; fiscal pressures that varied over time, and the modernization of medicine.[29]

France is not a federal state, so more decisions than in Germany are made at a national level, whether by the government or by other institutions. French interest groups are more fractured than Germany's: within any occupational category or industry there are likely to be competing employee organizations, often affiliated with competing political parties. The government then tries to divide and rule. But at the same time, because France has a strong tradition of political protest, confrontation tends to be more dramatic in France than in Germany.[30]

Like all other countries in this comparison, France has controlled medical costs more successfully than the United States, but less so than its payers would like. Marginal changes to improve cost containment are common. Yet the major differences between France and Germany and Canada have remained the same.

First, the system of sickness funds is far more concentrated than that in Germany (or Japan). All funds are national, and the largest has eighty percent of the members. Second, France has substantial copayments compared to Germany or Canada. Third, there are more exceptions to the fee schedule. Fourth, private insurance provides supplementary coverage for most of the population.

Financing French Health Care

The French pay for their health coverage through contributions to sickness funds, by purchasing supplementary coverage, and out-of-pocket.

SICKNESS FUND CONTRIBUTIONS. France groups the insured by occupational category. The main French sickness fund, Caisse Nationale de l'Assurance Maladie des Travailleurs Salaries (CNAMTS), for salaried workers and their dependents, includes about 80 percent of the population. Local governments provide some coverage for the 0.4 percent of the population that both does not fit the system's occupational basis and cannot buy in.[31]

The sickness fund approach means that, unlike in Canada, health care is financed mainly by dedicated premiums rather than from general revenues. But France's structure also creates differences from Germany. Eighty percent of the population pays the same contribution rate. Retirees remain members of the fund they belonged to when they were working, so there is no need for an explicit retiree contribution. There are no company funds. Some cross-subsidies among funds are still needed. Some of the small funds have shrinking memberships (such as the miners' fund). With fewer workers per retiree, they cannot support the latter at a bearable premium. A special commission therefore calculates transfers through a retrospective adjustment based mainly on actual costs.[32]

Employers contribute 12.8 percent of wages to CNAMTS and employees pay 6.8 percent. This split is different from the equal split in Germany, and the payments seem much higher but in fact are only slightly higher. Other funds have different rates, according to the political bargains made at the time they were created. The unemployed pay 1 percent of their checks, and pensioners pay 1.4 percent on their base pension and 2.4 percent on others. Thus their contribution rates are lower than in Germany.[33]

Health care is part of the larger structure of French social security (Securité Sociale). French social security is not part of the state budget, and most of its funds are not provided through the state budget process. For many years a shifting amount of more general, "health-related" taxes has been dedicated to the CNAMTS, but that has always been a small share of costs: 2.6 percent in 1984.[34] More important, since 1993 a separate "general social contribution" of 2.4 percent of *income* (a much larger number) has been assessed on both wage and investment earnings, and used partly to finance the sickness funds and partly to pay for family benefits.[35]

SICKNESS FUND BENEFITS. The French sickness funds cover almost as wide a range of benefits as the German: not just physicians and hospitals, but pharmaceuticals, medical aids, some dental care, and even spa treatment. The major difference is in cost sharing.

French coinsurance rates were raised an extra five percentage points in August 1993, as a conservative government introduced a new plan to control health care costs. So funds now pay 70 percent of physician fees and 60 percent of other nonhospital caregiver fees, for physical therapy, for example. They pay 75 percent of hospital charges for medical services.

Cost sharing is not, however, as significant as these figures suggest. Patients pay a flat fee (about ten dollars) for hospital room and board, and all cost sharing ceases after thirty days of hospitalization. Cost sharing is limited to fees for relatively simple surgery. There is no cost sharing at all for thirty medical conditions, either because they are too expensive (diabetes, cancer, AIDS) or because the state wants to encourage them (pregnancy). On application to a review panel, patients may also be given waivers for other degenerative conditions or disabling combinations of illnesses.[36] The exclusions for these conditions apply to ambulatory care expenses as well, including the cost of drugs.

The funds' contributions for pharmaceuticals vary from full payment for "essential and particularly costly" drugs to 65 percent for "regular" medications such as antibiotics and 35 percent for medications such as aspirin that treat nonthreatening problems. The French consume a huge amount of pharmaceuticals, but the base prices for all drugs subject to reimbursement are set by negotiations between the ministry and the producers, so are much lower than in Germany.[37] Spa treatment is covered but requires approval by the sickness funds' control doctors.[38]

SUPPLEMENTARY COVERAGE AND OUT-OF-POCKET COSTS. Two features of the French system could interfere with care for persons without much cash: cost sharing and its method of patient reimbursement. Except for hospital care, the system requires individuals to pay the bills and then apply for reimbursement. A number of measures reduce the possible negative effect of this payment mechanism upon access.

To begin with, the funds pay the reimbursements very quickly.[39] Even more significant, just as most Americans on medicare purchase medigap policies, over four-fifths of French citizens obtain supplementary coverage. Usually they obtain it from "*mutuelles*," which are descendants of the guild funds. Mutuelles pay for both cost sharing and some extra benefits. Hospitals and the private clinics bill a patient's mutuelle directly for coinsured inpatient care.[40] A few mutuelles run their own clinics, at which the patient need not lay out any cash for ambulatory care. Private insurance provides some of the same coverage. But private insurers do not have clinics; they risk-rate, and the government favors mutuelles with a range of tax policies. Therefore even some insurance company workers have their own mutuelles![41]

Because of fear of competition from pharmacies owned by the mutuelles, French pharmacists have agreed by contract to bill the CNAMTS directly for its share of pharmaceutical costs.[42] The very poor still might lose access to care because of their inability to share costs. For them, a local government (*département*) program called Aide Médicale pays mandatory contributions and coinsurance. They receive a membership card that they show to providers, who then bill the local governments. Because the vast majority of care is already covered through CNAMTS, Aide Médicale is much smaller than American medicaid.[43]

Overall, about 17 percent of French medical care expenses are paid out-of-pocket. Supplementary insurance covers about 8 percent of the total and more than 10 percent of hospital and ambulatory care.[44] The combination of catastrophic coverage and supplementary insurance can cover a lot. In one example, a person with catastrophic expenses due to a cerebral hemorrhage and complications paid 6,720 francs out of a total cost of more than 400,000 francs.[45]

French students cannot enter school without immunizations and must have checkups then, at age ten, and at entrance to technical school (age thirteen or fourteen) or to academic high school (age fifteen or sixteen). Family physicians and special centers provide free vaccinations, and there is a system of public mental health services. Local governments provide maternal and infant care. In the United States governments sometimes have difficulty ensuring that women seek prenatal care. The French solved this problem quite simply. They have a national program of "family allowances" that pays $150 per month to pregnant women. But they make receipt of the money conditional on having seven prenatal examinations.[46]

Paying the Providers

As everywhere, French methods of paying physicians have evolved over decades of conflict. The result as of the early 1990s was more similar to Australia's system than to others in this study.

LA MÉDECINE LIBÉRALE. French physicians are no more eager to cooperate with the government or other payers than their American counterparts are. Since 1928 their version of freedom—free choice of physician by patient and vice versa, fee-for-service practice, direct payment by patients to doctors, professional confidentiality, and clinical autonomy—has been summarized as "la médecine libérale" (free-market medicine). The AMA could put it no better.[47]

Fee schedules must by law be set by agreement among the sickness funds, the Ministries of Finance and Social Security, and physicians' unions. The process has two phases: negotiations between the unions and the funds, and state approval of the results.[48] As in other countries, physicians have the greatest voice in establishing relative values. The funds have the upper hand on the conversion factor, partly because they need agreement from only one of the three physicians' unions.[49] As compensation (of sorts) for restraint on the fee schedule, the government in 1980 created a new category of physicians called Sector 2. Patients who use physicians who join Sector 2 are reimbursed by the funds for the regular amount but have to pay the doctor his or her extra fee. In exchange for joining Sector 2, the doctors give up some social insurance benefits.

Before 1980 France had a small number of physicians who were voted by their peers the right to extra-bill. With Sector 2, the number increased dramatically. By 1993 more than 29 percent of all physicians and at least 40 percent of specialists could extra-bill. Because France, like Australia, has more generalists than specialists, it became relatively easy to find a GP who accepted the fee schedule, but difficult to find such a specialist—especially in large cities. With fees charged by Sector 2 physicians about 50 percent higher than the schedule, patients of those doctors might pay nearly half of their bills out-of-pocket.[50]

The proliferation of Sector 2 physicians created a serious political issue of equitable and adequate access to specialist care. Insurance for fees above the schedule is legal but not common. Between cost sharing and especially extra billing, 28.3 percent of physician fees are paid out-of-pocket.[51] In 1990 the government suspended the right to join Sector 2 but allowed existing members to remain, so access problems persist. As in Australia, persons who cannot pay more than the fee schedule amount will go to a hospital outpatient clinic to see a specialist, though availability and use of the services do not seem to be quite as extensive.[52]

The schedule fee in 1992 was about twenty dollars for a GP consultation and twenty-five for a specialist visit. Naturally, fee schedules that are binding and automatically adjusted to increased volume, as in Germany, control costs more effectively than those that are not, as in France. Yet slower growth (actually, a decline) of real prices is one reason why French costs have grown more slowly than American.[53]

French doctors have lower practice costs than American for the same reasons Canadian doctors do. But doctors evidently would prefer to charge more, and those who can, do. The fact that in France and Australia doctors whose skills are in shortest supply are much more likely to extra-bill, combined with the evidence from Germany that rising physician supply limits physician incomes, shows that although a rising number of physicians may well increase costs, it also puts individual doctors at a disadvantage when negotiating prices either separately in the market or together, with consolidated payers. A schedule probably enhances market pressures because it gives patients a standard for measuring how "excessive" a doctor's charge is (or, how much extra quality and prestige are associated with using that doctor).

All of that said, France still has had more success controlling hospital costs by budgeting than controlling ambulatory care costs by fee setting.

PAYING THE HOSPITALS. France has the third most expensive health care system in this study; but at 9.1 percent of GDP in 1991 (see table 2-1) it is much less expensive than America's, which cost 13.4 percent of GDP. In 1984 the government switched from day-rate reimbursement to a global budget process for public hospitals. William Glaser explains how this works with multiple payers:

Every French [public] hospital since 1984 continues to submit its retrospective cost report and its proposed budget to the local government rate regulator, who screens and approves it, pursuant to the financial guidelines and limits prescribed in Paris. In periods of austerity, the national government may fix a cap for all hospitals in a region, and the rate regulator can award individual hospitals more or less than the guidelines imply, so long as the regional cap is not exceeded. The sickness funds in an area share the biweekly installment of the global budget for each hospital, in ratios equal to their shares in all admissions there last year.[54]

The U.S. General Accounting Office estimates that the switch to global budgeting reduced spending at the end of three years by 9 percent from trend, and OECD figures show that French hospital care costs, after rising from 3.2 percent of GDP in 1977 to 4.2 percent in 1984, were 4.0 percent in 1991.[55]

Private hospitals are paid negotiated day rates and fees for some specific services. Physicians bill patients directly, and patients are reimbursed at 75 percent of the fee schedule.[56] The same rates are charged to non-sickness-fund members in either a private or a public hospital. They are distinctly lower than in the United States, as shown by an American's "tale of two eyes": One night in 1986, an American foreign correspondent in France started seeing spots. He went to the hospital; they made him stay overnight and the next afternoon mended his retina with laser surgery. He was billed $75 (at the exchange rate of the time) for the surgery and $180 for the semi-private room. A month later he returned for "a second zap of the laser, [which] cost another $75. Incredulous, I rechecked. I got a Gallic shrug. It's the same price for everyone, Monsieur." About three years later, in Boston, he started seeing spots in the other eye. He went to his ophthalmologist, who called the hospital and asked a technician to switch on the laser. Two hours later he was fixed up—for $1,556.85![57]

Delivery and Capacity in French Health Care

The French are twice as likely as Americans to visit a GP and only about 15 percent less likely to visit specialists. France also has a higher hospital admission rate and length of stay, as well as a much higher rate of pharmaceutical consumption.[58]

PUBLIC AND PRIVATE HOSPITALS. As in Australia, France has a system in which public hospitals, which are often linked to universities, compete with a separately financed system of private hospitals. "Many believe," Fielding and Lancry report, "that [the latter] facilities provide the most attentive patient care, and they are often used for routine operations, maternity care, and care for particular categories of problems, such as cancer." With fewer complicated cases, the private hospitals, with 37 percent of the beds and 42 percent of the bed days, account for just under a quarter of hospital costs.[59]

French public hospitals rely mainly on salaried physicians, especially eight thousand well-paid senior professors.[60] These senior physicians often are entitled to spend two half days per week with private patients and may use a few beds for private patients. But this system allows public hospitals to claim to offer an elite class of physicians, who have much less incentive than in Australia to favor one group of patients over another.[61] Because all sickness fund members may also use the private hospitals, those hospitals, unlike in Australia, do not provide a second tier of hospital care to a minority of the population.

CAPACITY CONTROLS. To finance capital investment in public hospitals, the French government capitalized a revolving loan fund. Hospitals borrow at low rates of interest and only with approval; their repayments, from their income, pay for future loans. Thus the sickness funds, through payments for service, pay most capital costs. "Enterprising hospital directors, service chiefs, and mayors might still extract subsidies from the national government," Glaser noted, "if the construction project made a notable contribution to medical education, to medical research, or (sometimes) to the political popularity of the President, Prime Minister, and Ministers in that region."[62]

Hospitals might also self-finance or borrow privately, but both public and private institutions are constrained by a law that says no hospital may be opened or beds added without authorization from the minister of health. This system of hospital licensing is more powerful than the certificate-of-need systems in the United States during the 1970s, because it is operated by the government rather than by committees dominated by providers, and it is enforced by criminal sanctions.[63]

When the government and funds clamped down in the 1980s, these measures were enough to control investment in beds in all hospitals and equipment in the public institutions. But the private institutions had plenty of beds; what they needed was equipment, and there was no law against that. Private hospitals began to merge and buy new equipment and therefore to look more competitive with the public institutions. The sickness funds have the power to limit capacity indirectly, by refusing to include specific services in their contracts with individual hospitals, but if services are desired by the public, using that power would be controversial.[64]

As discussed earlier, France has many more GPs per capita than the United States but is not so overendowed with specialists. Therefore access to GPs is easy; access to specialists is a problem for patients in areas where a large share of the specialists are members of Sector 2.

Conclusion

The French case provides further evidence about payment arrangements and cost controls. In France too, budgeting works better than limiting individual payments. France and Canada controlled their budgeted sector, hospitals, better than their unbudgeted sector, ambulatory care. Germany controlled physician expenses better than it did hospital costs because it had tighter budgeting for the former. In all cases, capital budgeting for hospitals contributes to cost control.[65]

France further confirms that continued expansion of physician supply at some point weakens doctors' bargaining power. That does not mean it is a good thing for payers. It does mean that when current physicians oppose limits on the training of new doctors, they undermine their own individual interests.

Private insurance has different functions in France and Germany. In Germany it provides special convenience to some persons who are willing to pay higher fees to providers. In France it provides some supplemental benefits and compensates for cost sharing.

Whether cost sharing threatens access depends on its extent and to what it applies. Is coinsurance limited to more elective activities, with some system to ensure that truly urgent care is not inhibited? And what is the *product* of the coinsurance rate and the fees? Twenty percent of $300 is more affordable than 10 percent of $1,000.

Unless there is no cost sharing or extra billing, fee levels affect not just the expense of the system but also its level of equity. In both France and Australia cost sharing, and especially extra billing, creates conditions under which some persons must use different providers than others: an outpatient clinic, for example, rather than an expensive specialist. Yet the effects of these inequalities depend on other factors, especially whether the delivery and financial systems create separate tiers of delivery. France is less likely to go down that road because its private hospitals are not funded by separate insurance. In each case a key is ensuring that the most prestigious doctors in the nation are available through the basic insurance system.[66] In both countries that means ensuring that the public hospitals maintain their leadership position. In the United States, that is more likely to mean ensuring the viability of and access to the academic medical centers.

Japan

Japan looked to Germany for guidance in much of its modernization, and health care is no exception. Yet the system evolved somewhat differently because Japan has neither states nor comparably strong unions. Absent those challengers, the national bureaucracy has been far more powerful and directive than in Germany or even France. In addition, Japan grafted western medicine onto an oriental (essentially Chinese) tradition of treatment that relied heavily on herbs and preparations. Japan therefore persists in a style of delivery that emphasizes drug treatment more than any other nation in this study.[67]

If the most basic official statistics were our only information, we would have to conclude that the Japanese health care system is the best in the world. In 1991 Japan had the longest life expectancies and was tied with Britain for the lowest expenses per share of GDP of all the countries in this study; and no country in the OECD matched its combination of life expectancy and cost.[68] We will see that evaluating Japanese health care is not so easy, but the system does illustrate some points about finance and cost control.[69]

Financing Japanese Health Care

Like Germany, Japan has hundreds of separate sickness funds linked to a person's employer, occupation, or geographic location. Each fund provides coverage for a person and his or her dependents. Unlike in Germany, there is no choice among funds, there are systematic differences in cost sharing, and both local and national governments provide direct subsidies. Japan has three categories of insurance: employer-based insurance, national health insurance, and health insurance for the elderly.

EMPLOYER-BASED INSURANCE. This category includes:
—"Society-managed health insurance," which in 1992 covered 26.2 percent of the population, through companies that self-finance. These provide standard benefits with substantial regulation and so are equivalent to German company funds, not to plans offered by American self-insured corporations. Total contributions averaged 8.254 percent of wages in 1992 but legally could range from 3 percent to 9.5 percent. Some employers agree to pay more than half of the contributions, so employee shares in the society-managed sector averaged 56.7 percent

of the total in 1991. The 1,823 funds (in 1992) receive a small subsidy for administrative expenses from the national government.

—Government-managed health insurance, in which the government creates a fund for employees of other firms. The plan is administered by 298 branch offices. Its premium in 1992 was fixed at 8.2 percent of payroll, divided equally among employers and employees. While society-based plans may offer extra benefits, government-managed plans offer only one package. In 1992 these plans insured 29.6 percent of the population. Because their members are generally lower-wage earners and less healthy than those in society-managed plans, the state in 1992 contributed 13 percent of benefit costs and all administrative costs.[70]

—Other occupational funds, for a total in 1992 of 10 percent of the insured. The state makes special contributions for seamen and day laborers, and the premiums vary slightly.[71]

NATIONAL HEALTH INSURANCE. National health insurance is run mainly by municipalities with substantial support from the national government and covers people who are not covered by the employer-based system. Examples include farmers, small-business owners, people who have retired and therefore left the employer-based funds, and doctors. In March 1992 there were 3,254 municipal plans and 166 separate national health insurance societies, which served separate craftspeople (for example, barbers). These plans enrolled 34.4 percent of the population in 1992. Premium rates vary from community to community and are based on both individuals' income and assets. In 1991 the maximum rate was about $1,850 annually.[72] In the absence of an employer, the state pays 50 percent of the costs under the municipal schemes and from 32 to 52 percent for the craft-based plans.[73]

HEALTH AND MEDICAL SERVICE FOR THE ELDERLY. Membership in this plan is for those over age seventy or, if bedridden, over age sixty-five. These persons may be in any fund, although they are most likely to be in the community version of national health insurance. The system for the elderly creates a pooled fund, to which each individual fund contributes as if it had the national proportion of elderly. This mechanism transfers cash from funds with fewer elderly to those with more. Seventy percent of the pooled total is contributed by the individual funds, 20 percent by the national government, and 10 percent by local governments.[74] A similar scheme transfers money from employer-based funds to the national health insurance community funds to help pay the costs of retirees before they become eligible for this plan for the elderly.[75]

These varied government payments and intrafund transfers are a more elaborate Japanese response to the same problem that arises in Germany: when funds are based on location and workplace, there will be large inequalities in their risk and income levels.

COVERAGE. All funds cover a broad range of medical services according to a detailed fee schedule. The covered services include hospital and physician care, dental care and pharmaceuticals, and even some transportation. The sickness funds also pay some cash benefits, such as for maternity leave; the society-managed funds generally pay greater cash benefits than national health insurance.

Health insurance covers little preventive care and for normal pregnancy provides only the cash payment (pregnancy is not considered an illness).[76] Large employers provide some preventive care, and governments provide very good prenatal and infant care, school-based care, and vaccinations.[77] There is a centralized, government-run ambulance system.[78]

All citizens except the elderly face substantial cost sharing. Unlike in France, it varies by status. In 1994 the elderly paid no more than 1,000 yen per month for outpatient care (about $5), and 700 yen ($3.50) per day for inpatient care.[79] The holders of employer-based health insurance pay 10 percent coinsurance for their care, but their dependents pay 20 percent for inpatient care and 30 percent for outpatient care. Retired employees within the national health insurance scheme pay 20 percent coinsurance, while the employed (farmers, barbers, lawyers, and their dependents) pay 30 percent.[80]

All funds pay 100 percent of expenses above about $300 per month. This cap is lower for low-income persons and those who have already paid the maximum for three months within a year.[81]

Analysts of the Japanese system commonly argue that because few people cite economic reasons for failing to see a physician, cost sharing is not a major problem and that Japanese fees are so low that it is hard to accumulate high expenses.[82]

Payment Regulation and Mechanisms

Japanese health insurance is complicated and inequitable in the sense that some benefits, the cost sharing, and premiums vary depending on a person's location and occupation. But everyone is part of the same delivery system, and payments are strictly coordinated. The rules for paying doctors and hospitals are identical for all plans, and providers are also paid in a centralized manner. Each month, bills are submitted to regional offices of two central funds, one for employer-based and one for national health insurance. Staffs of physicians review bills (which in practice mainly means spot-checking billings from providers whom they have some reason to suspect of excessive utilization). Thus there is utilization review, but it is both limited and conducted by physicians. Once approved, bills are forwarded for payment to the individual funds. Thus providers receive payment as long as two months after providing their services, but there is little administrative cost or confusion.[83]

One striking aspect of the Japanese system is its achievement of "low cost through regulated fees." These fees pay for most of what medical providers do whether in a clinic or a hospital.[84] Overhead must be paid out of the fees, although public hospitals receive some extra financing from the government, and some private hospitals are subsidized by their medical schools.[85] The fee schedule, then, largely determines the economic prospects of hospitals and doctors.

The schedule clearly favors physicians in private practice over hospitals. The former have dominated medical politics in Japan, in spite of the fact that they now are a distinct and aging minority of physicians.[86] The fee schedule is established by state authority after consultation with a twenty-member council (*chuikyo*) that includes eight representatives from providers (including five physicians) but no direct representatives of the hospitals. As a result the fees, which are extremely low to begin with, are especially low for the services that more advanced hospitals provide, such as surgery and intensive care.[87]

The ways that Japanese fee regulation limits costs cannot be separated from Japanese arrangements to deliver care. Each shapes the other.

Delivering Japanese Health Care

Japanese physicians practice either in a hospital, on salary, or separately, in their own clinics. Japan has lots of hospital beds by international standards. In 1988 just under 10 percent were in the national hospitals, which in many cases were affiliated with national government university medical schools (at least one per prefecture). Just over

20 percent were in local government (or other publicly owned body) facilities. The rest were in a wide variety of private hospitals, all owned (at least formally) by doctors or by "medical juridical persons," a form of nonprofit organization that must be managed by a doctor. Office-based physicians could have up to nineteen beds attached to their clinics.[88]

COMPETITION BETWEEN HOSPITALS AND CLINICS. Within this system, doctors who operate clinics do not have admitting privileges to hospitals. But, as explained above, the fee schedule favors services that those doctors can provide. Therefore hospitals compete with the clinic doctors by promoting their outpatient care. That promotion works for university hospitals in a very status- and technology-oriented society. Clinic doctors and lower-status hospitals counter by trying to buy prestige in the form of high-tech equipment such as imaging machines, even using them as "loss leaders." Japan therefore has many more of those items per capita than even the United States.[89]

The Japanese are no different from Americans in their interest in going to the "best," most prestigious facility.[90] But they have more reason to choose a university hospital outpatient clinic, because only doctors affiliated with the university hospitals' clinics are able to admit patients there; office-based physicians are not.[91] Those patients who choose to go to a university clinic often have to wait for two to three hours before being seen, for the hospitals do not schedule appointments. These waiting times are just one of many differences between the ways patients experience medical care in Japan and the United States.

INPATIENT SERVICES. By any calculation, the volume of surgery in Japan is no more than a third of the level of surgical activity in the United States.[92] Yet with at least twice as many inpatient beds per person in Japan as in America, much less surgery, and half as many admissions, Japan still has a higher occupancy rate. Japanese hospital beds are more likely to be full because the average length of stay in Japan is about five times as long as in the United States.[93] The average for university hospitals is about six times as long.[94]

Inside the hospitals, Japanese patients are much less likely than Americans to be placed in special areas for intensive care; of the 399 hospitals with more than 500 beds, only 252 have intensive care units.[95] The fee schedule, which does not reward surgery and intensive care, helps explain why Japan provides much less of these services than the United States. Culture is also a factor, but as one observer comments, "it is generally considered to be true that the average Japanese person would agree to have surgery if necessary. And the average American would avoid surgery if possible."[96] Japanese hospitals are not eager to perform money-losing procedures and hesitate to invest in the capacity to lose money.

Amenities in Japanese hospitals are far inferior to those in the other countries in this study. For instance, "Patients know that it is wise to provide their own soap and towels and that it is often necessary to hire a private nurse." Americans find facilities cramped, dingy, and extremely unprivate.[97]

PHARMACEUTICALS AND PHYSICIAN INCOMES. Japanese consumption of pharmaceuticals is very high. In the tradition of Chinese medicine, the Japanese use drugs not just to attack a disease but to restore physiological "balance." Drugs are frequently combined to obtain this balance, and dosages tend to be low and "gentle."[98] Yet Japanese levels of drug consumption, and the resulting high costs, cannot be explained by culture alone. "Blatant" overprescribing, two observers write, "has given rise to a popular expression 'kusuri zuke' (literally, 'pickling with drugs.')."[99] That expression hardly indicates popular approval. Instead, the Japanese consume huge amounts of drugs in large part because of economic incentives for physicians:

> Drugs are costly in Japan mainly because of the way they are distributed and sold. Japanese doctors not only prescribe drugs; they also dispense them. The doctors buy their drugs from wholesalers, who typically sell them at a discount to the official prices set by the Japanese government. Doctors are reimbursed by the government for the drugs they prescribe—but at the official price. This system encourages doctors to prescribe lots of expensive drugs—and pocketing the difference between the discount price and the official price has brought them handsome returns.[100]

Doctors are required by law to dispense limited amounts, but that suits them just fine; each time a patient must return for a new prescription, the physician earns a new dispensing fee.[101]

In its (successful) effort to limit health care costs during the 1980s, the Ministry of Health and Welfare slashed prices for existing drugs by roughly 50 percent. One result was that, by 1989, prices for the same drug tended to be much lower in Japan than in the United States.[102] Pharmaceutical reimbursements as a share of sickness fund expenses fell from 38.7 percent in 1981 to 28 percent in 1987.[103] Yet even in 1989, the Japanese spent as much on pharmaceuticals as Americans, while the system as a whole spent less than half as much.[104]

It is difficult to tell who has borne the financial brunt of the squeeze on drug costs, because medical incomes in Japan are rather opaque. Earnings of drug companies are heavily veiled no matter where they are headquartered. On balance, though, it seems that physicians have been able to maintain most of their income by prescribing more and charging higher fees for other services as part of a deal with the bureaucrats, while the drug companies have lost some from having to give even greater discounts than before to the physicians in order to maintain their patronage.[105]

PHYSICIAN SERVICES AND EARNINGS. Patients' frequent visits to their doctors to renew prescriptions help explain the high number of office visits per capita in Japan—more than one a month, a figure that only the Germans approach.[106] Given all those visits, substantially fewer doctors, and less reason for the visits, the average consultation with a physician is between three and five minutes long.[107]

Japanese physician training and accreditation differ from those of the six other countries in this study. A person can be licensed to practice after six years of undergraduate medical education, with no clinical training. The vast majority do at least two more years of internship but do not get much experience then either.[108] Many physicians receive further hospital training in a form of specialist residency; but there is no certification of specialists other than from the training institution itself. A senior doctor in a hospital will have been trained and vetted within that medical hierarchy, and there are some informal broader accreditation processes, but the system does not compare to specialist accreditation in the United States.[109]

The distribution of incomes among Japanese physicians is also unique among the countries studied here. Largely because of the pharmaceutical payment arrangements, clinic doctors, according to official statistics, earn twice the average for hospital doctors. Therefore even the best-trained specialists, except for chiefs of service, earn less than generalists.[110]

OTHER ASPECTS OF DELIVERY. A significant but uncounted number of Japanese health care services are not reimbursed by sickness funds and may not show up on national health care accounts. Families often help with nursing in the hospital, and that is neither a market nor a government transaction. Normal pregnancy care is paid for separately because it is not considered a sickness. There are also some under-the-table payments. A tradition of gratuities to physicians can turn into a very large payment to a chief of service in order to secure his special attention and treatment, and perhaps speed up admission.[111]

In short, the Japanese delivery system is very different from the one in America. Japan has very good public health coverage, especially for mothers and children. Frequent visits of about three minutes each may seem silly, but for purposes of keeping track of some patients, especially the elderly, they may be as informative and also as psychologically satisfying as less frequent but longer visits.[112] Long hospital stays should not do harm and may do good. The Japanese substitute other procedures for some surgery (we may do more cancer surgery, but they use a lot of chemotherapy), and American levels are surely too high. It might be hard to prove that overall Japanese quality of care is lower than in the United States, yet it is easy to say the two populations are buying quite different baskets of services.

Lessons from Japan?

One should be hesitant to draw any lessons from the Japanese case. The organization of delivery, and possibly the patterns of patient preferences, raise too many questions. For example, Naoki Ikegami reports that there are long waiting lists at two hospitals in Tokyo. He found that in the more prestigious institution more than half of the patients whose treatment was deemed "very urgent" waited more than a week for admission. Using a less subjective so more frightening measure, more than half of the patients with cervical cancer waited more than a month. But he notes that there are hardly any waits at some hospitals he did not study.[113] No system can avoid queuing by prestige; by definition, not everyone can use "the best." Is that the explanation for these waits? Perhaps.

Concern about the Japanese health care delivery system should not blind us to the fact that it seems to work for the Japanese, who live a long time and pay much less than any other people in this study, except the British. More important, the Japanese example provides evidence about economic incentives and health care costs.

If the persons receiving fees (such as physicians) also control the volume of services (say, prescriptions) they will normally respond to a reduction in fees by raising the volume of services to restore their income. That is why separation of ordering from income is generally important. But there are services for which fees can be cut drastically without making the supply of the services uneconomical. That is especially true for services that are only part of a provider's business, or for which margins are very high. In addition, some of the beneficiaries of prices cannot control incomes through volume: in this case, the pharmaceutical companies. These factors help explain why fee reductions without volume limits reduced the burden of Japanese pharmaceutical costs on the sickness funds. As an almost academic point, Japan shows that if the fees are kept low enough, fee regulation on virtually any service can control costs even without supplementary measures to limit volume. More significant, Japan highlights the potential effect of relative fees on delivery.

How does Japan get away with its unequal risk pools? One answer is that cost control is strong enough that the risks are not so great. In other words, *a high-cost medical care system must worry more about equity than a low-cost medical care system.* Another answer is, What is the alternative? When the Japanese or Germans or French talk about inequalities in payments, they mean as a percentage of income. In America, different people pay very different absolute amounts. The risk pooling in Japan does not allow the kind of burden on the working poor that is created by the pricing of American private insurance, because Japan still builds some redistribution into the premium structure. A third answer is simpler and seems relevant to the American debate of 1993–94. The government subsidizes low-income or high-risk funds from general revenues. American reformers tend to emphasize building on the nation's employment-based system. But American health care in 1994 was also financed by substantial general revenues. In that sense it was more similar to the system in Japan than to those in Germany and France, where payroll contributions to the sickness funds were supposed to cover almost all costs.

United Kingdom

The United Kingdom was the first country in this study to guarantee health care to all its citizens. The National Health Service (NHS), which began operation in 1948, provided universal coverage at a time when the sickness fund systems still did not include some large social groups.

"Socialized" (Really, Budgeted) Medicine

Britain's NHS thus was the prime target for the American Medical Association and other opponents of "socialized medicine." Over forty years later, this author heard Dr. Louis Sullivan, U.S. secretary of health and human services in the Bush administration, give a speech in which he claimed all universal systems were socialized medicine just like Britain's, and that if we went down that road we, like Britain, would have rationing, and old people would not be able to get dialysis.[114]

Kidney dialysis is the best-known case of a service that is in shorter supply in Britain than in the United States, and physicians are unlikely (though not forbidden) to prescribe it for the elderly. Dr. Sullivan failed to mention, however, that all Americans are entitled to dialysis through a federal government program, the end-stage renal disease (ESRD) program. The ESRD program does for kidney disease what Canada does for all health care: create an entitlement to treatment. In the good doctor's terms, it is socialized medicine.

As this example shows, government financing does not necessitate "rationing" any more than private financing of medical care guarantees plenty. Dialysis is paid for by government in both the United Kingdom and the United States, but less wealthy governments and people both buy less. It has been decades since Britain was rich and not in some form of budget crisis. Yet even with its shortages, the NHS has long been the second most popular institution in Britain, behind only the monarchy.[115] How, then, did the British manage to constrain both costs and services?

They did so by offering not insurance for care but access to a system of care. In an insurance system, the insurer pays for services that are bought from competing hospitals, physicians, and other suppliers. Cost control then requires efforts on three levels. There must be a process for limiting the cost of premiums, a way for insurers to agree with providers to keep costs within those premiums, and a process by which the government limits the supply of providers. An insurance system entitles people to reimbursement for whatever services someone is willing to sell them.

Britain's National Health Service made a different kind of promise. It said, in essence, "Your taxes have built an organization to provide you with care. That organization will serve you to the best of its ability." The difference between the two approaches is similar to the difference that budget analysts use to distinguish between two forms of government programs in the United States. They call programs that promise open-ended payment *entitlement* programs, such as medicare and social security. Programs that build an organization to deliver services are *discretionary* programs, such as the Federal Bureau of Investigation and the Department of Veterans Affairs medical services system.

Over the past three decades, federal entitlement programs have grown much more quickly than discretionary ones, for many reasons. The distinction between the two types of programs is deeply ingrained within Congress's budget procedures, also for many reasons.[116] But both rest ultimately on a logic of substance and politics.

When a government creates an organization that delivers services, it provides an intermediary that is responsible for the actual level of services. The legislature funds the organization, but its administrators must ensure that services are delivered. If the legislature wants to restrain spending, it can accuse the administrators of being inefficient and say better managers could do more at the given funding level. The government can also reduce funding for maintenance or capital investment, measures that show up eventually as restricted service but generally not quickly—especially because administrators, seeking to minimize criticism by keeping service levels up, will cut wherever immediate consequences are least.[117] Administrators can complain, but they are bureaucrats, an unpopular and mistrusted species to which the public rarely listens; and they risk their jobs by complaining.

To restrain an entitlement, such as health insurance, a government cannot simply reduce the budget of an organization. It must change a visible rule of payment, such as the price for a service, the services covered, who is covered, or cost sharing. In short, the government must admit who will suffer and how. The service providers are not government employees, so are in a much better position to protest.

In health care, this distinction between funding of entitlements and discretionary programs is not absolute, but the difference between a promise to reimburse for services and a promise to provide an organization to dispense services is extremely important.[118] As I have noted, cost control in most countries does involve limiting the capacity of and setting budgets for organizations wherever possible. This occurs mainly through budgeting of hospitals, as in Canada, France, and Australia. It includes capital investment limits in those countries and Germany. But before the current round of international reforms, the British National Health Service had two advantages.

First, the NHS was a more integrated system. Capital investment limits and fees for services were not established by different people; nor were there issues of cost-shifting between federal and state governments. Second, the NHS's budgetary reach stretched further. It covered not only hospital inpatient treatment but also the vast majority of specialist outpatient care (because it was included in hospital budgets) and a large part of primary care (because it was provided by general practitioners for fixed capitation fees).

Providing a direct service rather than insurance does not guarantee lower costs. Sweden, which has a similar system (though county-based) long ago had among the highest health care expenditures in the world. But it is easier to restrain spending in a direct-service system than in an entitlement system (and the Swedes did so during the 1980s). British budgeters further benefited from a strong conservative streak in British medicine.

British doctors do not go looking for trouble: if the patient does not report symptoms, doctors are unlikely to order tests on their own. A 1978 study showed that diabetes diagnosis depended more on symptoms, and less on routine testing, in Britain than in India, Poland, France, or East Berlin or on an American Indian reservation.[119] British cardiologists are less likely than Americans to prescribe angiography on the basis of tests, and more likely to do so in response to persistence of symptoms after maximum medical therapy. "You can't be diagnosed as having hypertension if nobody ever takes your blood pressure," Lynn Payer summarizes. "But," she adds, "even when blood pressure is taken, the British have a higher threshold for disease."[120]

This conservative approach has been reinforced by the heavy scientific orientation of the British medical profession. If a treatment has not been shown to be effective through randomized controlled trials, British doctors are unlikely to accept it. Therefore they prescribe fewer drugs than the French or Japanese, do less surgery than the Americans, and are more skeptical of innovations than either. The public has cooperated by "keeping a stiff upper lip."[121]

These cultural biases doubtless helped governments restrain the growth of medical capacity, especially capacity for invasive or intensive hospital care, during the 1960s and 1970s and into the 1980s. Limits on capital spending in the NHS budget, which became strict earlier than in any other country, help explain both the lower costs and the "rationing" that Aaron and Schwartz studied in the early 1980s. But the demand pressures created by trying to run a system with much less money than neighboring countries, its own ideological skepticism of direct government provision, and common criticisms of the NHS itself led to a series of reform efforts by the government of Prime Minister Margaret Thatcher in the 1980s, which culminated in the radical reforms promulgated at the end of the decade.

A January 1989 proposal announced that the NHS would "put the interests and wishes of the patients first." It offered NHS physicians and staff, "a new, exciting, and potentially rewarding challenge." And, it was said, the reforms would "enable a higher quality of patient care to be obtained from the resources which the nation is able to devote to the NHS"—that is, more output without more resources, especially taxes or deficits.[122] All these marvels would be gained from new forms of management and competition within the NHS.

Chapter 7 tells the story of the NHS reforms. As of 1991, the year on which all comparisons of performance in this book are based, the reforms could not yet have had any meaningful effect on the NHS's cost or quality, and they had had little effect as of 1994. I focus here on the "old" NHS, for two reasons. It is the service that opponents of guaranteeing health care to all Americans have used as a bogeyman for more than four decades, and many fundamentals of the old system remain in the new.

Fundamentals

From its beginning the NHS separated administration of hospitals, largely owned by the service and with salaried staff, from family practice, provided through contracts with GPs. Hospitals were directly budgeted ("cash-limited," in the government's accounts). Family practice costs were not limited because GPs received some fees for service and the system provided drug benefits. A third set of services related to health was incorporated in the personal social services (PSS) system, which has been funded separately by local governments, though policies have been heavily regulated from the center.[123] Record-keeping and some policies are complicated by the fact that the Welsh, Scottish, and Northern Irish versions of the system are overseen by their own ministries within the central government, while the Department of Health oversees only the English portions.[124]

Every Briton registers with a local general practitioner, who must guarantee care to all the persons she accepts on her list, twenty-four hours a day, 365 days a year. A GP makes about twenty house calls per week. In part to cover those hours outside the office, and with financial encouragement from the government, in the early 1990s, 90 percent of GPs practice in small groups. In 1991–92 the average GP in England had 1,947 patients.[125]

Choice of GP was limited not by rules, but by geography and custom. GPs could not be expected to make house calls at much distance from their homes or to take on too many patients. GPs also did not appreciate doctor-shopping and might hesitate to accept a switcher.[126] In order to coordinate the services of GPs and other providers, such as home-help nurses and midwives, the government encouraged doctors to practice in community health clinics by paying for the premises. But most physicians resisted the "perceived threats to the self-employed status of the doctor," and instead, many bought their own facilities and then rented to the community primary health care team.[127]

The NHS pays for most pharmaceuticals. A copayment per item (4.75 pounds, or about $8, in 1994) is waived for children, pensioners, and people with "special needs" such as diabetics, so over 80 percent of prescriptions are exempt from copayment.[128] The NHS also pays a portion of dental services, though at rates some dentists reject, and for optometric exams and glasses or contact lenses for some. Medical and dental examinations are provided through the schools, and the visiting nurse services include, for example, both pre- and postnatal home visits.[129]

In the prereform NHS, specialists saw patients at the hospital outpatient clinic at the written request of a GP. If the situation were urgent the GP might speak personally with the specialist instead. (This referral pattern is still the norm, but one of the goals and accomplishments of reform was to make specialists somewhat more responsive, as is described in chapter 7.) Known as "consultants," British specialists have had lifetime tenure on hospital staffs. They are paid a full- or part-time salary (full time is eleven half-day sessions). Specialists have resisted standards that might quantify the hours required. "Distinction awards," made by the minister with advice from the medical community, raised the pay of some specialists substantially.[130]

In this system, the specialists were king. They controlled allocation of services within the hospital, because hospital managers had few levers to influence them. And because they were salaried, they had little incentive to satisfy referring physicians. As one account summarizes:

> Before 1948 the voluntary hospitals and the consultants within them depended for their livelihood on GPs referring their paying patients to them. After 1948 the hospitals were directly funded by the state and the GPs became supplicants, seeking treatment for a patient on the consultant's waiting-list.[131]

Both managers and GPs therefore had incentives to support reforms that weakened specialists' hold on the system—though in the event, managers were a lot more enthusiastic.

Some private hospitals and private insurance persisted from the beginning of the NHS. Both grew in the 1970s and 1980s, because of the long wait for elective surgery through the NHS and the government's decision to allow private health insurance benefit increases during a period of wage and price controls. By the late 1980s about 10 percent of the population had some private insurance. Private spending on acute care constituted perhaps 5 percent of total spending.[132]

Private insurance nevertheless remained a much less significant factor in Britain than in Australia. Its role has been more like that of private education in the United States, except that there was no health care equivalent of low-cost, high-quality Catholic schools.[133] But given the long waiting lists for some elective surgeries, even strong advocates of the NHS could be tempted to go private, and the specialists were certainly suspected of steering patients to the private hospitals, where they earned fees above their state-paid salaries. Private patients were "paying to avoid waiting."[134]

The waiting-list controversy in Britain is subject to all the caveats about list manipulation that must be raised about any such argument. Yet there is little doubt that the waits endured by British citizens both before and after reform would be unacceptably long in the United States and are also not popular in the United Kingdom.[135] Waits for care are the major political symbol of substantive problems within the NHS, and the major indicator for the success or failure of the 1990 reforms.

The government's "Patient's Charter" announced a new right "to be guaranteed admission for treatment by a specific date no later than two years from the day when your consultant places you on the waiting list"; set new standards for waiting time for ambulance service, initial assessment in emergency departments, and outpatient appointments; and promised that local officials would create standards for waiting time for first outpatient appointments, treatment in emergency departments, and transportation home after treatment.[136] All of these promises reflected the system's real weaknesses.

The NHS remained popular both because the obvious alternative, *no* NHS, did not exactly sound more secure and because the system had real strengths. All Britons had a primary care physician, and the doctors made house calls. A system of visiting nurses also provided good pregnancy care. Pharmaceuticals were affordable. The most evident shortages were for "elective" procedures, the lack of which one might "grin and bear." For the money, by far the least among the countries described in this book, Britons received a lot of care.

Governments may be forgiven for suspecting that changing approaches in order to improve services would cost a lot more. Because governments were not likely to abandon the NHS in order to spend more money, public suspicion that the alternative would require more reliance on personal income, and therefore more inequality, was appropriate.

The 1990 reforms therefore promised only to improve, not remove, the NHS. How they work is still a matter for study. Before discussing them and the theories underlying them, I summarize what we have learned about the international standard.

6

Twentieth-Century
Health Care Systems

*T*HE detail about six different health care systems in chapters
4 and 5 might make them seem more different than similar—if we did not have the United States for comparison. But all have
much lower costs than the United States and virtually universal coverage. They achieve these ends with compulsory participation, contributions related to income, fee schedules, budgets, and capital spending limits.

At the same time, the evidence that their methods of financing
"work" leaves some open questions. Is the United States buying something for its money that is less measurable than the number of insured
and the costs? If American reform were to fit into the international
standard, what would be the most important choices *within* that framework? From the standpoint of longtime advocates of national health
insurance, for example, what compromises to the simplicity of the
Canadian model are worthwhile? And what are the basic dynamics to
which Americans must attend if they want to ensure that reform
works?

Performance Comparisons

This chapter begins from the facts presented by the tables in chapter
2. The United States spends much more for health care than any of
the six other countries studied here (or any other nation), and the gap
widened throughout the 1980s and into the 1990s. In the meantime,
American insurance coverage declined rather than expanded.

One might argue, however, that the U.S. system is better than it
seems. Perhaps access in other countries is worse even though they
have better coverage. Perhaps Americans have more choice of doctor.

Perhaps Americans have to buy more because the United States is a sicker society. Perhaps American medical care is of higher quality. Perhaps Americans are buying something else of value with all that extra money they spend on health care, such as a more pleasant experience when ill.

Many of these things cannot be measured precisely. But we can analyze them using the available evidence.

The analysis that follows emphasizes three logical points. First, arguments about cause and effect must take account of chronology. Second, comparison to Canada is the most reasonable basis for an assessment of what is possible in the United States. Third, any system of cost constraints has its own limits.

Time and Costs

There are many differences in cost control policies between the United States and the other six countries in this study. When certain features were strengthened—hospital budgets tightened in France and Germany, pharmaceutical prices restrained further in Japan, or volume adjustments for physician fees tightened in Canada and Germany, for example—costs grew more slowly. Such concerted efforts and resulting changes look like evidence of policy effectiveness. Similarly in the United States stricter fee regulation has been successful in slowing the increase in medicare costs. Between 1986 and 1991, that program's spending for physician services increased by 10.5 percent per year. After the implementation of the volume performance standard regulations, average annual growth fell to an estimated 3.8 percent between 1991 and 1993, and perhaps even less.[1]

Opponents of the common international measures assert that American costs are higher than other countries' for reasons not related to health care policy, such as more social problems, which create worse health. But many of the social problems in the United States are nothing new. An argument that emphasizes social factors can do so convincingly only if it can also show that American costs rose faster than other countries' in the 1980s while American social pathologies also increased more quickly. We will see that this test is hard to meet; indeed, it is unlikely that conservative opponents of universal coverage and "big government" cost control really want to show that the 1980s were a terrible time for the United States.

A more centrist argument emphasizes that costs have risen in America because spending on people in the last year or six months of their lives is so high. Expensive new technologies and invasive treatments are used to keep people alive longer. Therefore cost control requires a change in social values rather than in payment policies; indeed, it may require explicit rationing. Again, this argument implies something about time: if costs rise because more resources are used for people about to die, then a larger share of the health care dollar should be devoted, over time, to those patients—especially in medicare.

In fact, "the share of Medicare expenditures accounted for by persons in their last year of life remained virtually the same from 1976 through 1988." And less was paid for beneficiaries in their last years if they were older.[2] So increased costs could not be explained by a social choice to spend more on the dying elderly; Americans spent more on all medical care. More expensive technology combined with increased insurance did contribute to a growth throughout society in the proportion of health care costs concentrated on the most costly portion of the population throughout the 1960s and 1970s. But spending on the most expensive 1 percent grew from 29 percent in 1980 to only 30 percent in 1987, so spending more on the sickest patients cannot explain greater total spending during the period when American and other countries' spending trends diverged.[3]

It remains true that, as the population ages, health care costs as a share of the economy may be expected to rise. That is reason to be careful in setting targets for cost control and in estimating the long-term success of any set of measures. But the existence of long-term trends should not be a reason to avoid taking steps that will do good in the here-and-now. We all will die eventually, but that does not keep us from seeing a doctor when we get sick.

COST CONTROL AND COMPARISONS WITH CANADA. This book compares countries in order to argue that countries differ on certain dependent variables (such as cost and coverage) because they differ on certain independent variables (compulsory contributions, fee regulation, and the like). This chapter addresses claims that inferior American performance on the measured variables is misleading either because the financing and payment rules have negative effects on other dependent variables, such as quality, or because other independent variables, such as proportion of elderly persons in the population, explain the performance on cost and coverage.

A comparison of seven countries and many variables could be impossible to follow (or do), but it can be made intelligible by following some simple rules. One is to get the chronology straight. Another is to remember that the burden of proof should be on defenders of the American status quo to explain why the United States has to spend more than a third more than other countries to cover fewer persons and get worse aggregate health status statistics. The most important simplification is: when in doubt, focus on the difference between Canada and the United States.

The comparison with Canada is the most important for many reasons. As a practical matter, there is more information. We have to use the best evidence available, and the best evidence involves Canada. But there are also substantive reasons. First, Canada and the United States already have similar delivery systems. Therefore comparing the United States with Germany or Japan, for example, which separate office-based and hospital-based physicians, is more difficult. It is also less practical: American reform may ultimately restrict some choices substantially, but it is not likely to raise barriers between ambulatory and hospital care.

Second, Canada is the country most likely to be influenced by American notions of proper practice. Demand for services may be based on publicity about new treatments, personal acquaintance with recipients of services, and the dissemination of information among professionals. Canadians have wide access to American media, many travel widely in the United States and so know many Americans, and medical training is interchangeable between the two countries. Therefore Canada provides a better test of how well financing and payment institutions can restrain American-style demands for spending. As mentioned in chapter 4, the two systems had very similar profiles until around 1971.

Third, Canada has the second most expensive health care system in the world. The basic questions of this chapter may be rephrased as, "How much if anything do other countries give up in order to guarantee a basic standard of health care to all their citizens, while the United States leaves at least 16 percent behind? Who gives up what? And how much (if anything) do they give up in order to spend, in 1991, between 3.4 percent of GDP (Canada) and 6.8 percent (Japan and the United Kingdom) less on health care?" The problem with the last question is that the cost differences between the United States and the United Kingdom are so large that comparisons are unreasonable. It is possible to argue that one system could be so much more efficient than another—that Canada could get the same care for three-quarters as much money as the United States in 1991. But a prudent person should hesitate to believe that, whatever the failings of American institutions, some other system could be twice as efficient—that Japan and the United Kingdom could be receiving as much value while spending less than half as large a portion of their economies.

Therefore comparisons between the lower-cost countries and the United States pose two risks. If the variables other than cost and coverage are underplayed, the comparison likely overstates the possible savings from reform. Yet because systems do differ in quality and practice, these differences are too easy to exaggerate into statements about the risks of any form of the international standard methods of cost control. In fact, some opponents of health care reform during 1993 and 1994 chose to mix horror stories: to use British waiting lists and the shortness of office visits in Japan as arguments against creating a system like Canada's.[4] If different methods of cost control affect output differently, then it makes little sense to treat countries as different in their spending strategies as Japan and Canada as comparable examples of the evil effects of cost control.

The analysis that follows therefore treats countries other than Canada as supplementary evidence. Where the United States cannot show better performance than Japan or the United Kingdom for its money, one should be especially skeptical about the value provided by American institutions. But as a practical matter the only question is how far the United States could move toward Canada's level of health care spending, not whether it will or should spend even less.

LIMITS ON COST CONTROL. Readers should remember that no system of health care financing and delivery has unlimited capacity for efficiency. One system may enable lower administrative costs than another, but in any system there is some irreducible minimum of administration. One system might give payers more bargaining power than another, but providers must always have some power because they are needed to deliver the care. Limits on capital investment can lead to more efficient allocations of capacity, but it is always possible to have more real need than there is ability to serve it. One system might encourage more efficient use of labor, with the "right" proportions of nurse-practitioners (who cost less than general practitioners), GPs (who usually cost less than specialists), and specialists. But at some point efforts to reduce the cost of labor also reduce quality.

At the same time, populations in modern societies do tend to age, and as people age their medical needs increase. Moreover, medical advances provide new ways to address previously unmet needs. Therefore the demand for care should increase relative to other demands in society, and any set of arrangements must eventually reach the point where continued spending restraint creates popular dissatisfaction.

Nobody knows where that point is, in any system. And the fact that some people want a service does not mean that it should be guaranteed to all citizens through social insurance. At the same time, no country is likely to have a system of cost control that can hold costs steady forever, without forgoing some services that people want. One should not assume that when a country tightens its cost controls significantly, as Germany and Canada did from 1992 to 1994, satisfaction with health care outputs will remain as high as it was before that constriction.

Therefore, this chapter assesses the effects of cost controls as of 1991. That approach makes the differences between the cost-effectiveness and coverage of American and other countries' arrangements seem much smaller than they would with 1994 data. I would rather undersell the benefits of reform than oversell them.[5]

Nevertheless, the evidence will be clear: there are no arguments about choice, quality, or any other variable that can justify America's high costs and failure to guarantee decent care to all its citizens.

Measuring Quality from Mortality Data

The most obvious way to measure the quality of health care would seem to be to measure its outcomes. Unfortunately there are only two outcome measures for which there are remotely comparable international statistics, infant mortality and life expectancy (with its cousin, age-adjusted death rates). American performance on each is pretty miserable by the standards of the rest of the developed world. But the data reflect more than health care quality: they also reflect the social ills that cause a pregnant woman, for example, to be undernourished and bear a child who dies quickly.

Differences in how the United States and some of the comparison countries define outcomes may make the American infant mortality rate look higher.[6] But one should also remember that if, for example, infant mortality statistics are high because impoverished mothers are malnourished and do not get appropriate prenatal care, other social measures can be integrated with health care to address both problems. The French, for example, provide family allowances as income supplements for people with children, but require the recipients to get prenatal care. The American WIC (women, infants, and children) program is similar, but it does not reach all eligible persons and provides much less medical care because the mothers are not members of a system of national health insurance and the United States does not have a public health system that can provide wide-ranging pre- and postnatal care.[7]

Most of the differences in infant mortality between the United States and the other countries are probably due to measurement and social factors, but greater access to prenatal care early in pregnancy, especially for at-risk populations, would help.[8]

Basic data on the other standard measure, life expectancy, also put America at the bottom of the chart. Again, a wide range of social evils could be depressing American results—beginning with the social effects on infant mortality. But much of the effect of these factors should be reduced as the population ages. The victims of infant mortality drop out of the data quickly. People in their fifties are not as likely to be shot during drug deals as people in their teens and twenties. Table 6-1 shows life expectancy at birth in all the countries in this study and at ages forty-five, sixty-five, and eighty. It shows that the American disadvantage in life expectancy diminishes as the population ages.

As the table shows, the United States had higher life expectancy at birth in only one comparison, British females. American performance looks better at higher ages, and by age eighty it is in third place. Data for 1986 put the United States virtually tied for first with Canada.[9]

These data could mean that the American health care system kills off the weak more quickly than others, so our elderly are a hardier lot. But these data are also consistent with the general impression that the United States has a more interventionist medical culture than other countries and that this buys more lifesaving medicine for the elderly. The fact that U.S. life expectancies are not higher than Canada's, even for the elderly, also makes sense, because Canada is more directly

TABLE 6-1. *Life Expectancy by Age and Gender, 1990*

Age/gender	USA	Australia	Canada	France	Germany	Japan	UK
At birth							
Male	71.80	73.61	73.81	73.37	72.63	76.17	73.03
Female	78.80	80.05	81.11	81.76	79.16	82.05	78.68
Age 45							
Male	30.70	31.35	31.70	31.56	30.16	33.10	30.35
Female	35.90	36.67	37.83	38.53	35.79	38.29	35.26
Age 65							
Male	15.10	15.05	15.80	15.98	14.24	16.35	14.12
Female	18.90	19.05	20.69	20.69	18.18	20.11	18.00
Age 80							
Male	7.10	6.92	8.20	7.40	6.27	7.07	6.62
Female	9.00	8.80	10.99	9.52	7.98	8.91	8.46

Source: U.S. Congress, Office of Technology Assessment, *International Health Statistics: What the Numbers Mean for the United States-Background Paper*, OTA-BP-H-116 (November 1993), p. 49, table 5.1.

influenced by American patterns of medical practice than other countries are. The French are also reported to favor high-tech medicine (and trains, and telephone systems), a pattern that may allow France to stay ahead of the United States, but the difference between U.S. and French life expectancies narrows far more between ages sixty-five and eighty than does the difference in American and Canadian prospects.

There is reason, therefore, to believe that Americans are buying something for all their extra money: longer life for the elderly. This is not, however, an argument against national health insurance, because the elderly are the only Americans who have national health insurance. Nor does longer American life expectancy at higher ages justify spending more than Canada.

Someday someone may develop evidence that shows the U.S. health care system has done a better job of saving lives than others, and that social ills explain more than the observed differences in life expectancy between America and other countries. Yet the U.S. population is not riskier on all dimensions: alcohol consumption is higher in Australia, Canada, Germany and France; the percentage of American males who smoke has not been higher than in the other countries, on average, since the 1960s; and (according to OECD data) fewer American women smoke than in the other countries save for Japan and Germany.

Although there are international statistics on various health risks, such as income inequities and smoking, any attempt to build an index of all risks would require making arbitrary comparisons with lots of questionable data. But it is highly unlikely that the life expectancy data could be massaged to do more than show that the American health care system is equal to Canada's. In too many cases, American conditions are not worse, while in others the differences are small.[10] Testing at higher age brackets is biased in favor of the American status quo, because some of the people who die young would have lived longer if they had had insurance; the population for which the United States has the best statistics are the elderly, who are the only Americans with universal health coverage.

At a minimum, the mortality data suggest that if one wants to reduce mortality, providing decent health care coverage to all is more efficient than providing the American level of care to some. But is the American level of care for those with good insurance superior in some way to the norm in other countries? And, even if it is, is it worth the cost—the cost that is driving ever more Americans to the ranks of the un- or underinsured?

Access and Choice

Throughout the legislative struggle of 1993–94, opponents of the Clinton administration's and other universal coverage bills claimed that they threatened "choice." Many supporters, meanwhile, worried about whether even universal insurance would provide adequate access to care in those portions of the country that had few providers. The actual effects of any reform in the United States would depend on the legislation's provisions. But international experience allows us to consider the claim that universal coverage must limit choice, while forcing us to be realistic about what reform can achieve.[11]

Americans without insurance have very poor access to and choice of care, so the United States starts out behind all the other countries in this comparison. At the same time, none of the benefits packages in other countries cover too little by American standards. Some, like Canada's, cover as much as the American norm, and some, like Germany's and France's, cover more.

DISTRIBUTION OF DOCTORS AND FACILITIES. As the case of American medicaid shows, simply being insured for a nominally wide package of benefits does not guarantee access. Physicians and hospitals have to be willing to serve you, and between the understandable desire not to practice in some American neighborhoods and the low fees paid by medicaid, physicians in particular, as well as some hospitals, may not be willing to serve the poor.[12] Other countries do not expect doctors who work in more dangerous or lower-income neighborhoods to charge much less, and that may explain why the poor in other countries do not have as much difficulty finding a doctor. A poor person in Australia might have to go to a hospital outpatient clinic to see a specialist, but that situation is better than the plight of many U.S. medicaid beneficiaries, who have trouble finding a GP.

In all countries, there are many fewer physicians per capita in rural than in urban areas. This makes some sense: specialists and tertiary-care providers should be concentrated in population centers, where they have a critical mass of cases to keep up their skills. Nevertheless, inferior access in rural areas is a policy problem in all countries.

Foreign measures to attract or compel a more equal distribution of medical care are stronger than those in America. Payments per patient or case for physicians tend to follow local income levels in America; in France, Australia, Britain, and Japan they follow a national standard. Canada and Germany have both begun to restrict new practice in "overserved" areas, but as the combination of unemployed physicians and underserved areas in Germany suggests, it is hard to get people to go where they do not want to live. As the late political scientist Aaron Wildavsky once commented to me, "Even Stalin and Beria could not get doctors to move to the countryside."

By the most obvious measures of access, the number of office and home visits and hospital admissions, access is generally lower in the United States. The number of visits in the United Kingdom is similar to the number in the United States; it is at least 20 percent higher in the five other countries and more than double in both Germany and Japan. Hospitalization rates in the United Kingdom were 4 percent lower than in the United States in 1986. Japan's rates are much lower. But rates are higher everywhere else.[13] One cannot argue, therefore, that the distribution of facilities in other countries makes the promise of universal coverage deceptive. If anything, the access promised by America's partial system of subsidies for the poor, medicaid, is what is deceptive.

But many countries provide less access to certain treatments even as they make visits and hospitalization more accessible. The difficulty is in distinguishing between use and need. Clearly Americans receive an unusually high amount of elective surgery: is that because well-insured Americans have better access to needed care than citizens of other countries do, or because American arrangements encourage "too much" surgery? Americans receive fewer drugs than the Japanese: is that a failure of access? I address the surgery question below in the section on waiting lists. Here I note only that access to specialists is more restricted in both the United Kingdom and Japan than in the United States. In the United Kingdom family doctors function as gatekeepers to the limited supply of specialists. In Japan, the tendency of specialists to be located in the public hospitals creates barriers. We should add that access to "specialist care" is not necessarily the same thing as access to specialists. Having general practitioners handle routine pregnancies, with specialists in reserve, may in fact provide better-integrated care.

"CHOICE" AMONG DOCTORS AND FACILITIES. What about choice? Defenders of the American status quo talk a lot about choice. But in most ways the United States offers less choice than Canada, and somewhat different choices than other countries.

To most people, choice means choice of doctor or hospital: when they get sick, they want to be able to choose the providers they hear are best. There is no system in which everybody goes to "the best," because the best would be too busy to do a good job. But people want to be able to switch providers if they are dissatisfied and to go to the "best" doctor or hospital that has room for them.

Therefore opponents of national health insurance have long used the British National Health Service as an example of how a national guarantee would reduce choice: these opponents claim that the government will choose people's doctors. In fact the government has never chosen a person's family doctor in the United Kingdom. But people have had to select a local doctor in advance, physicians discouraged switching, and further services required the family doctor's approval. Traditionally other versions of a national health service, such as Sweden's, had similar restrictions on choice.[14]

But countries with national health insurance, such as Canada, Germany, and France, have always allowed patients to use any provider in the system under the terms of the insurance. It is American cost control through managed care, not Canadian or German cost control through managing payments, that most resembles the National Health Service approach.

Americans who are insured through their employer generally have a limited choice of insurance plans. Some insurers boast of their wide networks of providers, but many plans offer access to only some of the local physicians and hospitals. Or they offer a "point-of-service" option: beneficiaries may use other providers but must pay extra to do so. Of the other countries in this study, only the United Kingdom expects citizens to limit their options in advance, before becoming sick, by selecting a gatekeeper physician. Choice of a primary care physician is more limited in the United States than in the other countries.

But there is a real difference in the form of choices offered by the American and Canadian delivery systems and the norm in the other systems. The difference involves choice of specialist within the hospital. The Germans, Japanese, and French are less likely than Americans to be restricted in their choice of ambulatory care physicians, but once admitted to a hospital they are normally treated by the hospital staff as a group; in the United States and Canada hospital care is likely to be supervised by the patient's ambulatory care physician, who has admitting privileges to the hospital.

There are exceptions to all these patterns. In all systems the hospital staff provide emergency care, so ironically in the most serious cases there is no time for choice. Doctors have some admitting privileges even in Germany. In Australia doctors have admitting privileges, but care by one's outside doctor requires either paying more (having private status) or good luck (the hospital manages to assign him to your case). Even in the United States and Canada, much of the care for people hospitalized by admitting physicians must be provided by the resident staff.

There is no a priori basis on which to argue that reliance on hospital staff rather than admitting physicians raises or lowers quality. The former approach should lead to better coordination within the hospital but worse between sectors. But the difference between systems with and without admitting privileges should make reformers hesitate to claim that France, Germany, or Japan offers "better" choice than is available to people with private insurance in America. At the same time, Canadian physicians have hospital admitting privileges, and there are no restrictions on a patient's choice of doctor. Because choice of physician is clearly greater in Canada than in America, the charge that universal coverage and cost control must reduce Americans' choices is evidently false.

In the United States, high costs and the lack of guaranteed insurance for all citizens cannot be justified on the grounds that the insured have greater choice and access. But other countries have inequalities as well. Access to care in rural areas is a problem everywhere, and formal rules tell only part of the story. In all systems, those who are more aggressive, charming, or able to communicate with doctors and medical staff have a better chance of getting explanations or choices or attention. As Marilynn M. Rosenthal concluded from a study of these seven countries and five others, "The well-educated and assertive patient is best able to make a particular system work at some level of satisfaction."[15]

And reducing differences in access to health care will not eliminate differences in health outcomes. Medical treatments often fail. If some people are more susceptible than others to dangerous illness, then equalizing access will not equalize outcomes. But unequal access will only make the difference in outcomes worse.[16] International experience shows that decent national health insurance would not equalize health outcomes in the United States, but it would make outcomes more equitable.

Indirect Quality Measures

The American health care system does not appear to do a better job of preserving life than Canada's and may do worse than other countries' as well. It also does not offer superior access and choice. What, then, could justify its limited coverage and higher costs?

Defenders of the status quo must argue that the United States offers better care. Their first step is to dismiss the mortality statistics by pointing out their weaknesses. But that hardly provides evidence for a contrary claim that American medical care is superior, as the analysis earlier in this chapter shows. Absent statistical data to show higher American quality, defenders of the U.S. status quo may resort to purely impressionistic claims. For instance, they may say that U.S. doctors are "the best in the world." But why? The differences in training do not suggest that there would be differences in quality, save perhaps in Japan. And in Canada and the United States the training is identical.

One of the most common arguments against reform says that American medicine must be better because rich foreigners, such as Arab sheikhs, come to the United States for treatment. Whether Germans or Frenchmen come to the United States would seem more relevant than whether Saudis do. The fact that Saudis come to the United States tells us about Saudi health care, not French. The people who make this argument do not bother to find out whether foreigners go to other countries in this study, or whether in choosing America, language is a factor. In fact, foreigners do go elsewhere.[17] France provides medical treatment not just patients from other French-speaking countries but from other nations in Europe, to the point that "French kidneys for Frenchmen" has become a political and ethical issue.[18] America doubtless offers magnificent medicine for foreigners who can pay, but that tells us nothing about other systems.

PEACE OF MIND. Perhaps American medicine does a better job than other systems of relieving pain and discomfort. If so, the evidence is scarce. One gets relief by seeing a physician for minor aches and pains, for a diagnosis, or for referral to a specialist. In these cases access equals quality, and the United States does not look very good. Another aspect of relief is peace of mind; many Americans face much greater hassles and anxiety, especially dealing with the bills, than patients in any of the other six nations. Two witnesses provide evidence. One is a Japanese businessman, transplanted to Georgia:

You get separate bills for X-rays, for anesthesia, for surgery, for the hospital bed, for drugs, for service—there are so many kinds of bills coming to you. This makes it hard for you to know just how much you're being charged: new bills keep coming, day after day. Some wives developed a phobia of bills. Then after the patient has received all the bills, he has to consider how to obtain reimbursement from the insurance system. The medical insurance system itself is rather complicated and hard to understand. Our people learn from the insurance company how to utilize the system. Then other people say it is wrong, and conflicting advice comes in, making it more confusing.[19]

The other witness is one of the inventors of the "managed competition" idea described in chapter 7. As Alain Enthoven reports he told his elderly mother, "Anyone can handle their medical bills provided they have a son who is a professor of health care management in a business school."[20]

There is only one area in which the American health care system has any quality advantage over other countries: access to some high-tech, especially elective, services—especially surgeries. Are Americans "paying to avoid waiting"? And, if so, are they paying too much?

Elective Surgery and the Waiting-List Controversy

In terms of access and choice of physician, health care in Canada is clearly better than health care in the United States. A patient may choose a doctor outside the hospital and be treated by the same doctor inside it. There is no reason to believe that individual Canadian providers are of lower quality than Americans, since the training is identical and interchangeable.

American hospitals will usually treat an uninsured patient, but the uninsured are generally sicker than insured patients when admitted and are less likely to survive. Once admitted, the uninsured who obviously need treatment receive the same treatment the insured receive. But if there is doubt about the need for treatment it is less likely to be provided to uninsured patients.[21] Canadians do not postpone treatment because they cannot afford to see a doctor, and there are no financial barriers to equal treatment inside Canadian hospitals.

Many of these statements are also true of comparisons between Germany, France, or other countries and the United States. Yet there is certainly more surgery done in the United States. The question is whether that shows superior care.[22]

ELECTIVE SURGERY AS AN INDICATOR OF QUALITY. Because the American medical profession itself does not agree on when to perform surgery, the incidence of many procedures varies far more from community to community than could possibly be explained by differences in need.[23] Doctors in other countries do not agree with each other any more readily than U.S. doctors do, so variations by factors of two to four are common around the world.[24]

These statistics support the common assumption that someone other than doctors should "manage" care. Anyone who believes in managed care (which officially includes the leaders of all the large insurance companies that lobby to keep America from adapting the Canadian model) cannot logically argue that the United States has a higher-quality medical care system because we do more surgery. In fact, the inventor of the concept of "managed competition" argues that it would achieve huge savings by reducing the number of unnecessary procedures in the United States.[25] In short, skepticism as to whether more surgery shows that American medicine is superior is hardly confined to advocates of "big government."

Some procedures are truly elective, in the sense that different patients can be expected to make different choices. Prostate surgery reduces the risk of prostate cancer, but because that cancer progresses slowly, in many men it would not become life-threatening before something else did them in, and prostate removal has possible side effects that some men do not think are worth risking. For other procedures, the medical evidence is unclear and people's choices are influenced by their cultures.[26] Some choose an alternative treatment, such as chemotherapy or radiation, over surgery. When the benefits and cost of a surgery are matters of personal taste, or the evidence about outcomes is weak, it would be hard to show that higher rates of surgery represent higher-quality medicine.

Easier access to elective surgery also can produce lower quality, in two ways. First, anesthetizing people and cutting them open involves low but real health risks.[27] Second, wide access can mean that some of the many surgical teams available do not perform surgery often enough. One of the most robust findings in the medical outcomes literature is the high correlation between volume and successful outcome for cardiac surgery. As a result, the American College of Surgeons has recommended that each surgical team perform at least 150 operations per year. That standard often is not met, yet American hospitals continue to open more cardiac surgery facilities because they are "profit centers."[28] For all these reasons—real choice, alternative treatment, the general conclusion that U.S. levels of surgery are unjustifiably high, and the association of greater supply in some instances with lower quality per case—one should be skeptical of claims that American health care is of higher quality because the system does more elective surgery.

Yet by the same token, charges that other countries force patients to endure long waits for necessary care are one of the most popular arguments in defense of the American status quo. And this argument is not fully countered by the evidence that the United States does not need its current levels of elective surgery. Waiting lists in any country indicate at the very least a mismatch between what patients in that country want and what they are getting. Patients may be misled by their physicians into wanting unnecessary treatment, but that argument would be more convincing if it were the United States, the country that performs the most surgery, that had the waiting lists.

Waiting has not become an issue in France and Germany in part because of their delivery systems. Unless the United States changed its system of admitting physicians, Germany and France would always be able to have less waiting for use of the same amount of resources. For waiting lists especially, then, the right comparison is with Canada, which has admitting physicians and spends much more than the United Kingdom.

No one should imagine that the United Kingdom does not have real shortages. The United Kingdom spends less than is needed to provide what even conservative British doctors would consider proper levels of care. Economists can still find instances of excessive care. And the problems involve more than money.[29] But Britain's level of spending is so suspiciously low that it does not set a reasonable standard for American reform.

Where waiting lists exist, they are a major political issue, used by opponents of the national system as a sign of its inadequacy and by participants as an argument for more funding. The accuracy of these lists must be doubted because they are evidently manipulated by spending claimants and are subject to less politically motivated error. Physicians tend to put patients on several lists and on lists "just in case," and frequently do not remove them from those lists when they should. Often a popular individual doctor will have his patients wait rather than suggest they use a less popular physician, because in giving up a patient the first doctor would forfeit his fee. Given all these distortions, it should be no surprise that one hospital in Winnipeg discovered that, of 143 people waiting for cardiac angiography, only 56 were really candidates for the procedure.[30]

One set of anecdotes says Canadians go to American hospitals in order to avoid long waits for services in Canada. The U.S. General Accounting Office's analysis of the practice shows that it has been greatly exaggerated by those with an interest in doing so.[31] Yet Canadian governments have paid for some citizens to be treated in the United States. Canadian patients then get the services they need; and American providers have been willing to charge discounted rates in order to get the business. Canadians can argue that if America does not regulate its hospitals effectively and so therefore has excess capacity, and then in order to generate more business must sell services at a discount to Canadians, the Canadian provinces are not the governments whose behavior needs explaining. Rather, Americans should be angry about paying higher prices for excess capacity in their hospitals.

Canadian provinces use U.S. hospital services as a safety valve, when a mistake in planning or some other surprise creates unexpected problems. For example, in Ontario, waiting lists for open-heart surgery in the mid-1980s grew when physicians began to consider more elderly persons to be candidates for surgery; these older patients tended to use more resources than younger cases, because they were more likely to suffer complications, and by early 1989 waiting times "ranged from as little as four to eight weeks in some centers to six months or more in others. Discrepancies existed within the same city, and even in the same hospital depending on the surgeon."[32] A new unit was opened and capacity expanded in others; bottlenecks were addressed and bed allocations managed more carefully; but in the interim up to 300 patients were sent to the United States. By early 1991, after the changes had been implemented, waiting times averaged a few weeks for most surgeons.

In British Columbia a crisis was caused by bottlenecks and supply shocks. Shortages of critical-care nurses were aggravated in 1989 by a seventeen-day nursing strike; in addition, a shortage of cardiac perfusion technologists reduced operating room time; the provincially negotiated wage scales did not provide higher pay for work in critical-care areas, so recruiting for these more stressful jobs was difficult; and cardiac surgeons were competing with other physicians for resources such as recovery beds. By early 1990 more patients were waiting than the system could treat in any given quarter, though some patients in all hospitals were treated quickly. Waiting times varied greatly among the three hospitals and fourteen surgeons who did coronary artery surgery in the province. Two-thirds of the patients were waiting for only three of the surgeons.

While taking other steps to reduce the waits, such as increasing capacity and creating a registry of all patients, the Ministry of Health offered patients the opportunity to go to Washington State for care. Four Seattle-area hospitals contracted to do 200 relatively low-risk operations, for a total fee of 80 percent of their usual charges. Rather than rushing to Seattle, after a year, only 185 patients had gone to Seattle for surgery. It appears, as in Ontario, that some patients preferred to wait—they did not mind waiting, they wanted to use the doctor they knew, or their physicians discouraged them in order to keep their business.[33]

These are examples of waiting lists that the Canadians themselves, (with encouragement from publicity campaigns by Canadian doctors) decided were excessive. In each case the delays had less to do with decisions to constrain the supply of a particular service than with the consequences of overall constraints such as the number of beds available for intensive postoperative care and the provincial contracts with nonphysician staff. Some problems, such as the contracts, would be unlikely in an American context. But the more general problem, that a system with less flexibility cannot adjust easily to surprises such as a nurses' strike or change in the pattern of demand, is very important. Any system that wants to avoid waiting lists must be willing to support excess capacity most of the time—that is, to seem "inefficient" so as to be able to respond to surprises.

What do these examples tell us about the relative quality of Canadian and American medical care?[34] As we have seen, Canada does better than the United States on mortality measures even after all possible adjustments, and the quality of surgery in Canada is at least as high as in the United States.[35] But the lower level of surgery in Canada should have some effect on morbidity, with Canadians being more likely to suffer discomfort that surgery could relieve.

One comparison of medical utilization analyzed the differences between treatment of heart attack victims in the United States and Canada. In the days following the attack, American victims were twice as likely to undergo coronary arteriography, more than two-and-a-half times more likely to have revascularization procedures, and more than twice as likely to have a bypass or angioplasty. In the longer run the differences were smaller, but over a two-year period Canadian physicians performed about 55 percent as many of these procedures as American physicians did.

These different treatments produced no difference in long-run mortality: 22 percent of the Canadians and 23 percent of the Americans studied died over the following forty-two months. But more Canadian patients (33 percent) than American patients (27 percent) did have activity-limiting angina.[36] If one assumes that the difference in the incidence of angina was caused by the difference in number of invasive procedures, one would conclude that a much more conservative practice style in Canada, whatever its causes, is in this case associated with slightly worse morbidity statistics.

But the difference in morbidity is much smaller than the difference in volume of treatment. And the policy question is not whether America provides somewhat more of some forms of treatment, but how the overall quality of Canadian and American medical care compare. Any greater quality due to more extensive elective surgery could well be offset by reduced access to care for some Americans, less comprehensive and reliable care for pregnant women and infants in the United States, the dangers of excessive surgery, and relative constraints on access to ambulatory care even if insured.

A good example of the interrelationships among forms of care is provided by the case of breast cancer diagnosis in British Columbia and Washington State. In a study published in two parts, researchers first reported a much greater use of mammograms in Washington. One would therefore expect more early diagnoses in the United States. But in fact diagnosis was slightly more timely in British Columbia, apparently for two reasons: somewhat quicker access to the primary care physician, and fewer false negatives from mammograms.[37]

The General Accounting Office provided two more pieces of evidence about specific forms of care. The first study compared the availability, appropriateness, timing, and volume of allogenic bone marrow transplants (transplants from other persons) in ten countries for chronic myeloid, acute lymphoid, and acute myeloid leukemias. The researchers expected to find that the United States provided more of the service, thereby (a) confirming that the United States provided higher-quality care in some sense or (b) confirming that U.S. costs were higher because it provided excessive services. Instead, they found that the United States was in the middle of the pack for both availability and appropriateness, well behind France in numbers and either trailing or equal to Canada on both availability and appropriateness for all three diseases.[38]

Although this one study cannot be assumed to hold true for other examples of high-tech treatment of extremely serious disease, GAO did find that, "to a greater extent than was true elsewhere, patients in the United States for whom the treatment offered fewer likely benefits (for example, those in advanced stages of leukemia) often received transplants, while others who could benefit more did not."[39] And this finding would be likely for a system with great physical capacity, an aggressive practice style, but very uneven insurance: physicians and hospitals would be more likely to use aggressive care too late for those with good insurance but less likely to use necessary care for the poorly insured. Similarly, Germany's poor performance in the same study may be related to ambulatory care physicians' not giving up patients to the hospitals quickly enough, and perhaps low capacity for this care in the teaching hospitals.

In another study, GAO compared results of cancer treatment in Ontario and a representative range of states and communities in the United States for which there are especially good data. It asked what proportion of the population survived for each month after diagnosis. For three cancers—lung, colon, and Hodgkin's disease—Ontario began with very slightly worse results, but after a few years the lines crossed and Ontario did slightly better. For breast cancer Ontario did slightly and statistically significantly worse, though the difference narrowed over time. After ten years 50.7 percent of U.S. breast cancer patients and 48.2 percent of Ontario patients had survived.[40] A similar pattern, in which Canada has slightly worse outcomes immediately but slightly better outcomes over time, has been observed for surgical procedures as well.[41] Perhaps Canada's universal system provides more continuous and reliable care, making up for slight disadvantages from restricted capacity for the most expensive treatments. In the case of breast cancer Ontario clearly could do better, though the survival difference is still small.

The Canadian system is far from perfect. In specific studies for specific treatments it does very slightly better on some and very slightly worse on others. On balance, though, America's extra high-tech medicine is not saving more lives than Canada's system. It provides some extra comforts, but one must balance Canada's advantages in access, choice, ambulatory care, and simplicity of use. There are no gatekeepers or complex bills, and there is none of the anxiety that those things cause. It is easier for Canadians to go to the doctor, and they do so more often.

Waiting lists for elective surgery therefore do not justify a claim that the United States in 1991 had better health care than Canada. Instead, the two countries used their resources somewhat differently. But Canada had at least comparable quality of care, covered all citizens, and spent much less money. Americans could choose to spend more than Canada for elective surgery and other services. But they should not imagine that the current American level of spending is necessary to gain high-quality health care.

What America Buys for the Extra Money

This chapter has so far reviewed a wide range of arguments that claim, in essence, that American spending is justified by greater quality or choice. The evidence shows, though, that Americans are buying neither better outcomes nor more choice. Yet the money is paying for something. What is it?

CARE FOR A SICKER POPULATION. If Americans are sicker, they probably need more expensive care. Sicker people also consume *more* care, thus increasing total costs. But arguments about the population cannot explain why American costs grew so much faster than other countries' during the 1980s. What has changed since 1981? The most expensive "risk factor" is the age of the population, and its trend is not related to the gap between America's and other countries' costs.[42] Health care for immigrants may increase U.S. costs, but immigration has been quite heavy in France, Australia, and Canada (never mind post-1989 Germany) as well. And one would expect expenditures per immigrant to be higher in those countries because they have more egalitarian health care financing systems.

Gun violence and AIDS are far more prevalent in the United States. Unfortunately, it is difficult to find reliable figures on the former; estimates of the medical care costs of firearm injuries vary dramatically. At the lowest end, one study estimated that the 1990 figure was about $1.4 billion. But the authors emphasized that their data included many assumptions and that reaching any conclusions was like "shooting in the dark." Other estimates range as high as $14.4 billion in 1992.[43] Even that may understate the costs, by failing to account for expenditures such as long-term rehabilitation. And the United States clearly has much more gun-related violence than any of the other countries in this study. Yet the American rate of firearms-related deaths did not increase between 1980 and 1990. In fact, the rate of all "external" causes of death, which would include motor vehicle accidents as well, was substantially lower in 1990 than in 1980.[44] Death rates do not directly reflect medical costs, because the people who are saved are the expensive ones. To be blunt, a firearms suicide victim is not much of a burden on the health care system. But if violence caused any significant increase in the relative cost of American health care during the 1980s, it was more because medical treatments were successful than because of greater incidence of trauma.

Firearms injuries might have explained $10 billion to $15 billion of America's higher health care spending in 1991 but would not explain the faster growth of costs in the United States than in other countries during the 1980s.

Unlike gunshot wounds, however, AIDS is a new plague, and its higher incidence in America explains both some of the difference in total costs as of 1991 and some of the faster cost increases during the 1980s. The United States has had four times as many AIDS cases per capita as Canada.[45] In 1992, the estimated American cost of personal health care for persons with AIDS or who were HIV positive was $10.3 billion. Therefore, with the same level of cases as in Canada, the United States should have saved three-quarters of the total, or $7.8 billion. The United States also spends billions on AIDS research and other nontreatment expenses, which is included in the health care expenditure totals.[46]

The combined estimates of extra American costs from both gun violence and AIDS explain perhaps $25 billion of the health care cost difference between the United States and Canada as of 1992. Even that number assumes that Canadians paid for care in American prices, which of course they did not. And if health care had consumed the same share of the American as of the Canadian economy in 1992, American spending would have been $190 billion lower.[47] So even using high estimates of the effects of violence and AIDS, we can explain only a small fraction of the difference in costs between the United States and Canada.

AMENITIES. In addition to buying some extra and necessary care for a sicker population, the United States buys nicer amenities for some Americans. American hospitals and clinics compete with features such as impressive lobbies in order to attract middle-class, well-insured patients. The large public hospitals that attract mainly the poor, such as Cook County in Chicago and Charity in New Orleans, do not have money to spend on amenities and thus are not as pleasant. Better surroundings may improve mental attitude and, thus, even outcomes.

The most important amenity may be ward structure: the number of beds per room. Observers agree that in the United States a two-bed ("semi-private") room is the norm. In most other countries, the norm is a four-bed room, and in Japan six-bed rooms are common.[48] Reform is unlikely to change the ward structure (knocking down walls would not be cost-effective or popular), and the likely difference in costs would not explain the difference in cost trends during the 1980s; but ward structure is a reason to expect that American costs will always exceed other countries'.

HIGHER INCOMES FOR PROVIDERS. Americans are certainly buying higher incomes for their health care providers. It is safe to say that all comparative figures on physician income have large margins of error. Doctors do not have precisely the same job descriptions across systems; when earnings are adjusted for purchasing power or compared with wages, all sorts of funny numbers pop up, and comparisons normally use means when medians would be more appropriate (and similar). Sources do not agree with each other even when have been compiled by the same people.[49] National figures differ especially in how they combine the earnings of salaried hospital-based physicians and the earnings of office-based physicians in fee-for-service practices. And statistics on private practice income in some systems are not reliable.

All of these problems are likely to exaggerate the difference between American and other physicians' incomes. But it is still large. Even a comparison of medians, which says more about typical doctors, would not show that any country pays more than about three-quarters as well as the United States; comparing means, which shows how total costs are driven up by very high-earning practitioners, the figure is closer to 60 percent.[50] This difference in incomes is related, of course, to the even larger differences in fees. As we saw in discussions of individual countries, the United States generally provides fewer services, and for almost everything charges much higher prices.

So one thing Americans buy is more expensive physicians. Not only are American doctors paid more, but the compensation gap widened during the decade preceding the health care reform debate (1983–93). Faced with hard economic times some countries, such as Germany, have reduced individual physician incomes relative to the national norm (in large part because of big increases in the number of physicians). But in the United States, physician incomes rose even as their numbers grew and as the average citizen's income stagnated. From 1984, to 1990 median physician net incomes rose by about 12.4 percent, while the median for full-time employed women rose 6.1 percent, and the median for men fell 3.4 percent.[51]

American physicians do have costs that are uncommon in other countries. For example, they must pay much larger premiums for malpractice insurance and have much higher practice expenses for administration. But these higher costs are irrelevant to comparisons of physicians' net incomes after expenses. American physicians are more likely to have substantial debt upon finishing medical school, and that is paid out of their personal incomes. But the interest on that debt is much less than the annual average differences in income.[52] Physicians who become specialists delay their full incomes and perhaps incur more debt in return for higher incomes later. But most analysts believe the United States already has too many specialists. Policymakers should offer to pay for medical education in return for doctors' acceptance of measures to slow their income growth and to increase training of generalists.[53]

Would the United States want to reduce physician incomes to the Canadian level? Probably not, even if that were politically possible. But why should physician incomes rise faster than those of other Americans, from an already higher base? It is hard to see why they should.

Physicians, of course, are not the only recipients of higher medical fees in America. Drugs and equipment both cost more than they do in other countries. So American patients buy higher incomes for American providers of all sorts.

MORE PEOPLE WORKING IN HOSPITALS. Americans also pay for more staff in their hospitals.[54] "I worked in a 600-bed teaching hospital in Toronto that functioned beautifully with only 1,200 FTEs [full-time employees]—a staffing ratio of 2:1," one American hospital consultant reports. "That's unheard of in the United States."[55] Some of America's extra staffing is due to the costs of the payment system. For instance, in a comparison of fairly similar public hospitals in New York and Paris, the New York hospital had 40 percent more patient-care staff, 155 percent more non-patient-care staff, and 327 percent more finance and billing staff![56]

Yet the difference is not all in administration; some is in the efficiency of care. Comparisons with Canada suggest that a system with greater specialization among hospitals requires less staff in two ways. "A community hospital without a large number of specialists," an experienced administrator in both countries explains, "does not have the need for the same number of allied health services that a tertiary facility has."[57] Further, when hospitals buy equipment, they have to have the personnel to operate it. Thus controls on equipment purchases save money on both capital and labor.

"Canadian centralization, reliance on referral, and establishment of waiting lists," Victor Fuchs and Donald Redelmeier report, "result in less idle time for high-cost equipment and associated personnel." Their work suggests that American cost control efforts have had some perverse effects that probably increase personnel expenses even if they do not raise the number of staff. "The tremendous emphasis on early discharge in American hospitals creates a need for additional equipment and personnel ready to provide routine laboratory, radiologic, and other services on short notice. By contrast, the relatively long stays in Canadian hospitals are conducive to a queuing approach that probably results in better use of capacity."[58] The variable cost of keeping patients longer is mostly low-priced personnel such as orderlies (especially in America with its weak unions). So the United States is paying high-cost personnel (technicians) to save on low-cost personnel.

EXTRA ADMINISTRATION AND HASSLES. The last item Americans buy is the hardest to defend. Americans buy extra administrators and hassles.

Competition among insurers creates extra expenses in the sale, purchase, and administration of insurance. They pay staff to determine applicant risk and what to sell to those applicants. Competition creates extra expenses for employers who have to pay benefits managers to analyze and bargain about the choices and to monitor how insurers treat their employees. It creates immense expenses in the billing and administrative operations of the doctors and hospitals that must deal with the hundreds of payers and their different rules and prices.

The General Accounting Office estimated in 1991 that the American insurance system created costs of $67 billion over and above what the

United States would pay if it had Canadian-type institutions. That figure was about 1.2 percent of GDP.[59] Unlike other estimates of "waste," which involve necessary activities that supposedly could be done more efficiently, this estimate is much more credible, because it calls for eliminating activities that are themselves simply unnecessary.[60]

Summary: Value for the Health Care Dollar

Is it possible that all of the data are wrong and that policy analysts are mistaken? Would people in other countries prefer to live with an American-style health care system? Perhaps, but the polls show otherwise. In a 1990 poll of satisfaction with health care systems in ten nations, including all seven in this study, the United States came in tenth. Canada's system was the most popular. Many Americans expressed a preference for the Canadian system, while few Canadians would choose the American model.[61] Conservative parties in other countries go out of their way to inform voters that reform of health care systems does not mean they would be subject to the same risks and uncertainties that Americans endure.[62]

Ah, but aren't Canadians voting with their feet by coming to America for care? Not much. At large hospitals on the U.S. side of the border, near Canadian population centers, perhaps 1 percent of patients are Canadian. And some of those are there for services, such as cosmetic surgery, for which Canadian insurance does not pay, while others are being paid for by provincial health insurance plans.[63] No one has counted travel in either direction, but according to the *New York Times*, tens of thousands of Americans use Ontario's health care system each year.[64] In fact, thousands also go to Mexico in order to reduce costs. Pharmaceuticals are much cheaper across the southern border, and some companies, such as growers' associations, encourage their employees to use Mexican care.[65]

After reviewing the evidence, I must conclude that American health care costs are not justified. Americans are buying worse access and no better choice, on average, for the money. Americans surely receive a higher average quality of care than Britons but not than Canadians. The extra risks from factors such as violence and AIDS do justify some higher costs, but those explain only a fraction of Americans' extra spending.

How much could the United States save without giving up many of the things that most Americans value? In 1991 the difference between U.S. and Canadian costs was 3.4 percent of GDP. Any set of savings would require time to achieve. Prices, for example, would probably not be cut but would need to increase more slowly. Administrative savings would be realized over a period of years. But if Americans managed to save only half of the difference at the end of a period of implementation, by the year 2000 that would be 1.7 percent of GDP— almost exactly the Clinton administration's target in its proposal.[66]

Choices within the International Standard

International mechanisms for controlling costs were summarized in chapter 1: some limits on the medical arms race, standard fee schedules, and budgets where possible. Americans might save a little more from reform of malpractice litigation, though the data are not strong enough to count on that.[67] Changes in the delivery of health care might also increase value for money. There is already a transition to salaried hospital staffs in the academic medical centers; if the rest of the hospital system moves in that direction it might be possible to limit waits for surgery while spending less, as in Germany or France. Some other ideas for delivery reform are discussed in chapter 7.

The mechanisms for expanding access were also summarized at the beginning: compulsory contributions related to income, and collection of most of the money through either the general tax system or corporate payrolls. We have seen, however, that there are variations in both the exceptions allowed to these mechanisms and how these approaches are implemented. What variations suggest choices for developing an American version of the international norm? What aspects of other systems have not received enough attention in the American debate?

Single versus Multiple Payers

One choice is between single and multiple payers. What matters is not how many payers there are, but how well they are coordinated. If they provide the same plans, under the same rules, and negotiate as a group with providers, they will look just like a single payer to the providers, and they will control costs as effectively. There is no evident reason why the payers have to be nonprofit rather than for-profit, though in the countries examined here they are all nonprofit.

With multiple payers it is easier to maintain small differences in coverage within a national guarantee, such as the slightly higher fees paid by some German funds. It would also be possible to preserve some large insurers' business. That would cost some money, but insurers' profits are a small part of the costs of having private insurance.[68] As long as there is a standard plan and fee schedule, for-profit insurers can achieve savings by eliminating risk-rating and most of their plan design, and the big savings in doctors' offices and hospitals are unrelated to the ownership of insurers. Single is simpler, but multiple can work.

Cost Sharing

Cost sharing is a battleground between many economists, who believe it is necessary to save money, and persons more concerned about ensuring care, who worry that charges will deny care to persons who need it. Both use the famous Rand study to make their case.[69] Both are overdoing it.

Cost sharing might save money, but Canada and Germany spend much less than the United States with hardly any cost sharing. Cost sharing can restrict access, but Australia, France, and Japan still have better access than America. The effects of patient charges depend largely on the exceptions, such as a cap on catastrophic expenses; on prices, which determine the actual payments; and on the market positions of providers. They also depend on whether people are allowed to insure themselves for the difference.

One cannot maintain that cost sharing is outside the international norm, given that it is a significant feature of three of the six foreign systems discussed here. On balance, any system with cost sharing is likely to have slightly less demand for care, somewhat less equality, and higher administrative costs to cope with the collections than a system without it.[70] Whether to have cost sharing then is a matter of political choice, not necessity. On balance, less is more desirable than more: the Japanese or French level, in particular, would be much more burdensome in the United States, with its very high fees, than it is in Japan or France.

Fee Schedules

All countries in this study set fees for medical services, except when they set capitation rates or budgets. But that does not mean that the fee schedules are without exceptions. Substitute funds pay higher rates than primary funds in Germany, and private insurance pays much more. France has its Sector 2 physicians. Australia's fee schedule binds no one. From the patients' standpoint there is no evident reason for exceptions, but for policymakers who want to blunt opposition from the medical profession and other providers and to reduce ideological objections to use of state power, there are two issues.

First, is there a way to make fee schedules constrain most fees without being technically binding? Australia shows that there is: ban insurance for fees that are higher than the schedule permits. Some physicians believe that paying out-of-pocket creates a bond of trust between patient and doctor (or at least indicates trust on the patient's part).[71] At the same time, any reduction in what insurance can pay limits how much doctors can actually collect, because more payers choose to use lower-priced providers. The Australian approach therefore offers some fee restraint while not denying physicians the right to set fees the market will bear.[72]

Second, if a limited set of exceptions is explicitly allowed, how can it be managed to ensure access to care? One approach is to make sure that only a small portion of the market can pay for the exceptions (as is the case with German holders of private insurance). Another is to ensure that only a small portion can charge exceptional rates (a more restrictive version of France's Sector 2, perhaps through some deal with the medical profession). A third approach would ensure access to affordable care in some part of the system, as the Australian outpatient clinics do.

Because none of these approaches is infallible, reformers may want to set a binding fee schedule. But there is plenty of room for negotiation and flexibility between a fully binding schedule and no schedule at all.

A series of other issues can be raised about how the fee schedule is created and changed. In all cases, though, physicians should have the largest voice on relative values. They have that voice everywhere, even France and Japan, because it is not in anyone else's interest to object. But others, including other caregivers, should also participate in the negotiations. The negotiations over relative values and conversion factors should be separate. France, Australia, and Japan set conversion factors nationally, but they are set regionally for most funds in Germany and by the provinces in Canada. In Canada even the relative values are set in the provinces. In America a national relative value scale seems nearly inevitable, as *American Medical News* reported at the end of 1993. But the same report showed that procedures for calculating conversion factors will be more controversial, and whether they should be set at the national, state, or "health alliance" level is anything but clear.[73] And conflict between doctors and the government about resulting incomes is sure to flare up continually.

Systematic involvement of the medical profession in such matters faces a series of barriers in the United States. No physician organization enrolls all doctors, but splits among medical organizations have not prevented the French from setting up negotiating structures—disunity among the doctors is simply the doctors' problem. And limited membership in the AMA has not prevented the Health Care Financing Administration from consulting AMA bodies on a wide range of matters. At the national level the direct and legitimate involvement of interests in policy development (called "corporatism" by political scientists) is rare; but at the state level, the role of the medical profession in medical government through processes such as licensing is well established. If the United States wants to involve physicians and other professionals in negotiations about their fees, it can find a way.

General Revenues versus Dedicated Contributions

Within a system of income-related contributions, nations face a further choice: whether to rely upon general revenues or special health care–related collections. The latter do not have to be payroll collections but normally are. Canada uses mainly general revenues. Germany uses almost entirely payroll contributions. The German method has obvious political advantages: it does not have to call such contributions taxes because payments are made to someone other than the government. But because payroll contributions are related to employment, some critics say that they are bad for the economy.[74] Perhaps more important, they draw special fire from small businesses.

As a matter of economics, the advantages and disadvantages of various methods are likely to be oversold. Any system that collects in relation to income must have roughly identical distributional effects. If health care contributions represent an extra cost per employed person, employers might decide to limit employment. But that argument is exaggerated in many ways. If the charge is a percentage of wages rather than per worker, health care costs do not discourage hiring; indeed, employers should prefer hiring new workers over paying higher wages or overtime to current workers. Virtually all economists would argue that individual employees' wages are most affected by health care costs; for the most part, employers do not absorb the costs; if that is true, the health care costs cannot simultaneously be decreasing employment.[75] Other forced contributions also might reduce employment: for example, it can be argued that a value added tax reduces sales and therefore hiring. Ultimately money is money; it has to come from somewhere.

A dedicated funding source, including payroll contributions, does have implications for the adequacy of health care financing. A dedicated funding source directs attention to health care costs and so allows more focus on whether the public wants to pay more to get more. General revenue funding can lead to arguments about whether spending for something else should be cut to pay for health care. These arguments become particularly confused in federal systems, where the absence of a dedicated source of funds allows federal and state governments to blame each other for underfunding. The public is less likely to be confused about the cost of health care if its costs are reflected in separate, visible payments. Therefore I would support payroll-based financing. Yet if a person accepted social insurance for health care but was skeptical of other government activities, he might prefer a financing system that requires government to cut something else if it wants to pay for health care, while many liberals believe general revenue funding is more equitable. There is no international standard.

All of these differences and more provide much opportunity for conflict over how to implement the international standard of health care financing. But they should not obscure the importance of the obvious similarities, such as use of fee schedules and compulsory contributions, or of the two fundamental components of any system: hospitals and doctors.

Hospitals and Doctors

How any U.S. reform works will depend on the organization of hospitals and doctors. We have seen, for example, how the dual affiliations of Australian physicians increase the waits in public hospitals, and how the separation of ambulatory and hospital sectors decreases waiting for hospital care in Germany or France.

ACADEMIC MEDICAL CENTERS. Even more important is the relationship between hospital care and medical education, and so the governance of the academic medical centers. Of the six comparison countries, only Japan has a nontrivial number of teaching hospitals that are not directly budgeted by the government. Direct budgeting of teaching hospitals has a series of important effects.

First, the sector of hospital care that has most of the residents and interns is under public control (even if privately run, as in Canada). Therefore, it is possible to have policies that relate the level of outpatient services to gaps in the insurance structure, such as the higher fees for specialists in Australian cities.

Second, capital budgeting can work, in a rough-and-ready and unscientific way, by doing what comes naturally: distributing the most-advanced equipment to the hospitals that do the most research and teaching. Because state and local politicians like such facilities, they tend to be spread around the country. Because they have separate budgets based on education (and perhaps are even financed by the education ministry), they have extra funds.

Third, the state pays for physicians' education. State budgeters do not fully appreciate the advantages of paying these bills, and doctors do not love the state even when it pays for their education. But as we have seen, eliminating physicians' ability to argue that they need even higher incomes because of their debts is in the payers' interest. And once the government admits that it must pay for education, it need not worry so much about making special fee adjustments to compensate hospitals for the extra costs of teaching (which America makes in its payments for medicare services). If the state wants education it should pay for it.

Fourth, because the academic medical centers in other countries have most of the most advanced equipment and the residents, there appear to be limits on the inequalities that can be created by variations in fees and insurance coverage.

In short, a much more straightforward financing arrangement for academic medical centers simplifies management of the health care system immensely. Like any large organization built on knowledge, though, hospitals are notoriously difficult for outsiders to manage. The British adopted their reforms because many participants thought a purchaser-provider split would make hospital managers, or perhaps the senior specialists, more responsive to NHS policies. Australian states own the hospitals and still cannot manage to train enough orthopedic surgeons (what do you do if the current ones won't cooperate?). And no one knows how to train fewer physicians in order to slow the source of rising costs, yet still have enough residents and interns. At the very least, however, a reform that does not directly budget medical education (and thus much of what occurs within the AMCs) will take unnecessary risks with access and quality.[76]

COOPERATING WITH DOCTORS. How any reform works will also depend on building a mechanism that allows payers to work with doctors. Conflict is inevitable, the occasional explosion is dramatic, and resentment on both sides is likely to be deep. One should not expect friendship and peace. But there has to be some structure for consulting and disagreeing, and some expectations about how disputes will be settled. In William Glaser's words, "Organizing stable relations with the medical profession is one of the principal tasks in creating statutory health insurance."[77]

We have seen, for example, that all systems try to get doctors to handle most of the conflict about relative fees. Systems to reduce the amount of unnecessary care also require institutions of cooperation. Thus Germany, Japan, and France attach "control doctors" to the sickness fund payment system, and they review doctors whose practice patterns deviate from the norm. New South Wales has shown that it is possible to work with physicians on other matters of discipline and quality. Guidelines and protocols will be far more acceptable if physicians are involved in developing them, for then doctors cannot say bureaucrats are creating rules that are not in the patients' best interests.

Physicians are the heart of any health care system. Other professionals provide much useful care, and administrators make complex and vital institutions, such as hospitals, run well. But because physicians are still the major providers and supervisors of care, all nations pay them far more than the average national wage. Their training takes longer, and physicians everywhere view themselves as having a special place in society that entitles them to be paid very well and honored in return for providing high-quality care according to the high standards of the Hippocratic oath.

All other concerns—from cost control to quality assurance, capital allocation to access—raise questions about the role of physicians within the system. Governing health care in any country is not mainly a matter of building bureaucracies and writing regulations. It is a process of building a stable relationship between payers—which means all those served by the health care system—and physicians.

Ultimately, reformers do not have to worry much about insurance companies because a health care system can exist without them. But a health care system cannot exist without doctors. That is why doctors are the most important players in health care politics, with one exception: the citizens, who must decide, in a democracy, what kind of health care system they want.

Part Two
Competing Solutions

7

The Theory of Managed Competition

*T*HE evidence in the preceding three chapters suggests that
Americans should want a health care system more like that
in other countries and less like the one they have now. Yet in its plan
for health care reform the Clinton administration did not propose a
straightforward adaptation of other countries' approaches. Instead it
presented its proposal as a form of "managed competition." Other
proposals, such as those made by Representatives Jim Cooper
(D-Tenn.) and Fred Grandy (R-Iowa) and by Senator John Chafee (R-
R.I.), also emphasized this alternative approach.[1]

Managed competition is actually part of a family of proposals that
have different meanings in different contexts. Outside the United
States, the dominant form is the concept of an "internal market." In
this formulation, an existing national guarantee of health services—
usually a system of direct delivery such as the British National Health
Service (NHS)—is to be reformed to more closely resemble private
enterprise either because providers must compete for business or managers have more ability to act as entrepreneurs, or both.[2] An internal
market presumes, however, that trading occurs inside something: an
envelope of resource constraint. In essence, the "market" operates
within a budget.

The term managed competition has been applied to both kinds of
systems, those with and without budgets. Yet the substantive and
political consequences of the two approaches are very different. In this
chapter and the next we review the theories of managed competition,
British experience, and the "thought-experiment" offered through
analysis of the Chafee and Cooper-Grandy bills. This review shows
why the Clinton administration was correct in proposing "managed
competition with a global budget"—a form of internal market ap-

165

proach—rather than competition without a budget. But these chapters and the following chapter on the Clinton plan itself also show why even the Clinton plan did not meet its own goal. That goal was to combine the best of both the managed competition theory and the international standard.

The Attractions of Managed Competition

Adapting international approaches of ensuring coverage and limiting costs is hardly a new idea in the United States. In comparison with what America does now, it would be a significant improvement. The United States has had versions of all the international measures. State medical associations once set fees, and the Health Care Financing Administration does so now, for medicare. The private market is rapidly imitating medicare's resource-based relative value scale (RBRVS) schedule of relative prices. Some states have strictly regulated hospital rates. The United States once had a half-hearted, but in a few areas moderately useful, certificate-of-need system to regulate investments in hospitals. Public hospitals, including state university medical schools, are budgeted. All workers contribute a portion of their income to the subsidy structure for the care of the elderly and the poor, through taxes, and have no choice about it. And at one time American insurance premiums were set predominantly by community-rating schemes.

But these measures have been variously resisted, destroyed by market forces, and neutered, and they were always partial. Businesses that do not contribute to their employees' insurance costs naturally resisted doing so. Providers have objected to all forms of cost control (unless a worse alternative seemed more likely to be imposed on them).[3] People who could pay less in the market for insurance did so, and community-rating was destroyed. In short, America has never approached having a system built around the set of measures that provide the affordable health care found in other countries.

The torrent of cost increases in the 1980s weakened objections to the international standard. Some large businesses concluded that a greater government role is necessary to control their costs.[4] Most participants in the debate agree that there should be a standard benefit package and less risk-rating. Physicians are facing new forms of cost control that, to some doctors, make government regulation look pretty good by comparison.

Yet requiring participation and regulating costs simply does not fit with the ideological beliefs of Republicans and conservative Democrats and therefore seemed unlikely to pass in Congress even before the 1994 election. It is easy then to see why advocates would search for means to the same ends that might be more acceptable to the forces that resist adopting the international standard. Further, the international standard, while it has evidently worked far better than American practice, seems ideal to nobody. All countries are facing health care cost crises, and some are taking drastic measures in response. In the search for an ideal system, the same themes recur in health policy discussions throughout the world.[5]

The Search for Greater Efficiency

Simplifying greatly, there are two problems with the common forms of cost control. First, they do not seem to guarantee efficiency. More precisely, they do not promote efficiency in any way that is easily explained and measured. Because the scientific basis of medicine is not precise, analysts everywhere can find treatments that cannot be justified scientifically. Policymakers therefore dream of a system that reduces costs by selectively reducing unnecessary care. Among the measures that might attain this end, according to various theories, are:

—Cost sharing (or higher cost sharing) for services. Then, assuming patients have some idea how much they really need services, they might forgo those that are of least use.

—Greater price competition among providers of care. If they had to reduce costs, but still satisfy customers about quality (so customers would not change providers), providers might become more efficient.

—Better information about what constitutes necessary and high-quality care. That could help both patients and providers make more efficient and effective choices. By this logic, more research should be done to improve understanding, and the research should be summarized in accessible forms. The most useful form would be a treatment (or diagnosis) guideline or protocol: a list of steps to be taken given certain findings, either as advice (a guideline) or a requirement (protocol). Patients could consult outcome measurements to help them choose among providers.

—Greater visibility of transactions, so overseers who know what is efficient can tell whether providers are doing it. This is the logic of efforts to quantify everything providers do and relate that directly to diagnoses, as with diagnosis-related groups (DRGs); the desire for more detailed oversight also justifies pleas for "outcomes measurement" by hospitals.[6]

—Reorganizing care to better coordinate resources of hospitals, physicians, and other providers. If hospitals and physicians were linked in some sort of wider system, they might share an incentive to provide care in the less expensive (often ambulatory, rather than hospital) setting.

These ideas contemplate a more efficient system of health care delivery. In many cases they would supplement or depend on each other. An efficient system might require cost sharing within differently organized delivery systems, in which research, having been translated into guidelines, would be used to manage care and oversee the range of treatments provided. Financing reforms might be used to encourage development of this system.

The Search for More Extensive and Binding Budgeting

From another angle, the international standard is not an ideal form of cost control because its financial constraints are not binding enough. Capacity control provides somewhat greater efficiency, and fee regulation and budgeting where possible do reduce spending, but the fragmented nature of the system allows a variety of strategic responses. Care migrates to settings where regulators have not caught up with provider strategies.[7] Or those providers who can do so increase their volume of services to compensate for lower fees.

Over time, payers around the world have developed ways to bundle payments and reduce both cost-shifting and manipulation of volume. Medicare moved to prospective payment by diagnosis to eliminate the incentive for hospitals to multiply procedures, for which they previously could charge separately. In France and Germany hospital payment has moved from day rates that create the total to day rates that are made to fit the total—a budget. The German government has moved toward budgeting pharmaceutical costs. In America the government has spent two decades trying to induce more Americans to join health maintenance organizations (HMOs). All of these measures are ways to budget a larger part of medical care at once.

Budgeting and Efficiency in the ^へ
United States and Abroad

There are excellent reasons to believe that more-binding budgeting and more-efficient delivery go together. If one believes that health care professionals care about helping people, then one should expect them, if forced to set priorities, to eliminate less-useful care first. In medicine, this is known as triage and is taken for granted in emergency rooms and on battlefields. Whether the subject is British hospitals, or how American doctors treat uninsured patients, or Canadian cardiologists deciding among themselves how to allocate limited resources in a hospital, doctors tend to use professional norms and obligations to settle disputes among themselves about scarce resources and try to omit the least justified care.[8]

Yet it is easy in any system to find allocations that seem to have more to do with how things have always been done than with hard-headed analysis. Budgeting may encourage most budget holders to be more efficient, but it also encourages some to save money any way that they can get away with. Any provider that is not paid per service, whether a British NHS specialist or an American capitated HMO, has an economic incentive to do as little as possible for the money—no matter how large the amount.[9] Many outsiders—especially health system managers, economists, and legislators—therefore are unwilling to rely on physicians' professionalism to provide efficiency within a budget.

In a system that already has overall budget controls, such as Great Britain's, payers are not about to give that up. Instead, the British internal market reforms should be seen as efforts to change the delivery system in a way that promises greater efficiency and so provides political cover for continued stringent application of budgetary limits. In the United States, President Clinton proposed overall budget controls, but the best-publicized theoretical statement of managed competition did not. Each proposal, however, relied on increased budgeting within the health care delivery system.

Managed Competition as an Attempt to Leapfrog ahead of the Pack

As proposed by the Jackson Hole group of analysts and interests, managed competition offered all the features of the international reform agenda, without adapting other nations' institutions of cost control.[10]

A Synthesis of Efficiency and Budgeting

The Jackson Hole authors, Alain Enthoven, Paul Ellwood, and Lynn Etheredge, called their plan an initiative for a twenty-first century American health care system.[11] The plan was meant to leapfrog over the inadequacies of both the American and international approaches.

THE BUDGETING SIDE. Health plans would manage care and compete, through price and quality, for customers. Each plan would cover all the health care expenses that society decided should be guaranteed to all citizens, whether they were received from hospitals, doctors, or any other providers. Its premiums therefore would create a budget for all covered care for its members. Within each plan, the budget would be more thorough than those in any of the countries described in this book.

If there were only one plan, it could reduce costs by reducing care rather than by being efficient. Competition could limit that behavior only if customers had information about quality and care as well as price. The Jackson Hole analysts proposed creating intermediary organizations (what the Clinton administration called "health alliances") to remedy information problems.

Health alliances would provide standardized information ("report cards") to help customers compare plan performance. Because some plans might even prefer to have a bad reputation on expensive forms of care, such as geriatrics, so as to discourage high-cost customers, the alliances (or some body) would have to certify and decertify the competing plans.

In this structure every person's health costs would be inside a budgeted organization, but each budget would be determined by market competition rather than by a political process. The alliances would serve as referees to prevent cheating but not to determine the score.

FOCUSING COMPETITION ON EFFICIENCY. Managed competition advocates believed that some forms of competition should be "managed" out of existence. In their proposal every plan would have offered standard coverage at a set price to anyone who applied.[12] They agreed with other reformers that risk-rating makes insurance unaffordable or unavailable to many persons and is a major reason why the administrative costs of the American health care system are much higher than those of other countries. Further, unless all plans were required to offer standard benefits, comparison based on performance would be impossible. Their potential customers would have to make impossible judgments about whether they were more likely to need the benefits provided by Plan X than by Plan Y and account for those differences when comparing prices or other measures. Managed competition's designers also argued that if companies were allowed to compete by managing risk rather than managing care, they would do too little of the latter because it is more difficult.

The health alliance mechanism provides ways both to prevent and, if that fails, to compensate for, risk competition. Plans could be required to market through the alliance, which would distribute materials to all persons in an area, rather than selectively marketing to healthier customers. If plans intentionally or unintentionally ended up with different risk profiles, the alliance could operate systems of reinsurance, in which a central pool paid for extremely expensive cases. Or it might establish regimes to directly transfer money from plans with obviously less risky (for example, younger) to those with obviously more risky (for example, older) members. In short, the structure would allow versions of the cross-subsidies common abroad.

Eliminating risk competition also could greatly reduce the number of insurers. Small insurers could no longer compete by "cherry-picking" (choosing the most desirable beneficiaries) and could not afford the investment needed to manage care. The resulting consolidation of insurers should leave the remainder with larger market shares and so with greater bargaining power with which to get better terms from providers.

Incentives for Consumers to Spend Less

American insurers already compete on price, and that does not appear to have controlled costs. Managed competition's designers say this competition has not been sufficient because prices to individuals are disguised by the tax code and employer policies.

The tax code treats employer insurance payments as a legitimate business expense but not as employee income. An employer who buys insurance directly gets $1,000 worth of insurance for $1,000 because the money used to buy benefits is not taxed. In contrast, a person who gets a $1,000 raise and is in a 28 percent tax bracket can buy only an extra $720 in health insurance. Therefore employees, by having employers purchase their health insurance, can buy a dollar's worth of health insurance more easily than a dollar's worth of other goods, and by this standard employees buy too much. This argument suggests there should be no tax exclusion at all, but managed competition's proponents did not go that far. Instead, schemes proposed eliminating only the amount of subsidy that covered "excess" insurance. Excess could be defined in the market as, for example, any more than the lowest-priced plan certified by the alliance to cover the standard benefits. Then the premium for that plan would be a legitimate business expense, but larger amounts would not.

Managed competition advocates also wanted employers to pay only a fixed amount per employee, rather than, as in some benefit packages, a percentage of whatever plan the employee selected. In the latter case, if an employer covered 80 percent of the costs of two plans, one costing $4,000 and the other $4,400, an employee would pay only $80 more for making the more expensive choice. If instead the employer paid only 80 percent of the lower amount the cost difference would be $400.

COVERAGE. In the statements that established its place in the health care debate, the Jackson Hole group also emphasized the need to universalize health insurance. In Enthoven's words, "Nobody defends the proposition that people without coverage or money to pay should go without necessary medical care or should be allowed to suffer, be disabled, or die for lack of reasonable care." Further, "By putting market pressure on providers to cut costs, market reforms promoting competition—if not accompanied by universal coverage—could exacerbate access problems."[13] Any cost control measures would make providers less likely to provide whatever "free" care they already provided.

The Jackson Hole version of managed competition synthesized ideas in a way that should be considered neither left- nor right-wing. It showed an appreciation of the limits of both markets and bureaucracy. Its prominence in the American health care policy debate was no accident.

The Flaws in Managed Competition

Unfortunately, the theory in this form was not likely to work. "Work" here means provide universal coverage and cost control; more particularly, control costs well enough so that universal coverage could be achieved without large new taxes.

Some of the difficulties are inherent to the theory and some are unique to the American context. This chapter considers the inherent problems; the peculiar difficulties of implementation in the United States are discussed in chapter 8.

There are four basic difficulties: (1) Managed competition in some ways does not go far enough. (2) Competition might not have the required effects. (3) Success depends on managing care, but managed care is unlikely to work as well as its advocates suggest. (4) The best forms of managed care are not likely to be implemented quickly enough to realize major benefits.[14]

Not Going Far Enough

Managed competition as a theory of efficient delivery does not answer the question: who will pay to help whom? It would restore community-rating, but in the United States many, many people could not afford a community rate. Individual managed competition proposals could provide a financing mechanism, but the model itself neither provides nor justifies one.[15]

Further, one of the strongest arguments that managed competition will control costs is a better argument for alternatives. A smaller number of insurers may be able to win better prices than a larger number of insurers could, if all bargain separately. But if fewer payers is better, then one—or many payers bargaining as one—should be best. To the extent that some payers have more market power than others, the people who for one reason or another are in the less powerful pools lose. It is hard to explain why that is fair. But if people all move to the largest pool, there is no competition.

Reasons for Skepticism about Competition

Competition's ability to control costs depends on having enough competitors, on giving purchasers incentives to demand lower prices, on giving sellers incentives to provide them, and on ensuring that risk competition does not distort the process.

GEOGRAPHIC LIMITS. In large portions of the United States, competition in the contemplated form cannot exist because there are not enough competitors. The specialization of medicine means that many providers have local monopoly (or oligopoly) positions. If competition is defined as three or more competitors, then competition among integrated networks that include tertiary-care hospitals is possible for only 42 percent of the population. A larger part can support competition among multispecialty practices that use the same hospital, but then something other than competition with each other must control costs in the hospitals. Twenty-nine percent of Americans live in areas where there is not likely to be much competition among providers of a wide range of in-hospital specialties.[16]

INCENTIVES FOR "PRUDENT PURCHASING." Would managed competition cause purchasers to be more vigilant and demanding about costs? Its designers agree that patients are not in a position to bargain at the point of service, because they are sick at the time and because the topic is so complicated. Instead, the theorists wanted people to choose, while healthy, among plans based on costs and overall reputation; the plans themselves would then be the prudent purchasers for their ill members.

In short, by changing the choice from the selection of individual services to the selection of plans, managed competition's designers hoped to make consumers more cost-conscious. Much of their design involved new institutions within which employees would make more cost-conscious choices.

Having employees rather than employers make choices may be a fine idea, but it is unlikely to increase incentives to buy less expensive plans. In America in 1994 employers bargained for rates, offered their employees very limited choices, and paid most of the money. If they had not been very sensitive to costs, health care cost control would have been nowhere near as prominent an issue. In fact, all the innovative efforts to change consumer behavior were based on a ludicrous assumption, that employees, not employers, had the largest say in American health insurance purchasing.

Limiting the tax deductibility of health insurance benefits to a standard package may be a good idea as a matter of fairness.[17] But if the standard package were not bare-bones, savings from competition would be small. Some employers would have to provide more insurance than they do now, increasing the demand for care. Some would have the subsidies for their more generous packages, in the form of the ability to count their costs as business expenses, reduced. Yet the amount of "excess" coverage involved would not be so large. Remember, it is the *tax-subsidized* amount for *private-market* health care for plans that provide *more than a standard*—which means, provide the standard benefits in a more generous manner. The amount of extra subsidy, in one plausible estimate as of 1993, would be about 2 percent of total health expenditures.[18] That amount could not have a large effect on the system.

PLAN BEHAVIOR. Firms with a competitive advantage might lower prices to increase market share. But they also might decide to reap a higher profit margin from their efficiency. In that case the more efficient firm might engage in "shadow-pricing": keeping its price in the shadow of the price of the less efficient provider, just low enough to generate a comfortable amount of business.

Supporters of managed competition argue that it would eliminate current shadow-pricing by HMOs, but it is hard to imagine why that would happen. Again, suppose there were two plans, a fee-for-service plan for $4,400 and an HMO plan for $3,600. Imagine an employee whose employer, as many do today, paid a fixed share of the premium, perhaps 80 percent. At present, the employee would pay $720 for the HMO (20 percent of $3,600) and $880 for the average plan (20 percent of $4,400), which might be more attractive because it offered a wider choice of doctors.

Imagine that, instead, the employer paid 80 percent of the lower-cost plan. The employee would still pay $720 to join the HMO. But the employee would have to pay $1,520 (20 percent of the $3,600, plus the entire difference between $3,300 and $3,600) if he chose the fee-for-service plan. Undoubtedly, more employees would choose the HMO, but the HMO would have new incentives to raise its price, for example, to $4,000. Then employees would pay $800 (20 percent of $4,000) to join the HMO and $1,200 (the $800 plus the $400 difference between the two plans) for the higher-cost plan. At these prices the HMO would have a bigger cost advantage than in the original case from the employees' standpoint, and the HMO would also take in more money per employee. Whether total spending would fall would depend entirely on whether the effect of the HMO's price increase were canceled by the size of the shift from the more expensive to the less expensive plan or by a price reduction in the more expensive plan.[19]

Increasing the effective price advantage of one plan would allow it to raise its price. One certainly should not assume that its managers would forgo the opportunity—we do not assume that in any other market. When might a plan instead choose market share over margin? That would depend in part on how easily it could expand. Health plans are not factories that can put on a second shift, because plans cannot make patients come to the clinic at 3 A.M. And it is not as easy to recruit extra doctors as extra factory workers (normally). Expansion is especially difficult, as I argue below, for the seemingly most efficient current form of health plan, the group- or staff-model HMO.[20] And if the more efficient forms could not expand easily, their competitors would know that, so would be slower to lower prices to compete.

There are many other situations in which competition has led not to price competition but to price imitation. Providers have waited for another provider to make the first move in the steel and auto industries; banks do the same thing in setting interest rates. This informal collusion can be busted by new entries into the market—but in health care foreign competition is not very likely. Managed competition's efforts to limit costs through greater price competition are based on a very limited model of how firms behave.

RISK COMPETITION. Eliminating risk competition is not simple either. Banning explicit risk-rating is a start, but within a system of competing plans there are other ways to avoid unwanted customers. It is very hard to allow plans to select providers but prevent them from selecting patients. Yet selecting providers is central to most forms of managed care. Plans exclude or threaten to exclude providers who do not meet the plans' cost control standards.

A group- or staff-model HMO might choose not to build clinics in the ghetto. Other networks might choose not to contract with providers in those areas. A health alliance could threaten to decertify such plans. But beneficiaries of those plans would protest, and health alliances would need to have some plans around to provide care. Because threats to punish are not very credible when sanctions hurt the regulator as much as the regulated, the regulator winks at some amount of disobedience. Renaming regulation "management" will not eliminate the difficulty.

Unequal risk pools exist in the sickness fund systems of France, Germany, and Japan.[21] But the effect is mainly on the premiums, not the treatments, and is not desirable in any case. A person in a disadvantaged pool still pays the usual fees, and all providers are paid the usual rates for all patients. Those systems adjust for differences in need for services and ability to pay, in part, through transfers from other funds or from the general treasury. Managed competition contemplates some similar set of transfers to compensate for differences in the risk profiles of different funds' membership.

Designing these transfers is much simpler, however, in the sickness fund systems. Because all funds use the same delivery system, differences in members' health and incomes must explain different costs. Transfers can be based on observed differences in cost. Within managed competition, one fund might have higher costs than another because it managed care less efficiently. In order to compensate funds for more risky membership, that risk has to be estimated directly, without relying on actual observed costs. Transfers based on observed costs would punish the efficient and reward the inefficient.

This problem, risk-adjustment, has generated a huge literature with one simple conclusion: nobody, anywhere in the world, has developed a way to greatly reduce plans' incentives to "cherry-pick" or "cream-skim" that would be accepted as fair and avoid creating alternate perverse incentives.[22] The problem is inherent in all competitive schemes; two Dutch economists who have promoted competitive reform, for instance, argue that "a system of sufficiently refined risk-adjusted capitation payments is a necessary condition for reaping the fruits" of their proposed reforms.[23]

I would not go so far—after all, systems have existed with some levels of inequality for a long time. But advocates of managed competition should not imagine that plans would not continue trying to limit their risk. The rewards are too high: if even a small part of the most expensive patients can be avoided, the savings to a plan can be substantial.[24]

The Performance of Managed Care

Most of the weaknesses in the competitive side of the theory might be addressed by imposing the right kind of global cost controls. Yet even a global cost constraint could help managed competition work only if the managers in fact had ways to control costs to meet their targets.

This section reviews American experience with managed care. While advocates of managed competition argue that plans would do better, that is a large assumption. Necessity may be the mother of invention, but she is frequently barren.

OUTCOME MEASUREMENT. Managed competition advocates call for more guidelines, protocols, and outcome measurements, but that makes them no different from policy analysts in every other system. Progress is slow.[25] Wishing and hoping will not speed the process.

Although competition alone might encourage plans to devise ways to measure outcomes, so as to advertise their performance, plans if left to their own devices will choose whatever measures show them in the best light. Making the measurements truly comparable is very hard. A measurement that involves a mortality or morbidity rate must be adjusted for differences in the risk profiles of each plan's membership. A measurement that involves treatment success must control for possible differences in severity of illness. In all cases a plan's measurements are of limited use without benchmarks from the wider population. All of these problems are relevant to even the best efforts made to date.[26]

The difficulty of comparing outcomes leads to measuring inputs, such as the number of screening tests, and defining those inputs themselves as quality medicine. In some cases, such as level of pediatric immunizations, counting inputs is useful. Yet if quality care is defined by the level of certain inputs, rather than by outcomes, plans will have an incentive to spend on those inputs whether or not they improve outcomes. Any measurement scheme will divert resources to the services that can be measured, whether or not that is appropriate. Unfortunately, that can lead to paying attention to the wrong things.[27]

Even when good data exist, outcome measures may have little impact on consumer choices. Providers may vary little, as has been found in some hospital comparisons. Or they may vary on many matters; but if one plan is better on fifty items, and another is superior on a different fifty items, who can make sense of that? Any comparison of treatment success across enough different conditions to be representative will require making very controversial judgments about the relative value of different conditions and treatments. Is diabetes treatment more important than pregnancy care, or vice versa? How much more?[28]

At the moment, "there are tremendous deficiencies in the state of the art" in outcomes measurement, according to a designer of Kaiser Permanente's cutting-edge plan. Managed-care plans do not consider published outcomes an important part of competition;[29] nor do patients seem likely to follow report cards rather than their doctor's recommendation or the testimony of friends and acquaintances.[30] Where states create outcome measures, as they do for some hospitals, the data problems and other pressures mean that "information is not the objective determinant of choice and competition as market-oriented policy designers had hoped. . . . [It] is the result of political and bureaucratic exercises."[31]

Given the difficulties described here, it seems unreasonable to expect change quickly enough to fundamentally reduce the barriers to informed choice among competing plans. Many of the same information problems apply to developing treatment guidelines. It is hard enough to develop a standard of best practice for the normal case of a given condition. It requires years of research that adjusts for patients' underlying health and other factors. Some outcomes, such as levels of pain and mobility, are hard to measure. When research does not fit a group's preferences (think of studies that say cholesterol screening and mammograms are useful only in certain circumstances), the results become political controversies.

Developing guidelines is an important part of the advancement of medical knowledge and practice. Hospital staffs, for instance, can look at adherence to guidelines as a way to assess performance, as long as the guidelines are not too rigid. The effort to refine knowledge proceeds around the world, but competition is not likely to move that effort forward. For guidelines to provide competitive advantage, they must be proprietary and therefore could not be approved by the organized medical profession. As a result, doctors might not follow them (and juries in malpractice cases might not believe them). Competition might encourage adoption of protocols that were developed in a more public manner, but other payment systems can do the same at least as easily.

If managed competition is to make health care more efficient, then, it will not be through encouraging new and better measures. It is not relevant to that effort, and the effort is too difficult for any quick success. Instead, managed competition would have to increase efficiency through more intense application of the existing forms of managed care, which are usually described in terms of the form of contract between payers and providers. But it is more useful to think in terms of three basic forms of cost control.[32]

GROUP- AND STAFF-MODEL HMOS. The first is the group- or staff-model health maintenance organization. These systems, such as Kaiser Permanente, Group Health of Puget Sound, and the Harvard Community Health Plan, enrolled just under 15.7 million Americans at the end of 1992.[33]

As with any type of organization, there are better and worse examples. Health policy analysts generally agree that the better HMOs operate more efficiently than the rest of the medical care system, while providing care of at least equal quality. Standard estimates at the beginning of 1993 placed their costs at around 8 to 10 percent lower than those of indemnity insurance providers.[34]

This model normally uses a closed panel of providers.[35] With rare exceptions the plan's physicians work only for the plan, and the plan expects its patients to use only its physicians. A closed panel has many advantages when it operates well. The physicians work together, develop a shared practice culture, learn each other's strengths and weaknesses, and therefore can make decisions about treatments and resources collegially. The organization can develop larger roles for nonphysician providers, with the inevitable tensions worked out over time. Each customer can have a primary care physician who serves as a gatekeeper to other services. A closed panel has less need for detailed regulation and administrative reviews than more loosely structured groups: if a physician wants to make an exception to a conservative practice style, for example, she may work it out with her colleagues.

A pediatrician within one of these groups provided an example of the informal cost controls of a shared practice. Each of his colleagues does night rounds at the hospital four weeks during the year. They notice, for example, whether another doctor tends to admit patients to the hospital who do not need to be there, because that creates work for them. No doctor wants to be seen as creating unnecessary work for the others. The large group also provides security, predictable hours, and only one set of rules to worry about. Yet in spite of these advantages and the model's popularity with health policy analysts, group- and staff-model HMOs have grown more slowly than other forms of managed care over the past fifteen years. From the customers' perspective, the most evident objections are discomfort with the closed panel and the clinic setting.[36]

THIRD-PARTY MANAGEMENT THROUGH UTILIZATION REVIEW. The widest choice of physician can be offered in an entirely different form of managed care, third-party utilization management. An insurer contracts with a wide range of physicians and hospitals, which agree to accept some amount of utilization review. Rules about when services can be provided might be enforced either by requiring preapproval or by denying payment after the service is performed; in either case, reviewers second-guess a patient's health care providers.

Medicare, Blue Cross, and virtually all other payers now require some sort of utilization review, especially for admission to the hospital. Such review has contributed to a reduction in American hospital admissions and lengths of stay, though that is a worldwide trend and avoiding admissions does not necessarily save money. The doubts about third-party management are related to the logic of constraining medical care with rules. A given course of treatment may be best for a given diagnosis most of the time, but patients have different co-morbidities, their conditions are more or less severe, and some simply do not respond to the usual approach. Further, rules help only if a patient's condition has been diagnosed. These uncertainties are what make medicine professional, rather than purely technical work. When doctors object to detailed regulation of care, they are protecting not just their pride and income but in many cases their patients. Physicians do not want a nurse who has not seen a patient to overrule a doctor who has.[37]

The difficulties of utilization review are magnified when different payers try to enforce different limits. Physician practices and hospitals have to hire extra staff to negotiate with the plans, and providers must continually refer to each plan's rule book to ensure that they do not go over some limit.[38] As each plan searches for new efficiencies, the rules keep changing, creating ever more hassles.

In short, managing care through detailed third-party regulation has not worked very well. Its limited success, combined with the slow growth of group- and staff-model HMOs, helps explain the growth of a third form of managed care: risk-driven models.

NETWORKS OF RISK-BEARING GATEKEEPERS. In a group- or staff-model HMO, patients pay a fixed amount for all care. The plan itself then bears the risk if it provides more care than it has been paid for. Patients have to accept less choice than they might prefer, and physicians have to accept the constraints of a large organization.

In third-party managed care the plan is at risk and the providers are not, except to the extent that providers violate the rules and are not paid for specific treatments. This approach requires intrusive and expensive bureaucracies.[39]

Insurers therefore have been creating a third model, with many versions but two primary attributes. The insurer builds a network of providers that includes many more physicians per patient than a group- or staff-model HMO but excludes some portion of those in any area, on grounds of either credentials or a history of high costs. Then the organizer contracts to pay a set amount to primary care physicians, who are at risk if total costs for their patients exceed some target.

This approach provides incentives for the primary care physicians themselves to manage care. Each doctor's case-by-case judgment replaces some utilization review. Its logic is similar to the British and German reforms that have tried to increase primary care physicians' incentive and ability to manage the costs of other services. But the American version is likely to apply to a much wider range of costs (such as those for long hospitalization), and so puts the doctor at greater risk.

Experience with this model is too new to allow strong conclusions, but difficulties go with its advantages. Allocation of risk to the gatekeepers works for large group practices that contract with a variety of payers; the groups have enough volume to bear the risk, and if they already manage their practices efficiently, they will meet the standards.[40] Any large group practice that accepts capitation, however, looks much like a group- or staff-model HMO.

Other gatekeepers are less well positioned. In order to have more physicians per plan, each doctor must provide care through several plans. That means doctors are evaluated on a smaller number of cases, so are more likely to suffer from random variation. It also means that doctors must deal with the cost reports and other data from each plan as well as all the other utilization review—and the relevant data may be difficult to follow. The system puts doctors who are outside of large group practices at financial risk that they may not be able to control or even understand.

As with all versions of managed care, one should ask whether this variant cannot work better in a noncompetitive system. Some of the techniques of utilization review make more sense in a sickness fund system that sees a physician's entire practice; in a competitive system a reviewer might, by random chance, find that a physician is doing "too much." Similarly, if gatekeepers are to bear risk, they would be better off if all their patients were in the risk pool and they had to deal with only one set of rules and comparisons—as is the case in the United Kingdom and Germany.

THE PROSPECTS FOR MANAGED CARE. It is not obvious that either patients or physicians would be less constrained living with any of these forms of managed care than with a regulated fee-for-service system such as Canada's, France's, or Germany's. Nor do the savings from managed care match those achieved by established international methods.

In April 1994 the Congressional Budget Office issued its updated estimates, the political significance of which is described in chapter 8. But the substantive implications are clear enough. CBO explained that, for the geographic reasons described above, only the more effective examples of utilization review could be implemented in about 30 percent of the country. These forms could save about 3.7 percent of the costs of a system that had no review.[41] Otherwise, CBO reported that the most effective forms of managed care were the best group- and staff-model HMOs and forms of the risk-bearing gatekeeper approach described here. If these were implemented fully in the remainder of the country, the savings would be about 5.7 percent of "potentially manageable personal health care expenditures." Relative to the part of the system with the least management, medicare, savings could be 7 percent. Relative to total national health expenditures, savings would be 4.0 percent.[42]

CBO's figures were lower than its previous estimates and those made by some other analysts at the end of 1992.[43] The report explained that it used the existing partially implemented managed-care system, not an unmanaged system, for comparison, so the savings overall were lower than the effectiveness of the measures per se. But even doubling the CBO estimates would not approach the observed cost differences between the United States and Canada. Perhaps the most effective systems could add further savings by increasing cost sharing or reducing their operating margins. But the former would make them less popular, and there is no reason to count on their agreeing to the latter.

In short, experience with managed care simply does not support claims that it offers savings comparable to those achieved by the international standard forms of cost control.

Obstacles to Implementing the Best Forms of Managed Care

Even if patients and physicians were eager to join the policy analysts' preferred form of managed care, the group- or staff-model HMO, these systems could not be expanded quickly. Large capital investments would be required to build the clinics and buy the equipment. "There's a direct correlation," one consultant explained. "The more integrated the model, the more costly it is to put it together and run it."[44] And funds for expansion may not be available, especially for a business that the government is encouraging in hopes that it will have low profit margins.[45] Capital availability is one reason group- and staff-model HMOs grew more slowly than other forms during the 1980s. Because they are more expensive, they yielded less return on equity even though their operating margins, as a group, were as high as or higher than the alternatives.[46]

Expansion is not easy to manage. As any clinic-based plan expands, it goes from having too few members for its facility, which leads to high costs per person, to having too many members, which leads to worse service. Even more important, for a plan to work well, its physicians must work well together and accept the plan's practice style. The surest way to maintain a practice style is by selective recruiting.[47] The best HMOs carefully recruit doctors who will fit their practices. HMOs that grew quickly would be forced to add doctors who did not fit as well. (The situation is the same as if the National Football League suddenly created several new football teams, for example: most would not be as good as the current teams, because the best players had already been signed.) For HMOs, the challenge is not merely finding good doctors, but finding good doctors who also want to play the managed-care game. The difficulty of recruiting already-established physicians to join the group- and staff-model HMOs is exacerbated by the fact that they already have substantial investments in their own equipment and offices. Doctors who wanted to could join a network, but separate premises would prevent their building a shared practice culture.

Because of these constraints of both capital and labor, group- and staff-model HMOs are very unlikely to grow quickly. In the long run, prepaid group practices will probably become a larger part of our delivery system, with or without managed competition. As the form becomes more familiar, expectations about hours of work change, and setting up solo practice becomes even more costly, more and more medical graduates may be interested in working within a large group.[48] But the instruments of managed competition can do little to create a system of competing group- and staff-model HMOs.

NEVERTHELESS . . . "How can you say it can't be done?" a member of the Clinton administration's working groups on health care reform reports being continually asked by the groups' director, Ira Magaziner. "It's never been tried before!" One might reply that if something has never been done before, that is not the strongest evidence that something is possible. But when analyzed piece by piece, the case for managed competition without a global budget does not hold up. Both the competition and the management have been oversold.

Yet the best HMOs are institutions that the United States has and that analysts in other countries would like to build. In an international symposium, Alain Enthoven posed the question, "What can Europeans learn from Americans about the financing and organization of medical care?" "The obvious answer," he replied, "is 'not much.'" He went on, nonetheless, to suggest that versions of managed competition might make some European systems more user-friendly and efficient. In a response, Robert G. Evans and Morris L. Barer identified many of the problems with this idea, but they still agreed that the European (and they would say Canadian) systems are not perfect. They emphasized that no set of cost controls is ideal, that the international standard measures might be stretched to a point where they could become "less effective and/or more expensive to maintain," and that it would be desirable to find incremental changes in "the form of increased decentralization of decisionmaking, but within a continuation of the quite-tight centralized constraints that apply in one form or another in the successful European systems."[49]

Britain's version of "internal market" reform is one example of policymakers' attraction to this idea. Yet it shows how the same themes can refer to very different institutions in different contexts: Britain's "competitive" reform maintains the fundamental aspects of the international standard and diverges greatly from the American status quo.

Competition within a Budget: The New NHS

Britain's reforms are meant to create an "internal market" through a "purchaser-provider split" within a tightly budgeted system. In 1992–93, 79 percent of expenditures were paid by a fixed budget.[50] Instead of directly managing the provision of care, the NHS has moved to manage both sides of the market, which may contract with each other freely as long as the NHS managers approve.[51]

The NHS reforms are a moving target. Since the NHS and Community Care Act was passed in 1990 and implementation began in 1991, there has been continual institutional adjustment, partly from changing policies and partly from the working out of the new system's incentives. The government has had little interest in evaluating the reforms. In testifying on the proposals, the then secretary of state for health, Kenneth Clarke, "denied the need for formal monitoring and evaluation and expressed the view that calling on the advice of academics in this way was a sign of weakness."[52] Yet there are enough data and experience to provide a sense of the system's dynamics and potential.

Structure and Incentives

The NHS reforms did not change how money is raised for the system or how individuals become entitled to participate. In 1992–93, 81 percent of the services' income came from general revenues, 14 percent from payroll contributions specifically for the NHS, and the rest from charges for amenities, such as private rooms. The revenues are distributed from the national level out to eight regional health authorities (RHAs) in England and to separate bodies for Scotland, Wales, and Northern Ireland.[53]

PURCHASERS AND PROVIDERS. As implemented through 1994, RHAs dispense funds to three kinds of purchasers: District Health Authorities (DHAs), which buy institutional care; Family Health Services Authorities (FHSAs), which purchase ambulatory services from, for example, most general practitioners; and GP fundholders, which both provide care to patients on their lists and purchase some care on their behalf.[54]

There are four basic forms of provider: directly managed units (DMUs), self-governing NHS trusts, nonfundholding general practitioners, and GP fundholders. Institutions can be either DMUs or self-governing NHS trusts; hospitals are the most common and expensive form of institution, but this category also includes ambulance services, community centers, mental health facilities, and the like. Trusts were given more independence than DMUs in such matters as contracts, pay policies, and asset disposal but are still extensively regulated. DMUs and trusts are financed the same way: by "contracts" with DHAs, GP fundholders, or the private sector.[55]

Primary care services are provided by traditional GP practices or by fundholders. The reform requires that traditional practices refer patients to providers with which their FHSAs have contracts, while fundholders may, as before, refer patients wherever they wish. There are funding limits on "extracontractual referrals," and the DHA can refuse to pay the costs. Fear that those limits could interfere with their referral options was cited as a major reason for becoming a fundholder by the first groups of GPs who chose fundholder status, though such interference is reported to be uncommon.[56]

Fundholders receive supplemental budgets to pay for a range of services such as the costs of drugs they prescribe, outpatient diagnostic tests, and hospital care for some operations. These budgets are held by the FHSA (so fundholders do not earn interest on the balance), but fundholders draw on these accounts to pay for services and may pay for any of the covered services out of the total. Thus although there is a "notional" allocation for the purchase of hospital and community health services and one for pharmaceuticals, fundholders may pay for more of one and less of the other. Fundholders' budgets for practice staff are calculated using the same formula as for nonfundholders, but the latter need FHSA approval to hire, and the fundholders do not. Fundholders also receive an allocation for staff directly involved in managing the fund and for computing.[57]

INCENTIVES AND COMPETITION AMONG PROVIDERS. The reform also imposed a new contract on all GPs. It raised capitation payments from about 46 percent to 60 percent of their total compensation, so keeping patients on their lists has become more important, and GP care is now more thoroughly budgeted. In order to encourage preventive care such as immunizations and Pap smears, a system of targets and bonuses has replaced direct fees for service. Higher capitation fees thus give physicians greater incentives to keep patients happy and on their lists, while incentives for preventive care appeal both to public health professionals and to an ideological judgment of what patients should desire.[58]

Trusts and fundholders require management and financial capacity that not all prereform providers had. If any hospital could have decided to be a trust at any time, the results could have been chaotic, both for the DHAs, which would be continually reworking their plans and contracts, and within hospitals that did not anticipate the new management burdens. The NHS therefore created a system in which institutions would apply to become trusts, and GP practices to become fundholders, once a year. The "first wave" of conversions thus occurred in April 1991. After April 1994, the "fourth wave," about 95 percent of institutional services were being provided by trusts. About 36 percent of GP services were in fundholding practices.[59] Trusts won out so thoroughly over DMUs because, while both depended on contracts, there were no evident advantages to remaining a DMU, and there were at least minor advantages (such as setting one's own salary) for managers in setting up a trust.[60] The competition between fundholders and other GPs was more complex.

Fundholders appreciate having hiring flexibility and funds to create better computer services. They can use their ability to offer or withhold contracts to win either better prices or better service from providers such as specialists and laboratories. Fundholders also can manage their prescribing and referrals with an eye to what satisfies the most patients. Their incomes might increase from serving more patients.

On the other hand, becoming a fundholder presents any GP practice with new responsibilities and risks. The NHS reforms limited the risks by requiring the fundholders to have large pools and limiting their potential costs. First, fundholders were required to have at least 7,000 members (6,000 in Scotland). This measure ensures that risk is not allocated to just part of a solo practice, which is possible in the U.S. Allocating risk to the equivalent of at least three individual GPs' lists puts physicians at much less risk than in those American managed-care arrangements, but the practice size standard also constrains the implementation of fundholding to practices of that size.[61] Second, if the cost of hospital treatment for any patient exceeds 5,000 pounds, the district foots the bill. Third, the categories of hospital services for which fundholders are responsible constitute only about 15 percent of total hospital costs.[62]

Some analysts expected that fundholders would thrive in competition without being more efficient, either by "cherry-picking" less expensive patients, or because the government's extra financing to fundholders would exceed their legitimate extra costs. While there is controversy about the size of the government allocations they receive, the best guess is that the fundholders have not received "too much" extra money.[63] Instead, the passage of time seems to be convincing more and more GPs that the benefits of fundholding exceed the risks.

Operations and Performance

The most thorough review of the reforms' effects declares that "much of the direct research reported here indicates little actual change of any kind and even less that could be attributed to the reforms in key areas of quality, efficiency, choice, responsiveness and equity."[64] But the balance of available information does justify two conclusions. First, the creation of GP fundholding is more significant and useful than the creation of hospital trusts. Second, the reformed NHS bears little resemblance to American notions of competition.

OPERATIONS: NOT THE USUAL MARKET. The District Health Authorities and Family Health Services Authorities are planners and regulators as well as purchasers. As trustees for patients, they do not feel bound to accept whatever services the providers are willing to negotiate, and the purchasers have the authority, if necessary, to impose the terms. Further, NHS central management has direct authority over the purchasers. The law specifies that all contracts are subject to approval, interpretation, or if necessary imposition by the secretary of state for health or her designee.[65] As one observer reported, "Enough controls were built into the design of the market to give the Secretary of State fairly precise control over the degree of competitive behaviour that would be permitted."[66] There was a policy decision to ensure minimal disruption (and minimal political cost before the 1992 election) by managing the market to create a "steady state" in the first year of the reforms. This included limits, for example, on DHAs' "ability to move contracts from one provider to another or substantially alter the content and scope of their existing contracts."[67]

Profit-seeking behavior is as restricted as contracting. When trusts are established a value is set for their capital, and their prices are regulated to keep earnings at around 6 percent of capital. The state also still owns the trusts. In both these ways the trusts hardly resemble typical free-market firms.[68] Fundholders are not allowed to keep savings as income—that is, they may draw on the fund only to buy services. They may earn more only if through reinvestment they gain more patients. These rules force fundholders to pursue market share instead of margin, but any system that so limits realization of profits does not resemble (and may improve on) the normal incentives of a market.

Trusts do not have a normal firm's ability to make decisions about its labor force. In principle they may alter the terms of centrally determined employment contracts, but few have done so. Among other problems, the government has set overall limits for public sector pay increases. Because specialists naturally demand higher pay for less job security, and there is a shortage of specialists, few trusts have been able to get favorable terms. Trusts have more discretion in the allocation of jobs than in establishing rates of pay. They also have more discretion outside of direct patient care, such as with hotel services.[69]

In principle trusts may sell off buildings and in other ways manage their capital stock. In practice:

> The total amount of capital spending each year remains constrained by public spending controls. Within these overall planning totals, the Department creates regional shares of capital and central budgets to cover spending both in Trusts and other NHS bodies. Note that these are control totals; Trusts then have to fund their capital spending out of retained income from the elements in their prices which they are required to charge for the use of their existing assets, or from borrowing. Within the control totals, each Trust has an "External Financing Limit" set by the NHS Management Executive. This EFL controls spending by regulating the amount a Trust may borrow or draw down from its investments. Work is continuing on the administrative mechanisms to ensure that capital spending supports the strategic aims of NHS purchasers, while allowing Trusts sufficient freedom to develop their business.[70]

As the proper balance is sought, this regulation of capital investment "means that the independence and autonomy available to trusts is highly circumscribed."[71]

Hospitals have large fixed costs and cannot "downsize" easily. A hospital that loses a portion of its business within a market may have to raise prices, which will cause it to lose more business and perhaps eventually go bust. That often cannot be allowed in a system that already has capacity shortages. Thus in a highly publicized simulation to explore the dynamics of the regulated competition, the Regional Health Authority used its oversight of contracting to "freeze" the market to save a local university hospital.[72] When competition began to threaten London hospitals, the government intervened, first to avoid political turmoil during an election year, and second to create a planned set of closures to avoid substantive turmoil during the transition—a "managed rather than market solution."[73] In a further effort to direct the market, DHAs and FHSAs began forming "health commissions" and establishing other, less formal arrangements to coordinate purchasing of primary and acute care, and even to plan simultaneous purchasing by DHAs, FHSAs, and fundholders.[74]

In short, NHS reforms created an "internal market" in which entrepreneurs have very limited property rights and little ability to set labor contracts or to acquire or deploy capital; total spending in the market is determined by regulators, who may also set and impose contracts; market entrance by new suppliers requires approval; old capital plants can rarely be allowed to go out of business, and capital financing is so restricted that little new can be built. Other than for capital, labor, prices, entrance, and property, this is a perfectly normal set of market relationships. The defining advantages of competition are the features that conservatives usually emphasize—private property, the profit motive, free movement of capital, no restrictive labor market rules, prices negotiated between the ultimate consumer (here, patients) and the seller. The reformed NHS comes no closer to meeting those standards than does the health care system in any Canadian province.[75]

EFFECT OF TRUSTS. The Department of Health reports that the number of patients who had been waiting for more than two years fell from 51,000 in March 1991 to less than 1,700 in March 1992, and that the number of patients waiting over a year fell by more than 50 percent.

It proudly proclaimed a "new guarantee" that "no one should wait more than eighteen months for a hip or knee replacement or a cataract operation."[76]

This dramatic improvement is not, however, good evidence of the efficiency of trusts. There is a simpler explanation: output increased because the system got more money. The budgets for 1991–92 and 1992–93 gave the NHS its largest increases in over a decade: real growth of over 5 percent each year, including special funds to reduce waiting time.[77] As one report summarized, "With increases in resources of this magnitude, it would be astonishing if there were no changes in waiting lists or improvements in the range of services offered," quite independently of the reforms.[78] There was also what sociologists call the "Hawthorne Effect": regardless of other organizational changes, sudden attention to waiting lists led to special efforts, for a while, to reduce them. In Cambridge, surgeons even volunteered unpaid weekend work.[79]

Nor were these reductions in the number of persons waiting more than a year evidence that the system was more efficient. Sometimes, improvement in a publicized indicator is due to diversion of resources from a less-publicized but equally important area. It seems that in order to meet the political promise to serve those who had been waiting longest, more-urgent cases were delayed.[80] The number of people waiting increased slightly, so either more cases were being put on the list (indicating why waiting lists are a questionable indicator of services), or priorities were shuffled rather than output being increased.[81]

Even if one ignores the extra funding and accepts that fewer very long waits indicate greater efficiency, it is hard to ascribe improvement to the creation of trusts because, by the indicators used, DMUs became more productive as well. The first trusts did show slightly greater increases in efficiency measures than the DMUs. But the institutions that first decided to become trusts were already doing better than the others, and the differences are small.[82]

Britain is more densely populated than the United States, but the legacy of restricted capacity also meant that competition could not work well in much of the country. "Competition may drive quality up and/or prices down where purchasers have a choice of providers to buy from," the *Health Service Journal* said in an editorial. "But in most parts of the country, in most medical specialties, there is in reality only one local provider."[83] Even sources that emphasize the potential for competition reveal large limits. Thus in one study, "only" 38 percent of hospital patient episodes in the West Midlands region were in institutions with substantial monopoly positions.[84]

There is therefore little reason to believe that the switch of institutional care from direct management to trusts has or should have made care more efficient. Yet separating purchasers and providers relieves the purchaser of some managerial blame for provider performance, so can make purchasers (in this case, an RHA) more willing to use publicity against providers. Publicity is most easily used on simple, easily understood measures. Therefore the purchaser-provider split does seem to have encouraged a few, easily observable improvements. These include matters of convenience and patient satisfaction such as appointment systems at hospital outpatient clinics.[85]

EFFECT OF FUNDHOLDING. The evidence that fundholding has improved patient care is stronger than the case for any benefits from creating trusts. For some services, especially laboratory, there are enough options in the public or private sector that fundholders were able to shop around. In many cases fundholding gave the member practices more influence over specialists. The fundholder has some of the advantages of a private patient: it can make demands of specialists, who are interested in earning more than their base hospital income. Specialists have accepted contracts that guaranteed shorter waiting times, have agreed to hold office hours on Saturdays at the fundholder's office, and have communicated more with fundholding GPs.[86]

It is impossible to tell to what extent these advantages involve real efficiency increases, rather than the fundholding practices doing better at the expense of traditional practices. If the specialist is serving a fundholder's patients, he is not serving others. If he moves a fundholder's patients to the head of the line, he has moved other patients back.[87] This could be called "wait-shifting." It is analogous to the cost-shifting that happens to weaker payers in the United States. In the United States weaker payers would pay more; in the United Kingdom the patients of the weaker payers, traditional GPs, would wait longer. Traditional GPs clearly suspect as much, and it is only common sense to say that if all British GP practices were fundholders, they would not be able to favor their patients in the same ways that fundholding practices can in competing with nonfundholders.

Yet the fundholding approach still makes sense in the British context. As explained in chapter 5, creation of the NHS in 1948 made the specialists the key players in the system. Salaried specialists had to be courted by GPs who wanted good service for their patients. GP fundholding alters this power relationship. As a few observers told me, "consultants [specialists] send Christmas cards to GPs now." If all GPs were fundholders one would expect consultants to be more responsive in the simple ways that matter a lot to GPs, especially in their communications about patients' treatments. That would be better for patients as well.

What the Reform Does Not Do

GP fundholding offers some marginal improvements in patient services and in the long run a more responsive culture among specialists. These are worthwhile accomplishments. Yet the British reforms do not suggest that Americans can achieve the goals of health care reform without adapting some version of the international standard measures.

On the financing side, the NHS is still funded mainly by general revenues. People contribute to a system according to income rather than by buying separate insurance products in a market transaction. Everybody must participate.

Costs are controlled through a stringent budget. GP fundholding expands the budgeted part of the system by including pharmaceutical costs and some other expenses for patients within fundholding practices, while the new GP contract expanded budgeting by raising the share of GP costs paid by capitation. As with many "efficiency" reforms, then, the budgeting creates more certainties. There is no competition among GPs to get patients by lowering prices, and there are no financial incentives influencing choice of GP, and thus competition is not a form of cost control. At best, competition in the reformed NHS is a measure to provide a bit more care within the existing budgets and so reduce demands for more spending.

A Caveat: Different Capacity Might Allow Different Policies

One difference between the United Kingdom and United States might allow competition to be a more significant force for cost control in the United States—the difference in capacity to provide hospital services.

NHS managers dare not allow competition to restructure system capacity. For many years they have relied on capacity limits to control costs, and they fear that if they allow a proliferation of equipment, it will be hard to resist applications to use it. So they do not want to give trusts a free hand to buy. Yet the result of years of capacity control is a situation in which competition cannot be allowed to drive institutions out of business, either (inner-city London excepted).

The United States has far greater hospital capacity for most services, which means there is less risk in allowing competition to proceed unfettered. Competition should be better at eliminating existing excess capacity in the United States. If, for example, the government were to try to close down five of the cardiac surgery units in Michigan, there would likely be a political uproar, including arguments about due process and discrimination and the like. If individual insurers just happened not to contract with those five, nobody could be blamed.[88]

And in an ideal model, competition would not risk overinvestment—the bane of unregulated systems. Hospitals that compete for physician affiliations and patronage in the United States tend to overexpand and then blame others for their lack of business. In a system of competing integrated plans that included hospitals, every dollar spent for investment would have to be justified by sale of premiums. The public would get the capacity it chose through the market.

Unfortunately this scenario requires many leaps of faith. The first would fly over the likelihood that plans would, nevertheless, overexpand, as they tried to satisfy physicians in order to attract patients. Why should plan managers be different from hospital managers? The second leap involves equity. Plans that charged more would be able to build more; how, then, would adequate services for people with less money, presumably in plans that charged lower premiums, be guaranteed? The third leap must clear a barrier mentioned earlier: the fact that, in much of the country, competing plans would not be able to own their own hospitals, so some regulation of hospital capacity would still be needed.

Even in the United States, competition that eliminated capacity without regulation could create shortages—and once they occurred, and the public faced waiting lists, it might be too late to fix the problem. Loss of one service could endanger the rest of an institution's services, something individual plans would be unlikely to address.[89] Most important, a large part of the health care system, the academic medical centers, fit poorly into a system of competing integrated networks. Their research and training activities add costs for which plans would not wish to pay. Plans need not value those functions, but the rest of us should, so no country is likely to let competition determine the fate of the AMCs.

A health care system must do many things besides deliver quality care efficiently to specific patients. If these tasks are performed by the same institutions that deliver care, the role of competition must be limited.[90] If a country chose to ignore these issues, and created a system of competition that were stringent enough, then competition might overly reduce system capacity. The Jackson Hole proposal seems less likely than previous legislation to create that effect, but it might have begun in a few American markets without either reform. Whether the cost control benefits of drastic and uncontrolled system downsizing are worth the likely effects of that process on both access to and the equity of health care is, of course, a matter of judgment. Here we can say only that British experience cannot help Americans make that choice.

Conclusion: Finance and Delivery

The strongest argument for managed competition as a form of cost control is that it might force a drastic and unprecedented restructuring of America's health care providers. That is the only scenario in which it could exceed the international standard for achieving cost control. Many health economists would applaud. But it is an extreme agenda hidden within familiar, comforting language.

Both management and competition sound very American. Businessmen believe that managing and competing is what they do. The term managed competition is a superb example of persuasive labeling: it says, here is the moderate, centrist, uniquely American plan for health care reform.

Yet for both patients and providers, managed competition, if it worked at all, would require bigger changes and be riskier than adopting the international methods. Early in this book I distinguished between reforming the financing and the delivery of health care. The major purpose of the managed competition model, to the policy innovators who invented it, is to revolutionize the *delivery* of medicine in the United States by creating competing large, integrated, managed care plans—what I have called "competing Kaisers."[91]

I have no personal bias against group- or staff-model HMOs. When I was a member of Kaiser Permanente I was satisfied with my care; unfortunately, in the current American system of health care financing, I had to leave that system because my employer limits the available plans and it stopped offering the Kaiser coverage. I personally like the fact that in the Clinton proposals, for example, I would have been able to choose Kaiser again. When I use Kaiser Permanente as the model I do its proponents a favor, identifying their ideas with the most successful prepaid group practice in the country, one that in many ways, such as its outcomes measurement effort, is a leader. But not all group- and staff-model HMOs are Kaisers, and the idea that reform could create a world of competing Kaisers in any reasonable amount of time, with savings comparable to those from adapting the international standard of cost controls, and be acceptable to most Americans, flies in the face of what we know about managed care, about group- and staff-model HMOs in particular, and about competition.

Cost control in the six other countries discussed in this book uses institutions that enable the consumers of care, either through the government or through insurers grouped together, to work out terms of payment with providers. Payers do not compete with each other, because doing so would weaken their bargaining position. Yet neither do payers separately try to run medical practice. This process of co-operation to manage payments, rather than competition to manage care, can be awkward and conflictual. Yet it mainly requires new activities at the top levels of organizations, such as creating a fee schedule. The international standard does not require that doctors and patients change how they do their business (although providers could greatly simplify their billing).

Creating an internal market in the NHS was difficult enough. But the NHS reforms began from a system in which GPs already were everybody's gatekeepers. The reforms do not rely on new restrictions on patient choice to create savings, and the major reform of GP practice, fundholding, does not restrict GPs' ability to choose where they refer patients. In the United States the elimination of fees for service would be a much more radical undertaking.

If reforming delivery were the only hope for cost control, the gamble might make sense. But that is less true in the United States than in any other country in the world. When dealing with a fundamental aspect of daily life, I would rather try what has worked before and is least disruptive. The best approach would be to reform financial arrangements in ways that create cost control while leaving room for the evolution of preferable delivery systems. Ironically, this has not been defined in America as the moderate approach. Instead, in the American political battles of 1993–94, moderation was defined as either a purist or a watered-down version of managed competition.

The watered-down version, in the form of the Chafee proposal and many later dilutions, was at least truly moderate in the sense that it would not accomplish much. The purist version, in the form of the Cooper-Grandy bill, would have done more, but much would not have been good. Each suffered from the weaknesses of managed competition as theory. The Chafee proposal weakened the theory in order to satisfy powerful interests. The Cooper bill was weakened by the Congressional Budget Office's well-founded skepticism about its savings projections.

But both were made even less plausible as solutions, though not as political vehicles, by the institutional inheritance of the American health care system. Ironically, internal market reforms may be easier to implement in the countries that already guarantee health care to all their citizens than in the United States. Chapter 8 uses the attempts to draft managed competition legislation to demonstrate its weaknesses in the American context.

8

Drafting Managed Competition

*T*HE obvious theoretical issues raised by managed competition are matters of economics. Its supporters offer incentives they claim will change costs by changing behavior. As chapter 7 explained, both evidence and argument raise doubts as to whether intensified management and revised competition could have the intended effects. The problems with the theory, however, exceed those discussed in chapter 7. There are (at least) three further major obstacles to using managed competition to ensure health care to all Americans at a reasonable cost.

The first problem is political. "Managed competition" sounds more ideologically acceptable than "government health insurance," but it involves extensive compulsion and regulation. Thus it may not buy many votes. The second problem is administrative. Incentives that work in theory must also work in practice, and implementing managed competition's core ideas would involve immense administrative challenges. If those challenges could be met at all, there is little doubt that meeting them would require a level of administration that would not satisfy opponents of "big government."

The third problem involves coordination. Managed competition is a theory about cost control, not access. Its theory of cost control, however, would require the creation of institutions that would be difficult to coordinate with the normal measures for increasing access.

In this chapter I consider these problems by discussing two federal proposals: those introduced by Representatives Jim Cooper (D-Tenn.) and Fred Grandy (R-Iowa) (the Cooper-Grandy bill) and Senator John Chafee (R-R.I.) (the Chafee bill). Many of these obstacles would present themselves at the state level as well, if a state tried to set up an independent managed competition system (see the appendix for some of the more complex technical detail).

By the time Congress got down to serious votes on health care reform, both the Chafee and the Cooper-Grandy bills had faded from the policy agenda. They faded because, in each case, the sponsors decided to reach "right," diluting their own proposals. Nevertheless, these two bills represented distinct prototypes of managed competition. The watered-down approaches that their sponsors endorsed toward the end were no longer managed competition bills; instead, they fell into the category of incremental approaches, which I address in chapter 10.

Offered by a combination of conservative Democrats and Republicans, H.R. 3222, the Managed Competition Act of 1993, was closer than the Chafee (or any other) bill to a version of the Jackson Hole proposal. Its primary sponsors were Jim Cooper, Mike Andrews (D-Tex.), and Fred Grandy in the House, and John Breaux (D-La.) in the Senate. It was commonly called Cooper-Grandy to emphasize its bipartisan sponsorship. The Health Equity and Access Reform Today Act of 1993 was introduced as S. 1770 and H.R. 3704. Its prime sponsors were Senator Chafee and Representative Bill Thomas (R-Calif.), but it was drafted in the Senate and commonly known as the Chafee bill.[1] It was a compromise between managed competition and an incremental approach.

The two bills reveal the limits of each political strategy. What they teach about individual provisions is even more important. The difficulties discussed in this chapter and the appendix—such as how to set a benchmark premium, how to administer the limit on tax deductibility, and the administrative burdens of any system of means-tested individual subsidies—would be faced by any other bill that attempted to implement similar measures.

The most fundamental failure involved cost control. The sponsors of both these prototypes and many other bills would have preferred to believe that universal coverage could be financed by the measures of managed competition. Their problems began with the fact that the Congressional Budget Office (CBO) did not agree.

The Deficit and CBO

The CBO analysis was crucial because the politics of the federal budget deficit are so sensitive. The budget battles of the 1980s produced congressional budget procedures for raising points of order when legislation threatens to raise the deficit above what is known as the current law baseline—what the deficit would be without new legislation.[2] In Congress's lexicon, programs must obey the "Paygo" rule—that is, they must be "pay-as-you-go." In the Senate, sixty out of the one hundred senators must approve a motion to waive the point of order.

Any health care reform bill that did not pay for itself, through spending cuts, new revenues, or a combination of the two, would be out of order. In principle, sixty votes are required to defeat determined Senate opponents of any piece of legislation, because sixty votes are needed for cloture on a filibuster. But to uphold a filibuster, forty-one senators must endorse obstruction and risk blame for preventing Congress from even taking a vote on an issue that affects all Americans. To enforce the point of order, forty-one senators must endorse obeying Congress's own rules and keeping the deficit from getting any worse.

Paygo would have little effect if it were possible to simply increase revenues to pay for expanded coverage. Here again, we need only note that if raising taxes were not difficult, the deficit would not be an obstacle.[3] Although "sin" taxes (taxes on alcohol or tobacco, for example) and payments by the newly covered would raise some revenue, much of the expense the federal government would incur by expanding coverage would have to be paid by reducing the costs that the federal government would incur for its existing health programs, such as medicare, if there were no legislation at all. And the burden of new obligations would be lessened if it included effective cost controls for the new obligations.

So any health care reform bill had to meet the Paygo rule largely by controlling costs. Participants and observers might disagree about whether a bill met the requirements, but the final determination would be made, as at a ballgame, not by the players or spectators but by an umpire, in this case CBO.

CBO cannot avoid accusations of bias but tries to limit criticism by following professional norms of budget estimation.[4] These norms include erring on the side of caution and seeking consensus. CBO bases estimates on what can be known from previous experience. Its analysts ask what inputs might change, what specific savings can be expected, and particularly what happened when similar things were tried before. CBO cost estimates are generally in the ballpark of respected outside estimates, if they exist. In the case of managed competition, no neutral outside analyses projected that it alone would provide the savings needed to finance universal coverage with benefits resembling the international norm within a reasonable amount of time.[5]

The most frequently cited example of a plan that has achieved large savings, the California Public Employee Retirement System (CalPERS) looks more like the international standard than like most theoretical versions of a plan for managed competition. CalPERS enrolls 900,000 persons through family members who are employed by the state; these families choose among a wide variety of health care plans. In 1992 and 1993 CalPERS significantly reduced its costs relative to trend, but it did so not by increasing competition among insurers to increase efficiency, but by bargaining. CalPERS managers began by freezing new enrollments in the Kaiser Permanente HMO (health maintenance organization) and threatened to pull large numbers of subscribers out of other plans unless those plans significantly lowered their bids. If managed competition is a matter of raw market power exercised by the alliance, then CalPERS is the prototype—but that is not what most managed competition supporters had in mind.[6]

Because of the effects of health care costs on the federal budget, and a strong suspicion that his office would have to estimate a lot of different bills during the next few years, CBO director Robert Reischauer had his staff begin studying cost control issues long before the election of a president committed to historic reform.[7] CBO was skeptical about all the proposals, but especially managed competition, because the theory relied on the market's doing something that had never been seen before. The last time anyone made budget estimates on such grounds, about the tax cuts of 1981, they had not proven true.[8]

Basic Issues and Structural Choices

Any health care reform must address questions of whom to subsidize and how much, what to cover, and how to do good without raising the deficit. Managed competition also requires its designers to structure health alliances and devise the incentives for competition among plans.

Managed competition sounds unbureaucratic, yet Cooper-Grandy required an immense new federal bureaucracy to process millions of subsidy applications, evaluate probably thousands of plans, and at least try to define the benefits and to some extent the taxes of all

Americans. The Chafee bill appeared to avoid growth in the bureaucracy by failing to create systems to perform tasks that it required (such as risk adjustment) and by creating organizations (such as voluntary purchasing groups) but giving them little power or purpose. Both bills required one crucial task, administering a cap on tax deductibility, adequate performance of which seems nearly impossible. Another task, the creation and administration of a system of individual subsidies for the costs of premiums, both creates huge administrative burdens and risks creating incentives that would discourage employment. Because CBO insisted on basing its estimates on available data, it was unable to say that either bill would provide universal coverage.

Alliances and Incentives

Managed competition would create alliances in order to affect market practices without directly using state power. But such alliances would be criticized by advocates of private authority on the grounds that they would have too much power to manipulate the market, and by supporters of public authority on the grounds that the alliances would have too much power for an agent that was not under direct democratic control.

In defining the alliances' authority, each bill therefore had to balance effectiveness and political support. Alliances that could negotiate prices with health plans, like CalPERS, would be more effective but would be opposed by the insurers and by anyone who disliked regulation in principle. Alliances that included a large share of the population in any area, on a compulsory basis, would be better able to manage risk adjustments and have more market power in any negotiations, but would seem more like a government.

Each bill had to answer questions about incentives and boundaries. If the tax system were used to encourage purchase of less expensive plans, whose taxes would be targeted, employers' or employees'? How would a "benchmark" premium beyond which expenses were not tax deductible be set? In limiting risk competition, what exceptions to community-rating could be allowed, and how would differential marketing be controlled?

A Structural Overview of Both Plans

Under Cooper-Grandy, only "accountable health plans" (AHPs) could qualify for favorable tax treatment. Small businesses and individuals would purchase the AHPs through health plan purchasing cooperatives (HPPCs), this bill's term for alliances. Many regulatory and administrative responsibilities would be lodged in an innocuously named health care standards commission (HCSC).

The Chafee Health Equity and Access Reform Today Act was a diluted version of managed competition mixed with ideas propounded by other Republican factions.[9] Its alliances were not mandatory, and it did not include a national organization with powers comparable to the HCSC (partly because it failed to specify who would exercise certain powers).

Both bills required employers to make insurance "available" to their employees, but neither one required that employers pay any of the cost. Making insurance available then really meant allowing employees to pay for it through a payroll deduction. This seems at least as large a benefit for insurers as for employees: it guarantees premiums will be paid on time, which is good for insurers, and an employer might "offer" only some of the many plans available in the private market, which deprives employees of some options. It is equivalent to employers' collecting for the United Way campaign and no more enables people to buy health insurance than United Way enables people to contribute to charities.

Each plan did provide new subsidies so individuals and families with low incomes could buy insurance. Each proposed to fund these subsidies with cost savings from cuts in existing federal programs and the benefits of competition, and through a revenue increase generated by limiting the amount of insurance premiums that could be deducted for tax purposes. Their sponsors did not advertise this as a tax hike.

CBO could not report enough savings to pay for health care for all Americans. Violating the Paygo rule was politically impossible. Cooper-Grandy therefore did not formally promise universal coverage, while Chafee promised it so far in the future and with so many conditions that one could hardly call it a guarantee.

Responding to the same pressures, neither bill specified what would be covered. Instead, that would be determined later, when a "benefits commission" (Chafee) or a health care standards commission (Cooper-Grandy) submitted a proposal to Congress, which Congress could not amend. This rather strange procedure was proposed in a number of other bills and amendments as well. (International readers should understand that it seemed vaguely plausible to Americans who do not trust politicians to do anything important.)

There were other, less "principled" reasons that neither bill specified the covered benefits. Anyone who specifies anything but a huge benefits package will have a host of importunate health care lobbies accusing them of causing endless suffering. Given CBO's likely positions, sponsors of managed competition plans could only pass the Paygo test by producing a less generous benefit package than the Clinton or McDermott-Wellstone bills.[10] Not only would the benefits look worse, but a lower benefit package means a lower cap on tax deductibility, so lower benefits mean larger tax hikes. Politicians understandably do not like admitting these sorts of things.

Both bills would have made it hard for states to isolate populations in the inner cities from the wealthier and likely healthier people in the suburbs, by requiring either alliance areas or, in the Chafee bill, "health care coverage areas" (HCCAs) to include all of any metropolitan statistical area and at least 250,000 persons.[11] A state could have anywhere from one to as many areas as this constraint allowed.

Managed competition requires that somebody determine whether a given plan provides the standard benefits and therefore is eligible for tax-deductible purchase. In Cooper-Grandy, the health care standards commission (HCSC) had to approve the accountable health plans (AHPs), and could only approve plans that were "accessible to each enrollee, within the area served by the plan, with reasonable promptness."[12] Without this regulation, the plan that sets the standard for tax deductibility might ration by inconvenience. But with it, the HCSC had the first of many regulatory jobs: to evaluate the capacity of thousands of plans.

The Chafee bill avoided criticism for having a large new bureaucracy by fragmenting and even abandoning authority over plans. "Qualified general access plans," for small employers, would be certified by the states; "qualified large employer plans" would not be certified by anyone; they would be regulated, depending on the issue, by the secretary of health and human services or the secretary of labor or both.[13] Because a plan might be certified as a qualified general access plan yet also sell to large employers, some of its features might be simultaneously regulated by the state and by both secretaries.

Both bills restricted alliances to employers with a hundred full-time-equivalent employees or fewer, though Cooper-Grandy allowed states to raise the figure, as long as no more than half of all employees in any state would be insured through alliances.[14] As a result each bill relied on large employers' choices of what to "offer," rather than employees' choices of what plan to join in the alliance, to drive the market.

Chafee, in an attempt to seem as nonregulatory as possible, weakened alliances further. States, not alliances, would provide information about all qualified general access plans in a coverage area to small employers, and employers, not alliances, would have to provide their employees with that information.[15] Large employers could limit their offer to one plan.[16] States would charter "purchasing groups," with membership limited to individuals and small employers. These groups could operate in more than one coverage area, their membership would be voluntary, and there might be no group in a given area.[17] Groups could market plans, but only if the plans agreed.[18] Plans could market however they wished. Therefore plans that wished to avoid selection by the riskier sets of employees within a group could do so by refusing to be marketed through the group and selling directly to companies with less risky employees.

The Chafee bill's "voluntary" alliances would be very much like something that already existed, called a "multiple employer welfare arrangement" (MEWA). MEWAs, and voluntary purchasing groups, have a few weaknesses. If insurers can choose whether to sell through a group, and can market separately to its members, the group structure does nothing to prevent poaching of low-risk employers and employees. If employers are not paying for the group as a whole, it is even more likely that group members who choose to buy insurance will be those who are more likely to incur expenses, giving insurers a strong hint that they should not market through the MEWAs. Experience with current MEWAs has been rife with fraud, in part because they provide an extra level of transactions outside of normal regulation.[19] Standardization and regulation of benefits packages would likely reduce fraud, because purchasers would have a better idea what kind of coverage the MEWA was offering. Yet there was little reason to believe such voluntary measures would have more than a small effect on the level of insurance: numerous state experiments as of mid-1994 had extremely small payoffs.[20]

As in many other matters, the Chafee bill thus adopted some of the language of managed competition with little substance. The Cooper-

Grandy authors made a much more serious effort to ensure lower administrative overhead costs and eliminate risk-rating, so required membership in exclusive alliances. But they had a problem: how to have enough market power to project savings but not so much as to lose support from large insurance companies.

They therefore gave alliances no negotiating power, limited their size, allowed large employers to self-insure by setting up "closed" AHPs, and allowed them to limit their offerings so that employers, not alliances, would bargain with plans. This approach turned the original Jackson Hole theories about competition upside down. In the original version, plans would compete for employees' patronage; Cooper-Grandy had the plans competing for employers' patronage. But plans already compete for business from employers, so that was not a change. In particular, "large" firms with little market power (those with, say, only 120 employees) would be as weak as before.

Because they were not changing who purchased insurance, Cooper-Grandy drafters were staking their hopes for new savings entirely on two other aspects of the original Jackson Hole scheme: limits on risk competition and changes in the tax code.

The Difficulty of Regulating Competition

These regulations and incentives for competition required huge administrative bureaucracies to perform tasks that may be impossible to perform well. Both bills' designs for capping the tax-deductible amount of health insurance revealed that making the cap work in a defensible manner would be a nearly impossible task.

Big Problems with a Tax Cap

Cooper-Grandy limited all tax deductions and exclusions to the "reference premium rate" for the insured person's class of premium within an HPPC area. The reference premium had to be the lowest rate charged by an AHP in that area, as long as that plan enrolled "at least such proportion of eligible individuals as the Commission shall specify."[21]

If an employer paid more for an employee, the *employer could not treat "excess" insurance contributions as a business expense.* Thus if an employer provided a $5,000 insurance policy to its employees in an HPPC area where the reference rate was $4,000, the employer would pay a 35 percent excise tax on the extra $1,000, an extra $350. This provision fit Cooper-Grandy's reliance on employer, not employee, choice to limit costs. It also was as tough as a tax incentive could be. If the employer reduced its contribution and gave the employee wages for the difference, then the employee would be taxed on that income (though normally at a lower rate). So there would be no way around the limit.[22]

Chafee limited individual, not employer, tax deductibility to a different standard, the average of the premiums of the bottom half of standard packages offered in a health care coverage area. If an employer paid more, then it and the employee would have to report the difference as employee income, and the employee would be taxed on that amount.[23] This provision was less stringent but also fit the basic managed competition theory.

There are two basic problems, both explained at greater length in the appendix. First, there is no good way to set the benchmark premium. If that premium is based (as in the Chafee bill) on what plans are "offered," rather than on the plans in which substantial numbers of persons enroll, then insurers can manipulate the list, lowering their price relative to the benchmark, by creating extra, high-priced plans. But if the benchmark premium is based on actual enrollment, then whoever sets the standard must judge three things: the proposed price of each plan, whether the plan meets the quality standards, and how many people will enroll in it. Unfortunately, only the price can be known in advance. Therefore individuals could be forced to pay taxes for choosing a plan that is more expensive than the benchmark, *when the "benchmark," in fact, turns out not to meet the standards.*

The second difficulty is, once the benchmark was somehow determined, administering the cap on tax deductibility would be extremely difficult. There would have to be hundreds, even thousands, of different caps, based on where people live, their family type, and their age (in both the Chafee and Cooper-Grandy bills). Keeping track of the appropriate caps would be hard enough if people's status did not change during the year, but it *does* change, as people have birthdays and give birth, get married and divorced, and change residence. Both the burdens and confusion would be extensive for individual tax filers, employers, and the Internal Revenue Service. Henry Aaron had it right: "Attempts to make these rules work would give new meaning to complexity in tax administration and compliance."[24]

If there is a solution to these problems, nobody had found it by the end of the 103d Congress. *Capping the deductibility of health benefits according to competition in individual markets would be nearly impossible* without huge and unpopular hassles. Like most administrative issues, this passed almost unnoticed in the press and Congress, but it clearly affected the Clinton administration's deliberations. Thus when attacked by Alain Enthoven for not including the cap, his erstwhile coauthor Richard Kronick, who had become a central designer of the Clinton plan, replied:

> If it were possible to implement a tax cap set at the level of the lowest-price plan available to each person, then one could at least argue that only those persons who voluntarily choose more-expensive plans would face additional tax liability. However, even with large alliances, it is not possible to implement such a proposal.[25]

In response to testimony to his Senate Finance Committee about the administrative difficulties, Senator Daniel Patrick Moynihan (D-N.Y.) quipped, "It's difficult only if you want to be fair."[26]

Compromising Limits on Risk Competition

Any theory of managed competition must, at a minimum, restrict risk-rating. Both bills would have limited risk-rating, but each compromised its ability to do so, though Chafee to a far greater extent, in response to their sponsors' distrust of regulation.

All managed competition plans, including Clinton's, promise to find new and accurate risk-adjustment formulas, but none can say how. At this level all plans are flawed. They can be distinguished, however, by their preemptive controls, such as limiting price variations and requiring wide marketing. Plans also differ as to whether even flawed risk-adjustment formulas can be administered within a bill's structure.

Cooper-Grandy established four classes of enrollment: individual, couple, individual and one child, and individual and more than one family member (couple with child(ren), individual with two or more children); Chafee had two classes, individual and other. In each bill a commission would establish "reasonable age bands." Each also had provisions to directly limit exclusions for pre-existing conditions.[27]

The bills differed in the price variation allowed among categories and how limits on risk competition would be enforced. In Cooper-

Grandy, the relative prices for each demographic category were to be the same in each plan. Plans would also have had to set standard premium rates within any HPPC area. Open plans (those available through the HPPC) with service areas smaller than the HPPC area would have had to deny membership to outsiders uniformly; a plan that claimed it could serve only a limited number of persons would have had to accept applicants on a first-come, first-served basis. Open plans also would have had to accept a risk-adjustment system devised by the health care standards commission and enforced by the local HPPC. Within the confines of the theory, Cooper-Grandy did as much as possible to limit the difficulties created by possible mismatches between plan service areas and HPPC coverage areas.[28]

But the Cooper-Grandy plan had one gaping hole: "closed" plans that chose not to market to small employers could then have chosen not to market to large employers with less healthy workers. Higher rates were banned, but cherry-picking and cream-skimming were not. There was no risk adjustment in the large-employer sector.[29] Because insurers could not charge more but could refuse to sell to any employer with 101 or more employees, high-risk groups might have been forced to self-insure (create their own "closed" plan). Employers at the lower end of "large" would then have been at great risk from just a few catastrophic illnesses.

In trying to limit the power of the alliance as a regulator, Cooper-Grandy therefore eliminated some of its usefulness as a risk-management system. At some point an employer is large enough not to worry about random variation breaking a self-insured system, and some are so big and rich that we do not care if they are discriminated against in the market because of their risk profiles. The former number is surely smaller than the Clinton administration's original cutoff at 5,000 employees, but it is much larger than a hundred.

The Chafee drafters compromised their system's usefulness in other ways. They did not force plans to market themselves to small groups through an alliance structure, so plans could direct *all* their marketing away from more risky clients. The bill also allowed premium differences "based on identifiable differences in marketing and other legitimate administrative costs." That statement seems to justify charging smaller businesses more. Other language suggested that some restrictions would be, as was often the case in that bill, left to administrative determination.[30]

Nor did the Chafee bill provide methods for risk adjustment, even though the bill text explicitly required it.[31] There were no answers to questions such as who would collect and distribute money, and how. The risk adjustment was also limited to the individual and small-employer world, so plans would have been able to limit their exposure by simply marketing only to less risky large employers—and this bill defined a company with 101 employees as a large company.

Once more, the desire to provide a less regulatory version of managed competition, in order to respond to the political objections to regulation, made the system unlikely to work as advertised.

Summary: Politics and Administration

As soon as one tries to reduce managed competition to working institutions, it becomes apparent that this "nonregulatory" approach requires *somebody*, a public or private body, to constrain powerful existing institutions, such as insurers and employers. Two problems emerge.

First, the kind of regulation required would be very difficult to implement. That would be true of the tax cap, for example. In contrast, setting a fee schedule is simple. Fees can be negotiated or imposed in advance and prices posted; payers then enforce the schedule by following it.

Second, even regulation that is simple to formulate will be resisted by the regulated interests and attacked as bureaucratic. Cooper-Grandy compromised with those special interests less than Chafee and included many well-thought-out provisions. But each compromised enough to threaten serious failures in the operation of their proposed systems.

Managed Competition and Universal Coverage

All questions of coverage and subsidy could be addressed in the United States by eliminating the entire existing structure and replacing it with a coherent new one, such as the McDermott-Wellstone single-payer plan (sponsored by Representative Jim McDermott (D-Wash.) and Senator Paul Wellstone (D-Minn.)). When a political decision is made to build on or around existing institutions, as contemplated by all of the plans that invoked managed competition, choices are more complicated.

Medicaid Puzzles

With the elderly taken care of fairly adequately through medicare, that program might be left alone. So the first question about income subsidies in any plan is what to do about medicaid.

Medicaid is really two main programs: one for poor families with children and one for people who need long-term care and have been bankrupted by its expense. From the standpoint of care for poor families, the obvious reform is to abolish medicaid and put the poor in the same system as everybody else. But that approach would not take care of long-term care unless that care were provided on the same terms as all other, without a means test. Eliminating the means test for long-term care would be extremely expensive. It could not be achieved within the Paygo rules without large new taxes.

Because states pay some of the costs of medicaid, national reform that abolishes that program and replaces it with something else has to find a way to continue state contributions (unless, again, Congress wants to violate Paygo or raise taxes substantially). In addition, the medicaid list of covered services is very generous; but states' low payments and other factors have led to low provider participation. A reform that folded the medicaid population into the regular system would improve access to the standard benefits, but unless it created a supplementary program it would end the limited access to the current extra benefits (such as coverage for eyeglasses).

Chafee allowed states to provide the standard medicaid benefits through the "qualified general access plans," as long as the states did not require and did not pay for membership in a plan that cost more than the benchmark. But each state that did so would require federal approval, and membership would be phased in slowly. As part of Chafee's cost savings, federal contributions for medicaid acute-care services would have been capped through a formula determining payments to each state.[32] States would be punished if they reduced eligibility from the 1994 baseline.

States therefore were put in a box: if need increased or costs rose quickly, they would lose because of the cap on federal spending. In response, the Chafee bill gave states the option of putting more of the medicaid population into managed care.[33] In this way Chafee paralleled many state proposals that required managed care within a budget for the poor but not for everybody else.

Rather than create such a two-tier system, Cooper-Grandy abolished medicaid entirely. Its plan was for the federal government to replace the acute-care portion of medicaid with subsidies for that population to join the accountable health plans. Having relieved the states of acute-care costs, Cooper-Grandy drafters assumed (but did not require) that the states would choose to maintain the long-term care component with their own funds.[34]

The alternative is to maintain the long-term care program and create a formula for continued state contributions to subsidies for the poor in the alliances, which is what Clinton proposed. Then the challenge is to define the formula.[35]

Financing Subsidies

Cooper-Grandy and Chafee both would have expanded coverage through federal subsidies according to family income. Cooper-Grandy called for the government to pay an AHP the reference premium (if all went right) for families with income at or below the poverty line. Above the poverty line, families would have lost 1 percent of their subsidies for each 1 percent increase in earnings, so the subsidy would phase out when family income reached twice the poverty level. Chafee would have provided its benchmark premium up to the poverty level and then phased it out, eliminating it when family income reached 240 percent of poverty.

Both Cooper-Grandy and Chafee (like the Clinton plan) projected savings from various sources, such as the tax cap, medicare, and medicaid. But those savings might not materialize as hoped. Then what? In an easier world, the deficit would just go up. But in the world of Paygo it was hard to allow that risk, and the sponsors of both Cooper-Grandy and Chafee opposed it in principle. Therefore, both proposals limited federal expenditure to the amount of federal savings. The Chafee bill then provided a choice between delaying subsidies and cutting the standard benefits to make up the difference. Cutting benefits would be the equivalent of a tax hike for the middle class, because it would lower the allowed "reference premium" for tax deductibility, so delaying coverage was much more likely.

The Cooper-Grandy designers were more committed to expanding coverage. They also sought to address the possibility that the poor might not be able to find and join a plan that cost the specified premium amount or less. The drafters' solution was ingenious, but it would not work without the mandatory coverage that they insisted on avoiding. In essence, Cooper-Grandy would have required insured persons to pay the difference between the government's savings and the cost of subsidizing the newly insured (described in more detail in the appendix). That means that those who chose not to buy insurance would also not have to pay the subsidies. Therefore persons with lower risk would be especially likely to drop their insurance coverage altogether. CBO concluded that this approach could "rapidly undermine insurance markets," creating a version of the "death spiral" that destroyed community-rating for American health insurance.[36]

If subsidies depend on savings, and must be limited to that amount, and cost controls are weak, the system is not secure. Chafee was willing to give up on coverage either by covering fewer people or offering lower benefits. Cooper-Grandy tried to avoid reducing coverage by dividing the cost of subsidies between general revenues and insurance premiums. But because insurance coverage, and therefore premiums, was voluntary rather than mandatory, contributing would not have been guaranteed, and the insurance system itself would have been at risk.

Delivering Subsidies

Paying out individual subsidies is as difficult as collecting the money in the first place. As a family's or an individual's subsidy is phased out, the reduction in the subsidy for each dollar of new earnings is much like a tax. Under Cooper-Grandy's provisions, assuming a family of three and a (very inexpensive) $4,000 policy, the marginal tax from reducing the health care subsidy above the poverty line would be 33.7 percent.[37] Combined with the payroll tax, income tax, and phasing out of the earned income tax credit, the phasing out of health care subsidies would add up to the equivalent of a 70 percent marginal tax on each dollar of earnings above the poverty level.

A marginal tax rate of 70 percent (and it could well be higher) is unfair and does little to reward work. The disincentive could be limited by providing a smaller subsidy, but the subsidy would then be less adequate. It could also be limited by phasing out the subsidy more slowly, as in Chafee—but then the subsidy would cost more.[38] With that inexpensive $4,000 policy, Chafee only has a marginal tax rate of 60 percent. That is a lot for a family with income of, say, $15,000 per year.

One group, however, would not have to worry about work incen-

tives: bureaucrats. They would be responsible for accepting and veri-
fying applications from all the individuals who thought they qualified.[39] Even if beneficiaries of the main income assistance programs
were included automatically, there would be millions of applications
each year.[40] Individuals' incomes and needs for subsidy would change
during the year, creating further difficulties (see the appendix). Such
a subsidy program would require a choice between three unpleasant
options: having a huge bureaucracy (to process all applications quickly
and accurately), a smaller bureaucracy that was thorough but made
people wait, or a smaller bureaucracy that was less thorough so as to
reduce waits and that therefore made lots of mistakes.

The work disincentives and administrative overhead of a system of
individual subsidies can be reduced by making the system less adequate. Chafee did so by implementing its subsidies so slowly that it
would only have reached the Cooper-Grandy proposal's population
by the year 2003. Even that depended on the medicaid and medicare
savings, and the phaseout of medicaid was both slow and optional, so
the Chafee bill ensured that there would be many fewer subsidy applications and many more people with no or inferior coverage.[41]

Individual Subsidies versus the International Standard

Any nation could choose to live with both the administrative burdens and the work disincentives of a system of individual subsidies.
It could also accept the consequences of not requiring participation.
But none of the other countries in this study have done so. I have
reviewed the difficulties at this length in order to make the choice
clear.

The international standard relies to only a small extent on subsidies
targeted to specific individuals. Such payments may be made to cover
cost sharing where cost sharing exists, or subsidize premiums that are
only a small part of costs and so are low to begin with, as in British
Columbia. In those instances the costs of error are low: waiting two
months for help with a $72 contribution is not the same as having to
wait for assistance to pay $400 per month. Only in Germany is a
substantial part of the population given a choice about whether to
contribute to a system of cross-subsidies. And many of those people,
the top 20 percent or so of the income bracket, participate because the
system is good and they do not want to risk exclusion if their risk
should rise.

The international standard finances whole systems, not individuals, in a redistributive manner. It proceeds in the following steps:

1. A system is created. It may have many pieces (as Japan does) or one basic organization (as the United Kingdom does).
2. Everybody (or almost everybody) is required to participate.
3. For the system as a whole or for specific subsystems (such as sickness funds), someone figures out how much money is needed.
4. A rule is made about how much everybody should contribute. This is defined in relationship to income: (a) In a sickness fund scheme, payers contribute a percentage of payroll (or other income, such as pensions); (b) if financing is through general revenue the decision is made in two stages. First, a national or provincial tax structure collects roughly in proportion to income, and then a budget determines what proportion of that revenue goes to health care, and thus what proportion of personal income is paid for health costs.[42]
5. The contribution rate is set to pay for expected costs, because there is no doubt about who will participate.

Any further adjustment, such as for cost-sharing assistance, is small. The key determination—how much money is needed and what a fair contribution rate is—can be made at the level of the system or fund rather than as a distinct figure for each household. The system is therefore quite simple to implement. If people are paying the right rates, the system will work.

Both the international standard and means-tested individual subsidies seek to adjust families' health insurance payments to their ability to pay. But the two approaches start from different premises about insurance. Individual subsidies start from the premise that each person chooses whether to be insured, and some choose, perhaps as a matter of charity, to help out others. The international standard presumes that everyone wants health care when sick. It then asks how people can organize themselves as a group to ensure that care. The notions of justice are similar, but the relationship of the individual to the community is different.

If Americans want to emphasize individualism, that is their choice. If they have any doubt, they should decide on practical grounds. By collecting contributions directly as a share of income, through pre-existing compulsory systems (general revenue taxation or a broader social security structure), the international standard risks little error, is simple to implement, and provides a stable insurance system. Any system of direct subsidies to individuals has none of these features, yet still, if it is to be adequate, requires the same net transfers from people with higher incomes to people with lower incomes.

The International Standard and Managed Competition

Proponents of systems with individual mandates might not be aware of the practical difficulties, or might choose to accept them. But the sponsors of the bills described in this chapter had one more reason to accept the difficulties of individual subsidies.

In the other systems described in this book, separate individual subsidies are either small or unnecessary because the rules of contribution, by requiring more from some people and less from others, already relate payment to ability to pay. In that approach, beneficiaries contribute to a system. They do not pay a price for personal insurance; they do not shop; they contribute.

The theory of managed competition presumes that beneficiaries shop. It seeks to reduce the level of insurance by imposing price constraints on individuals (or employers). They are supposed to *choose* to buy less. They will be able to do so only if their contributions are not determined by law, and if those individual contributions are large enough to be noticed. If they are large enough to be noticed, some people will not be able to afford them. Therefore, *managed competition inherently requires individual payments and thus some process of individual subsidies. It requires an inferior financing arrangement.* The Clinton administration's exceedingly complex plan for financing health care reform must be understood as an attempt to combine the cost-consciousness of managed competition theory with the advantages of the international standard. That is not easy.

Wishful Thinking in Chafee and Cooper-Grandy

This chapter has reviewed the major choices involved in setting up a system of managed competition without a global budget, by looking at two bills that adopted some of the theory of managed competition. In order to appeal to the same forces that object to adapting the international standard, these bills would have weakened the regulation necessary to govern the competition. In the case of some provisions, managed competition would have created grave administrative difficulties.

Chapter 7 argued that there is good reason to doubt that managed competition alone could provide affordable universal coverage. One may then wonder why anyone would think watered-down versions of managed competition, especially one as diluted as the Chafee bill, could do the job. A plausible answer is that some portion of those who backed Chafee or Cooper-Grandy, and some supporters of diluted proposals at the state level, wanted to upset entrenched interests as little as possible while still appearing to "do something." Making insurance "available," as defined in both bills, was an extreme version of favoring the appearance of action over action. But many sponsors surely wished to believe nonconflictual measures could work; they would be guilty more of wishful thinking than of any willful deception.

Both bills include measures that were also part of what chapter 10 describes as the "incremental" approach to reform. These were ideas that, good or bad, would not do as much good as their advocates claimed. Each bill encouraged the gathering of more information for consumers, the streamlining of data processing, and the development of more protocols and guidelines. These are all good ideas and appeal to the common desire to believe that technology can solve all problems.[43] But as I explained in chapter 7, there are many obstacles to developing adequate consumer information, and it cannot accomplish much. Each bill also included some extra preventive care benefits and strong incentives to encourage primary care residencies. Again, these are popular ideas endorsed by most health policy analysts, but they would do nothing to improve access to hospitals for people who are already in need.[44]

Both bills also included reforms of the malpractice system, designed to make lawsuits less likely. These included caps on noneconomic damages and on attorneys' fees as a share of damages. Such measures would make attorneys less likely to take cases for clients who could not pay on an hourly basis, and make them more likely to pursue cases for those with earning power (such as thirty-year-old MBAs) than for victims with little future earning potential (such as sixty-four-year-old housewives). Other provisions on the liability reform agenda included processes for mandatory arbitration; requirements that unsuccessful complainants pay or even post bond for court costs; and even, in Chafee, that plaintiffs' attorneys "at the time of entering into the agreement with respect to such hiring disclose . . . the estimated probability of success on the action" and expected billings. The latter proposal might force attorneys to be conservative in both their estimation and their levels of work in order to avoid being sued for malpractice themselves.[45] Such measures might have substantial effects on the malpractice litigation system. Yet, as I discussed in chapter 3, the argument that malpractice litigation significantly raises American health care costs is not supported by evidence.

Both bills sought medicare savings. A few of the measures were not controversial, such as making "temporary" savings from previous legislation permanent. Others, such as requiring higher cost sharing and charging higher medical benefit premiums for the wealthy elderly, were simply benefit cuts.[46]

The Clinton bill sought similar savings, but with a significant difference. Both Cooper-Grandy and Chafee risked creating situations in which prices rose more quickly in the private insurance than the medicare sector of health care. If that were to happen, providers might begin to refuse the medicare business, creating a two-tier system with the elderly on the lower tier. The Clinton bill's cost controls were more credible, so would be less likely to create medicare access problems. In short, more comprehensive cost control was safer for medicare beneficiaries than the partial measures in the Cooper-Grandy and Chafee bills.

As we have seen, the evidence for skepticism about managed care, combined with the Paygo rule, led to Cooper-Grandy's not promising universal coverage, Chafee's promising it far in the future if at all, and neither bill's specifying a benefit package.

At one level, the failure to specify a benefit package was just a deception: both Cooper-Grandy and Chafee included statements about the broad categories of benefits that would be covered, but by leaving their different commissions to determine any cost sharing, they enabled those bodies to make any coverage mean very little by requiring high enough out-of-pocket payments.[47]

But leaving benefits to be determined by a commission also appeals to some Americans' wishful thinking that a matter as important as health care reform could be determined without relying on "politics." That is a bad enough idea in principle.

Because the standard benefits would determine the tax treatment of health insurance, leaving that decision to a commission, if that could work, contradicts the basic constitutional provision that the legislature controls taxes, as well as the American Revolution's principle that taxation should be based on representation. But the largest problem is that the odds of a commission's actually operating without "political influence" are extremely low.

Establishing health benefits is very different from closing military bases, the model on which the commission process in the Chafee and Cooper-Grandy bills was based. Base closings are an issue of distribution: given that some will close, which districts and states will lose? A commission can choose a list of losers, who are a minority of Congress, and their colleagues can say, "don't blame us, the commission did it." But the potential losers from a health care benefit package would be in every district. They would also include many middle-class people who would lose from a more limited benefit package. Both the president and individual legislators would have plenty of incentive to disapprove the package offered by the commission and propose one of their own. Less generous benefits may be good for the budget, but they also raise taxes on the middle class. One should not assume that the political appointees to any commission would propose dramatic cuts in people's standard benefits.

Failing to specify the basic benefit package is an example of politicians trying to avoid responsibility. It may be popular with citizens who do not trust politicians with any responsibility, but is still a truly bad idea.

Conclusion: The Difficulty of a Synthesis

Chapter 7 explained why managed competition is an attractive idea and why it probably would not work. This chapter has reviewed the administrative and political vulnerabilities that make it even less likely to succeed.

The benefits of the international standard methods of cost control and coverage are proven; the benefits of managed competition are theoretical and highly unlikely. Yet, in spite of all its exaggerations, the case for some aspects of what managed competition proponents desire still has merit. The international methods are not perfect. America has, in its large group practices and its good HMOs, institutions that may offer savings and performance advantages even within a broader system that adapts the international standard. Trying to force people to join those institutions is not appropriate, but preserving them, and giving them a fair chance to grow, seems desirable.

Yet it is not easy. The conflict between creating financial incentives that favor more efficient plans and having an efficient and simple contribution system is illustrated by the one proposal in Congress during 1993–94 that explicitly accepted the international standard as the template for reform: the McDermott-Wellstone "single-payer" proposal.

McDermott-Wellstone guaranteed free choice of physician to everyone, had physicians in any one area all charging the same fees, and got its cost control from fee schedules and institutional budgets. It also provided for "comprehensive health services organizations" (CHSOs), which would have to have open enrollment up to their capacity. States could pay these plans by capitation or establish budgets for them. If the CHSO used an institutional facility that it did not own, it would have to reimburse the state for an appropriate part of the institution's budget (much as funds pay shares of hospital budgets in France). CHSOs could charge "reasonable" premiums for services not included in the national standard and would be subject to the same capital planning processes that other providers were. Each state would include a figure for CHSO spending in its annual budget.[48]

But why would anybody join? People could choose CHSOs over other plans for some combination of lower premiums, less cost sharing, and more extensive benefits. In the McDermott-Wellstone framework, no one would pay premiums, there would be very little cost sharing, and the benefits would be extensive. Under these circumstances it is hard to see what an HMO (or "CHSO") could offer customers that would seem to justify accepting a limited choice of providers.

There is another puzzle. This bill included capital budgeting, but it is not clear why that is appropriate for something like a CHSO. As long as those integrated plans accepted the basic payment structure, the state has no reason to care about their capacity. If a capitated plan spent more on capital one year and less on operations, people who objected could leave the plan. Conversely, if a CHSO managed to expand capacity in a way that attracted more customers, the state would have no reason to complain as long as its payments did not rise.

These examples suggest two points. First, group- or staff-model HMOs are more likely to prosper if the standard benefits include cost sharing for pharmaceuticals and other services, so the HMOs (or CHSOs) could attract customers by reducing or eliminating such charges. Second, it would make sense to exclude those HMOs from any capital regulation, as long as they were required to pay their fair share for the use of other capital facilities (for example, a capital contribution charge in addition to operating cost charge for use of hospitals that the CHSO did not own), and their total costs were controlled by a budget. A well-managed plan might then be able to provide better benefits to patients. If there is any legitimacy to the argument that care can be managed, it also might be able to pay providers more for their services than the fee-for-service sector. For example, the efficient and patient-friendly use of nonphysician practitioners could lower the cost of some services, allowing higher payments to the physicians who provide the other services.

The Clinton administration's proposal was comprehensible only as an effort to combine the good parts of managed competition with the international standard. Chapter 9 discusses the Clinton plan; chapter 10 discusses what Americans might do instead. For both Americans and international readers interested in a synthesis, however, one irony must be emphasized: if HMOs by any name are to compete with a system that adapts the international standard, patients must have reason to choose the former. That means something must be "wrong" with the latter from the patients' standpoint.

It is relatively easy to imagine an American reform that, with high cost sharing or insufficient subsidies, left room for competition from closed panels. In the NHS, restricted capacity clearly gives fundholders a chance to compete. It is much harder to imagine why voters in systems without cost sharing, with wide choice of provider, and with broad benefits, such as Canada and Germany, would be interested.

9

The Clinton Plan:
Managed Competition with a
Global Budget

ON September 10, 1992, the *New England Journal of Medicine* published health care reform statements from then-secretary of health and human services Louis W. Sullivan, representing the Bush administration, and from then-governor Bill Clinton. In his statement, the Democratic candidate for president listed the following "key elements" of his health care plan:

A national health board would establish a "core benefit package that must be available to every American" and "national and state budget targets." Provider networks and other insurers would offer "health care within the global budgets." States would "establish consistent rates outside managed-care networks as a backup mechanism to meet the global budget targets." Universal coverage would be "phased in by building on the public-private partnership that is uniquely American." Medicare would remain independent. Employers would purchase private health benefits directly or through "publicly sponsored alternatives." In addition:

Insurers, physicians, and health care institutions will be given strong incentives to collaborate in developing local health networks. . . . They will compete for patients enrolled in private or public health plans on the basis of both cost and quality. This structured form of competition will yield results far more productive than today's competition to avoid covering the sickest. Moreover, collaborative networks of health-care providers operating within global budgetary constraints could shelter the provider-patient relationship from some of the intrusive methods of many of today's efforts to control costs.

Clinton said there would be special provisions for small employers. There would be medical malpractice reform through alternative dispute resolution and development of guidelines, but the plan made no mention of lower contingency fees for lawyers or caps on noneconomic damages for victims. More money would be spent on and more effort put into preventive and primary care and health education. There would be some expansion of long-term care within the medicare program. Price increases for prescription drugs would be slowed through some form of regulation.[1]

Within the context of the choices posed in this book, Bill Clinton already knew where he wanted to go. In most significant ways, the bill introduced into Congress on October 27, 1993, was the plan he described during his campaign.

Most important, candidate and later President Clinton proposed "managed competition with a global budget." Rather than rely on competition alone to control costs, Clinton added that total premiums could not exceed a budget cap. Second, the system would be employer based, with some set of options. Individuals and employers would purchase insurance. Therefore it would not be a tax-based system. Third, candidate Clinton envisioned competing, integrated networks and built all-payer rate regulation of a fee-for-service system ("consistent rates") into the design as a "backup."

Bill Clinton never endorsed the Jackson Hole version of managed competition. He rejected Alain Enthoven's posing of the ideologue's choice of "an overall strategy based on reformed incentives and organization in a decentralized private market system, or . . . centralized, top-down government control."[2] As candidate and president, he sought a division of labor that he described in a speech on September 24, 1992:

> I want to keep consumers with a variety of choices, including access to local health care networks put together by insurers, hospitals, clinics and doctors—managed care networks that will receive the money they need to meet a consumer's full health care needs over a life time. By limiting a network's total spending, without interfering at all with its practices, the state by state budgets that I recommend will create real incentives for hospitals, clinics, doctors and consumers to reduce bureaucracy, eliminate unnecessary duplicative technology and practices, and cut waste on their own.[3]

Translating the campaign position into a legislative proposal required addressing a wide array of issues: how the health systems of the Department of Veterans Affairs, for civilian dependents of the military, the Federal Employee Health Benefit Program, and the Indian Health Service would fit into a new system; what the benefit package should include; how to structure malpractice reform and new long-term care benefits. In addition, new and expanded public health initiatives and all the apparatus of new quality and consumer protection provisions had to be designed. Each of these matters is important to many people, and they engaged many of the famed "five hundred experts" who gathered to prepare options and drafts of a plan in the winter and spring of 1993.[4]

But the really tough choices were who would subsidize whom, how the money would be collected, and how costs would be controlled. The Clinton adaptation of managed competition would have to address the issues described in chapter 8. What would be the roles of alliances: their geographic boundaries, the proportion of the population enrolled through them, and their powers to negotiate prices? What would be the incentives to purchase less expensive plans? How would the goal of eliminating risk competition be pursued? How would funds for subsidies be collected and then distributed? In a system of managed competition with a global budget there were further issues: how to set, allocate, and enforce the budget.

To explain the administration's Health Security Act I first summarize its basic logic and then analyze its most important individual provisions.[5]

Clinton's Combination of Competition and Regulation

Even if President Clinton believed competition would suffice to control costs quickly enough to pay for universal coverage, the Congressional Budget Office did not; and the administration's bill, like all others, had to satisfy the Paygo (pay-as-you-go) rule.

Regulating Premiums and Fees

The Clinton plan therefore provided for a national budget for the covered spending, allocated among alliances, and then enforced at the level of plans' premiums. Plan managers would know the target average premium in each alliance and that if they chose a higher figure, the new national health board might force them to accept a lower one. Either by anticipation or regulation, plans therefore would fit their prices into the budget.

Creating and enforcing an overall budget would short-circuit the questions about plans' competitive behavior that I raised in chapter 7. If necessary, the more expensive plans could be simply forced to lower their premiums. There could be no process of "follow the leader" in which competitors raised prices in tandem; and less expensive plans might be prevented from choosing higher profit margins by raising prices. Even better, CBO would credit the savings from premium controls. But these controls were obviously a form of regulation and did not fit into the administration's strategy of emphasizing the competitive, private market aspects of its plan. The administration therefore refused to admit that the caps were anything more than a "backup" that would probably not be necessary.[6]

The dream of competing integrated networks is made less practical by the fact that much of the country is sparsely populated, by public distaste for the necessary restrictions on choice, and by the difficulties of building such systems. In response to these problems, the administration's plan mandated, in every alliance area, the existence of at least one fee-for-service plan. Fee-for-service plans would be open to any provider who wished to participate. There could be no gatekeepers. Instead, their costs would be limited by a system of all-payer fee regulation. The fees and any volume adjustments could be negotiated between payers and providers within the alliance or legislated by a state government.[7]

The combination of premium regulation and these fee schedules meant that believers in the Jackson Hole version of managed competition viewed the Clinton plan as, in Alain Enthoven's words, "a single-payer system in Jackson Hole clothing."[8] Many of the Clinton administration's policy designers believed that the experiences of other countries and medicare showed that regulation was acceptable and the two approaches could and should be combined.[9] But again, the administration wanted to emphasize the competition and seemed embarrassed by the fee regulation. Explaining the plan in a special issue of *Health Affairs*, two central designers, Walter Zelman and Richard Kronick, never mentioned the fee schedules.[10]

The administration thus trapped itself in its own rhetoric. Other plans compromised in the wrong direction in order to meet objections to the necessary regulation in managed competition. The administration rightly filled the holes in competition with regulation, *but would not admit what it was doing, because it too wanted to appeal to people who distrusted government by emphasizing the plan's reliance on "competition."* Because opponents of reform were happy to point out the Clinton plan's offending provisions, the administration's strategy amounted to failing to defend its own plan.

Competing Plans within Alliances

The Clinton plan provided for one alliance per region, with mandatory participation. Only employers with five thousand or more employees could opt out of these regional alliances; those employers would establish "corporate alliances." The boundaries were restricted in much the same way that they were in the Chafee and Cooper-Grandy designs, so as to inhibit isolation of poorer populations in separate alliances.[11] The Clinton plan's alliances would have no real power to negotiate premiums—they would be price takers. Instead, premium regulation was left in the hands of the national health board.

But the Clinton alliances would be the main regulators of risk competition. They would do so in part by controlling plan marketing: plans would market mainly through the alliance structure. The regional alliances would also run a risk-adjustment process, according to a formula that would be devised by the board. The alliances would be able to administer the formula (however accurate) fairly easily, because they would receive the premium payments and then risk-adjust the amounts they sent on to the plans. Only the corporate alliances thus would be out of the risk-adjustment structure. It could be presumed that only corporations with lower than average risk would bother setting up corporate alliances. But given the small number of eligible employers, and requirements that they transfer some extra funds into the regional alliance system, this exception was nowhere near as significant as the holes in the Chafee or Cooper-Grandy processes.

INCENTIVES FOR COMPETITION. Political pressures from unions that would be big losers, and the huge practical obstacles described in chapter 8 and the appendix, caused the Clinton administration to abandon the idea of a cap on the tax deductibility of benefits.[12] Other measures would still have provided some incentive for employees to choose the less expensive plans.

All employers would be required to contribute to health care in a way that would pay for 80 percent of the local budget for employees and their families.[13] Employees would be expected to pay the difference between their preferred plan's premium and 80 percent of the target for their family type within that alliance. Prices could plausibly range from 80 percent to 120 percent of the target, so given the minimum employer payment, employees could pay from 0 to 40 percent of the target premium.

If employers chose to pay more than the standard, employees could take the difference in cash rather than insurance. Would employees prefer the cash, which could be taxed? Nobody knew, but the difference between the administration's incentive for employees to choose less expensive plans and the effect of the Cooper-Grandy or Chafee tax caps was less than it seemed even to people in the administration.[14] The incentive to choose the cash would be a significant change from the status quo. It was also an administrable proposal, unlike the tax deductibility cap.

Governing Institutions

The national health board and regional alliances would be the key new organizations in this scheme. But the board would rely on the Department of Health and Human Services (HHS) for much of its staffing, and that department's secretary, not the board, would have most of the enforcement powers at the federal level. Regional alliances would be in all fundamental ways creatures of the state governments.

STATE ROLES AND OPTIONS. Other proposals, such as Chafee's, gave many responsibilities to the states, but the Clinton administration was more careful to specify what was required. Each state would establish the alliance boundaries, establish the alliances, certify all health insurance plans, monitor plans' compliance with the criteria, regulate fees in the fee-for-service system, and require some plan or plans to cover an entire alliance area. States could allow alliances to set up all-payer negotiations with providers to negotiate the fee-for-service fee schedule.[15]

The plan also gave states the power to pursue different means to the ends of universal coverage and cost control. The case for encouraging different forms of health care reform in different states is especially strong since the ability to implement managed competition varies greatly by geography. The Clinton plan explicitly allowed creation of a single-payer system.[16] It also gave states the flexibility to blend competing networks and fee regulation in a way that looked more like a European all-payer rate regulation system than like competing networks. In order to allow a single-payer option, the Clinton plan established rules under which medicare patients (and their funding) could be included in a state's alternative system. To make all-payer regulation possible, the Health Security Act included provisions to alter or allow interpretation of the antitrust laws so as to allow bargaining between groups of insurers and providers, and waive the ERISA (Employee Retirement Income Security Act) restrictions on state regulation of self-insured corporate health plans. It therefore offered states far more flexibility than did proposals that claimed to emphasize the federal government less.

NATIONAL HEALTH BOARD. The Clinton plan called for this board to have seven members, with staggered terms and a chairman appointed by the president. Only its central responsibilities are considered here.[17]

The board would interpret the benefit package and recommend legislative changes. It would similarly interpret or develop rules of eligibility and certification. The board would set the national budget for spending on covered services and divide it into state and alliance budgets. These budgets would have to reflect the relative health care needs of different areas (risk), and the existing base of health care expenditure (some areas have higher prices and utilization than others). The draft legislation established the allowed percentage increases from year to year, all other things being equal. But the board would have to determine the baseline (spending in 1993), and would make adjustments for changes in demographics and for reform's effects on demand for services.[18] It would develop the risk-adjustment formulas to be applied both in its own budget making and to the risk adjustment among plans performed by the alliances.[19] These tasks would be very politically sensitive.

If states did not comply with requirements to participate in the system, the proposed national health board could impose sanctions.

If noncompliance were severe—for example, if the state simply did not implement a system—the board would notify the secretary of health and human services that she should establish the system in that state under federal authority.[20]

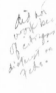

Given a regional alliance, plans, and budget, *the board would enforce the premium cap upon the plans.* (The board would also establish methods to set targets for corporate alliances, but enforcing them would be the secretary of labor's problem.) I explain that process in the analysis of crucial parts of the Clinton proposal.

Other federal departments would have significant responsibilities. HHS would administer a wide range of changes in the medicare program, the quality improvement and information dissemination systems, and public health and work force initiatives. If states failed to exercise their own responsibilities, HHS would run the regional alliances itself. The Labor Department would have basic regulatory authority over the corporate alliances.[21] The Treasury Department, naturally, would deal with revenue measures, and the Justice Department with antitrust reforms.

Benefits and Coverage

The Health Security Act would have guaranteed health insurance for all citizens and other legal residents of the United States effective January 1, 1998. It thus contemplated a three-year phasein of universal coverage. Persons would be enrolled in plans in four statuses: single, couple, single parent, and "dual parent."[22] There would be no age categories. The bill provided rules for combinations of residence and employment, such as a person having two jobs, two persons in one family being eligible for different alliances, veterans, and military personnel.[23]

BENEFITS WITHIN THE ALLIANCES. Candidate Clinton had suggested allowing the board to define benefits, but his bill was as precise as one could reasonably expect through legislation. Aside from basic hospital and physician services, the plan covered a wide array of other benefits, possibly including abortion.[24] There would be benefits for hospice care, home health care, and extended care similar to those for medicare, though with some specific limits in the bill.[25] Pharmaceuticals, rehabilitation services, and durable medical equipment would be covered but with special cost-sharing provisions. The bill listed covered clinical preventive services, with schedules for how often they would be provided.[26] Mental health benefits were defined in terms of types of treatments and with specific limits—for example, "Prior to January 1, 2001, psychotherapy and collateral services are subject to an aggregate annual limit of 30 visits per individual." A major expansion was scheduled for the year 2001.[27] Vision and dental care were limited to specific types or beneficiaries (to children, for example), though also were scheduled for expansion in 2001.[28]

Most important, the administration defined its cost sharing in its draft law. There would be three versions: low, high, and combination. All three would limit individual out-of-pocket payments for a year to $1,500, and family out-of-pocket payments to $3,000. Plans with lower cost sharing would have required no copayments for inpatient services and preventive care and low flat fees (for example, $10 for outpatient visits) for other services. Plans with high cost sharing would have required coinsurance of 20 percent for most services and had a system of deductibles.[29] Combination plans would have charged essentially the lower rate for in-network services and the higher rate out of network.[30]

The package was better in some ways and worse in others than what was already available through employers in the United States.[31] Persons who chose to pay more would get better benefits in the form of lower cost sharing. Even the schedule for high cost sharing did not require higher proportional contributions than in France. But the much higher prices in the United States would make that coinsurance more of a burden in America, and, as described in chapter 5, most of the French have supplementary insurance. On balance, the Clinton benefit package was in the ballpark of other countries but, at least until the expansions in 2001, on the low end of the scale.

According to the bill, families with incomes below 150 percent of the poverty level could apply for subsidies to help with the cost sharing so that, even if they could not manage to enroll in a plan with low cost sharing, they would pay the lower rate. The much poorer families receiving aid to families with dependent children (AFDC) or supplemental security income (SSI) would pay only 20 percent of the low cost-sharing rate (thus, $2 for an office visit and $5 for a trip to the emergency room).[32] The administration required that everyone contribute something out-of-pocket as a matter of principle, a belief that the act of payment increased individual responsibility.

CHANGES TO MEDICARE AND MEDICAID. The plan would not have insured the elderly through the alliance system unless they qualified as employees or spouses,[33] or their state received a waiver to fold medicare into the state system.[34] Medicaid would survive as a long-term care program only, with some modest changes.[35] The Clinton plan created a new program to continue medicaid's extra benefits for qualified children.[36]

Like Cooper-Grandy and Chafee, the HSA included tighter medicare cost controls to help pay for coverage expansions. Unlike those bills, it used some of the money for countervailing expansions in medicare itself.[37] First, medicare part B would add a pharmaceutical benefit.[38] Second, the bill created a new federal program for home- and community-based long-term care. It would be operated by the states, which would receive payments from the federal government according to a formula within a cap.[39] That budget would rise from $4.5 billion in fiscal year 1996 to $38.3 billion in fiscal year 2003. This program also would have cost sharing and would be means-tested as well.[40]

Thus programs for the medicare population would be expanded while spending for its basic package was being constrained. The plan also explicitly banned extra billing.[41] On balance, then, the HSA was better for the elderly than any plan except McDermott-Wellstone's single-payer system. But it left the elderly with fewer benefits than the general population. The new pharmaceutical benefit was not as good as in the alliances, and the elderly's hospitalization benefits would still be capped.

Medicare is less adequate than the standard package in any other country in this study. The fact that it would be made only marginally better testifies to the power of the deficit constraint, which prevented even fair expansions of benefits to the most powerful interest group in the country.

Financing the Health Security Act

COLLECTING THE MONEY. The Clinton plan left much of the government health care spending and revenue intact, such as for medicare and veterans' and medicaid long-term care programs. States, then, were required to maintain their previous effort in support of the medicaid acute-care population.[42] They would pay this money to the alliances, which also would be receiving money from employers, individuals, and the federal government. (See the appendix for more details.)

PAYMENTS TO THE ALLIANCES. We can think of the money flowing into an alliance as going into three separate accounts. The employer account would be expected to cover 80 percent of total costs—the "alliance credit amount"—for families covered through employment, and it would receive funds mainly from employers.[43] In contributing their portion of the funds, employers *would not* be paying 80 percent of the costs of insurance per employee, because workers in two-income families would not need full payments from each employer. Another fund, the employee or individual account, would pay for the other 20 percent of costs for employees and be funded mainly from individual payments. A separate subsidy account would receive money from the federal government and states and use it to pay for insurance for nonworkers and for transfers to cover shortfalls in the other two accounts.

Thus when a person ordered insurance through the alliance, the alliance would assume that 80 percent of her target premium was paid for from the employer or subsidy funds.[44] The alliance would pay this "alliance credit amount" to the plan she selected without regard to whether she was actually employed or how much her employer contributed on her behalf. The alliance's only concern would be that the total of employer and government contributions to its funds was enough to pay total credits. Thus, as in a sickness fund system, the focus would be on defining contribution rules that bring in enough money and on ensuring that contributions were made.

But individuals and families would be personally responsible for the balance of their premium costs, and the alliance would keep track. Because the alliance could refuse to offer any plan that cost more than 120 percent of the average, and there would be no point in charging less than 80 percent, families would choose to pay somewhere between 0 and 40 percent.[45] The average would equal 20 percent.

This design created a price constraint, but it eased subsidy administration because, if a person's status changed, the alliance credit would not be affected. If she were paying a $450 premium per month, and that were also the target, the alliance would pay $360 and the family $90. In Chafee, Cooper-Grandy, or the current system, when a family's sole breadwinner loses a job, the family suddenly has to make both its own personal contribution and the former employer's, so $450. But in the Clinton plan, the family would still be responsible for only the $90. An unemployed person might still need help, but the consequences of either delay (for individuals) or error (for individuals and the government) would be a fifth as large.

There were some further protections for individuals, but the total of all individual subsidies in the Clinton bill was much less than in a system of means-tested subsidies for the full cost of insurance. Therefore, in comparison with Cooper-Grandy or Chafee, the phaseout of assistance in the Clinton bill involved a much lower extra marginal "tax," so was fairer and created fewer work disincentives.[46]

THE EMPLOYER MANDATE. This system to create price incentives for individuals without the administrative difficulties and policy perversities of entirely individual payment depended on having a separate flow of funds from employers. That employer contribution, aside from encountering resistance in principle, also raised a wide range of issues about the relative contributions of employers.

First, how would the plan ensure that employers could afford their contributions? Under its basic contribution rules, an employer who was required to contribute on behalf of a previously uninsured employee with children could easily be paying more than 20 percent more for that employee than without the health care contribution (see the example in the appendix). If employer payments were defined as a percentage of each employee's wage, no employer would have seen his wage bill increase so dramatically, but that evidently seemed too much like a payroll tax for political purposes. Instead, the bill limited the extra compensation expenses required of any employer by capping each employer's obligation at 7.9 percent of total payroll.[47]

That approach requires some extra record-keeping (adding up total payrolls) but would have been easier to administer than what the administration did next. In a bid for support from small business, the administration provided lower caps on a sliding scale for employers with fewer than seventy-six employees and wages below various limits. For example, employers with fewer than twenty-five employees and an average annual wage per full-time-equivalent employee of $12,000 or less were to pay no more than 3.5 percent of total payroll. Such discounts would reduce the funds in the employer account and so require more funds from other sources. The plan provided subsidies for low-wage companies far greater than the very large subsidies inherent in any system of percentage of payroll premiums. Differential rates would also have provided incentives for companies to try to gain those rates—for example, by setting up separate units with low-wage employees. "The outsourcing of employees," administration estimators acknowledged, "is a primary concern of the administration, both fiscally and economically."[48]

A second issue was how to treat employer-provided benefits for retirees. Many large employers paid such costs. If employers were told to maintain their existing contributions, writing rules to determine which employers should pay how much would be very difficult. Plans varied; most employers did not pay; in the ordinary course of labor bargaining provisions do change; requiring employers that currently provided partial coverage to instead pay for full coverage would punish them for previous good deeds. What would be done with new retirees? Where would the money even go? On what basis would the alliances collect it and budget it? Could retirees be expected to pay a contribution from their pension or other retirement earnings if they had not been making such payments before?

Any answer seemed either to impose an unfair cost or to provide a windfall benefit to someone. The administration chose to base employer contributions on employment and to exempt retirees who were over age fifty-five and had met medicare's work requirements from contributing to the employer account.[49] So employers who already paid for retirees would pay much less (if anything), and the retirees would not have extra costs (save their 20 percent).[50] As politics this was a bid for support from smokestack industries and from their workers: a core Democratic constituency. As economics the policy was a subsidy to important industries burdened by especially high health care costs. It would be criticized as a subsidy to big business, but none of the countries in this study expect large corporations to pay separately for their own retirees.

Third, what would be the distributional effects of having two forms of alliances? Restricting corporate alliances to very large employers meant fewer would opt out of the regional alliance pool in order to take advantage of the lower cost of having healthier workers. Conversely, creating regional alliances would allow large corporations that currently had less healthy workers to enter the system and pay less than they were paying before. The Clinton plan therefore limited the advantages of staying out by providing a 1 percent of payroll surcharge on all corporate alliances. It phased in the advantages of joining the regional alliance for any employer that had an expensive pool of employees, by requiring extra contributions for seven years.[51]

OTHER SOURCES OF FUNDS. All of these distributional issues related to the employer mandate involve only one flow of funds, the one from employers. The flow of funds from the government (subsidies) had to be large enough to cover shortfalls in both employer and individual contributions. The vast majority of that money would come from existing revenues, mainly those used for medicare and medicaid. Relative to the status quo, the reformed system would gather new revenues from some employers' contributions to the alliances and from the premiums paid by newly insured individuals. These sources would not yield quite enough money to cover the new costs. The proposal therefore would have increased taxes on cigarettes by 75 cents per pack and on other tobacco products by "approximately the same amount per pound of tobacco content." Other measures included plugging some potential loopholes, requiring all state and local employees to pay the medicare payroll tax and the tax on extra wages if employees chose them instead of surplus insurance.[52] Because the bill also included some new tax preferences, such as raising to 100 percent the amount of insurance payments that could be deducted by the self-employed, and for long-term care, the net extra revenue was fairly small: $29 billion in 1999.[53] Still, the revenue was necessary to pass the Paygo test, and all the increases could be justified as related to health care; they did not have to be called new general taxes.[54]

CONCLUSION. The Clinton administration's financing proposals were complex and controversial. The complexity followed from three choices: to maintain some form of price incentive in line with managed competition, to avoid a straight percentage-of-payroll contribution scheme for the employment-related, mandated contributions, and to give further subsidies to "small business." The controversy was unavoidable: no matter how a plan was designed, somebody would have to spend new money to finance new benefits.

Because the Clinton plan relied on employer payments, small employers were the most fervent opponents of reform. But relying instead on such middle-class taxes as a value added tax would not have been any more popular. Relying on individual payments is no answer at all, because some people cannot afford to pay. There was no politically safe, and perhaps no passable, road.

Analysis of the Clinton Plan

In practice, the Clinton proposal turned out to be yet another prototype: something that would not be enacted but that illuminated the choices involved in its basic approach: managed competition with a global budget and the necessary financing for universal coverage.

Suggestions for compromise during the legislative process weakened the prototype by turning crucial provisions into options; for example, the budgeting would not happen unless voluntary cost controls failed, or the employer mandate would not go into effect unless voluntary methods did not meet an enrollment standard by a preset date. Both of these compromises contemplated some sort of "trigger," but no trigger could have been pulled automatically, without protest. Similarly, alliances could be made "optional" rather than required, but states would then be left with responsibility to perform the alliances' basic functions.[55]

Any measures that left choices for later, or up to the states, still would require that policymakers eventually engage the issues raised by the Clinton design. The key issues fall into three categories: the roles of alliances, budgeting, and plans and providers.

Alliances in the Clinton Plan

Clinton's regional alliances would have collected funds from employers, beneficiaries, and the government and forwarded payments to each plan. They would have enforced risk adjustments by paying each plan a "blended plan per capita payment amount" that accounted for risk (as best as possible) and for membership by SSI and AFDC beneficiaries.[56]

SIZE AND BOUNDARIES. Clinton's boundary provisions were similar to those in the Chafee and Cooper-Grandy proposals. Making the alliances mandatory for all employers with fewer than five thousand employees was very different. There are no compelling reasons to choose five thousand rather than, say, three thousand or seven thousand. Chapter 8 explained why a number much higher than one hundred, with mandatory participation, was advisable. Walter Zelman summarized the administration's reasons:

A significantly lower cutoff would leave thousands of employers outside the alliance. This would dramatically decrease portability of insurance coverage and increase administrative costs and complexity as individuals and their families and dependents moved between regional alliance and nonalliance circumstances. Moreover, making certain that nonalliance employers were delivering the guaranteed benefits would entail a major regulatory effort, especially if self-insurance were allowed. Such an apparatus might be a worthwhile investment if there were any evidence that mid-size employers can genuinely reduce health care costs. But little, if any, such evidence exists. In most cases, the best such employers can do to reduce costs is to obtain better risk-based, short-term deals. But over time, all concerned—families especially—are better off if guaranteed more security through maintenance of a fair price guaranteed over the long term.[57]

ALLIANCES AND SUBSIDY ADMINISTRATION. The set of subsidies and transfers built into the Health Security Act represented a daunting administrative burden. Though the subsidies to individuals would have been smaller than in Chafee or Cooper-Grandy, they still would have required substantial new bureaucracy, as would risk adjustment and the calculations of employer limits. It is easy to criticize the decision to allocate those responsibilities to a semipublic body such as the alliance. Unfortunately, all the possible candidates to operate a subsidy system have evident disadvantages (see the appendix). The design in the Clinton plan might be the best option, yet three points are clearly important for future debate.

First, it is easier to administer subsidies if there are fewer of them. Special subsidies to some employers greatly complicate the task. Second, the major difficulties from state administration stem from the conflict of interest between the states and the federal government. If the federal contribution were fixed, as in Canada, state administration would not threaten the federal budget. Last, if one is going to have individual subsidies, the problems finding the right institution to administer them are yet another reason to try to limit individual premium payments to only a small part of total costs, and thereby limit the consequences of error.

INFLUENCE ON COSTS. In spite of their size and mandatory character, Clinton's alliances were not price makers in the mold of CalPERS (the California Public Employee Retirement System). Aside from refusing to contract with any state-certified plan that charged more than 120 percent of the target premium, an alliance had no negotiating power. If a plan and alliance did not agree, "the final bid submitted by a plan . . . [would] be considered to be the final accepted bid." The alliance could not reject a bid and had no inducements it could offer or sanctions it could impose.[58]

The administration could not trust the market to create premiums that fit budget targets, yet also did not want government agents to have any discretionary power over plans. A regional alliance that could negotiate like CalPERS would pose serious questions of governance: on what basis could alliance boards have that kind of life-or-death power over plans? Legal challenges as to arbitrariness or due process would have been likely. The search for a less discretionary but certain limit on premiums led to a process governed not by the alliances but by the bill's national health board. Its problems are discussed below and in the appendix.

Budgeting American Health Care

Any attempt to budget the costs of health care must first define the budget's proper scope. A budget should apply only to costs for providing the standard benefit package to all Americans, because that standard defines the difference between care that must be guaranteed as a matter of social decency and the further care that constitutes discretionary consumption. There is no more reason to limit discretionary health care consumption than any other consumption good. And if an item is viewed as nondiscretionary, it should be in the standard package, guaranteed to all.

Budgeting for the costs of the standard package then involves three issues. First, what is the proper total? Second, how can that total be allocated within a geographic area? Third, how can it be enforced?

CLINTON'S TARGET. Chapter 6 argued that, based on comparison to costs and services in other systems, the cost control goals of the Clinton health care plan seemed modest. At the end of 1993 the administration projected spending 16.9 percent of GDP in the year 2000; without any legislation, according to CBO's "baseline" estimates, total American health care spending would have been 18.2 percent. The difference of 1.3 percent of GDP was just over 7 percent of the total.

As Uwe Reinhardt wrote, "It is a remarkable comment on our health system—and on our political system as well—that this rather modest program of cost containment is decried as sheer fantasy."[59]

Yet so it was. The experts were all over the map on this issue. Reinhardt supported the target. Stuart Altman, codirector of the administration's transition task force on health care reform, declared that "the reductions suggested by the Clinton plan seem unrealistically tough."[60] Henry Aaron referred to "the ferocity of the implied cost containment."[61] Jack Hadley and Stephen Zuckerman, however, called the administration's savings target "a relatively modest one," and "the principle of using cost savings to achieve universal coverage . . . sound."[62]

Supporters of the target were looking at the spending totals, comparing them with other spending totals, and asking if the goals for the change in totals were reasonable. In chapter 6 I asked, in essence, how much of the difference in costs between the United States and Canada could be explained by factors that could be eliminated (administrative costs) or slowly shaved (fees), and concluded that over time the savings contemplated by the administration were quite plausible. The international comparison builds in a control for the costs of expanding coverage, because other countries already have universal coverage.

Skeptics saw an existing trend in costs and a proposed change in the trend, and the latter seemed "tough" or "ferocious" to them. This conflict in perspective can be resolved if we distinguish between a system during and after the reform period.

Absent structural change, holding cost increases per person to the growth of the consumer price index is stringent cost control. Even holding total health care cost increases to the rate of growth of GDP, which includes both price increases and productivity growth, can be difficult.[63] But major reform involves structural change, and as that is implemented a system can realize some one-time savings. In moving to a single-payer system, one-time savings would include reductions in administrative costs from simplification of insurance. From a managed competition perspective, they would include the savings from people moving into lower-cost plans. In either case a time comes when further savings are unlikely: administrative costs are down to a reasonable level, or everyone who is likely to accept greater managed care has done so. But during the restructuring the process of realizing one-time savings allows a slower growth of costs than in a stable system.

Analysts who compared the Clinton targets to rates of growth per capita in other OECD nations during the 1980s were comparing to systems that were not benefiting from such restructuring.

Second, growth in costs per capita is not the right standard for stringency of cost control in the context of an expansion of coverage. Who, after all, is hurt by cost control? Providers. What is hurt? Their incomes. Although reform may reduce their incomes per insured patient, it also increases the number of insured patients. Most providers would probably prefer to do less work for higher fees, but increased volume would compensate for at least some of the financial pain of lower prices per patient. It would mean that fixed costs for capital equipment were amortized over more uses, and some of the increased work would be for people who are otherwise idle—for instance, the overstaffed MRI (magnetic resonance imaging) and other diagnostic units discussed in chapter 6's comparison of Canadian and American hospitals. *Criticisms of the Clinton administration's targets for the first five years failed to adjust for both the one-time savings from restructuring and the fact that during the transition premiums from the larger number of insured persons would compensate providers substantially for the restrictions in premium increases.*

After reform was completely implemented (in the year 2000), the Clinton plan would have limited increases not to the growth of consumer prices but to the growth of gross domestic product—a target that Germany and Australia, among other countries, met for most of the 1980s. And the bill also called for the national health board to recommend alternative standards.[64] The targets were sensible in the short run and reasonable and appropriately flexible in the long run. Similar targets would be appropriate in any reform with cost controls based on experience rather than speculation.

ALLOCATING THE BUDGET AMONG REGIONS. Dividing the total among alliances would be more difficult. Would Congress really accept a risk-adjustment system that would affect the distribution of funds to every state and district? Perhaps, because changing a formula is hard—but only perhaps. As long as the national health board set the original formula at something close to the existing distribution of costs, its allocations might pass muster. Unfortunately, nobody knew the existing costs in each state. Surrogate figures, such as shares of current medicare spending, might be used as a basis for dividing the pie. Yet it is hard to imagine Congress staying entirely out of a distributional fight when the data are not totally credible (it got heavily involved in adjustments to the 1990 census, for example).

Devising an allocation is not impossible. Congress does so successfully for other grant programs. Yet the difficulty should alert readers to an alternative.

If the federal contribution were limited it could still be redistributive, as the federal grants in Australia and Canada are. And as usual, Congress would fight about how it was distributed. States, however, could set their own budgets. They could then complain about their subsidies, but not that the national government was claiming to know more about their health care needs than they did.

ENFORCING THE BUDGET AT THE LEVEL OF THE HEALTH PLAN. However the budget is allocated among regions, that difficulty would not compare to the problems of translating the budget into premiums for plans.In its effort to limit the discretion of federal or other officials, the Clinton plan relied on the national health board to manage and adjust a bidding process, so it would punish plans whose bids were too high in a nearly automatic manner.

Again there is more detail in the appendix. Here we begin with the standard. Spending in any alliance would depend on how many families of which premium types (single, couple without children, one adult with child(ren), couple with child(ren))[65] signed up for plans at their different prices. The average of all these premiums, weighted by the proportions who signed up for each plan, would be the *weighted average premium*.

The weighted average would have thus depended on two things: the plans' premiums and how many people signed up for each of them. The regulatory structure would have had to estimate the product of those two factors, and then force reductions in the premiums of plans whose prices were by some standard "too high."

In the Clinton design, this process ostensibly gave plans a choice to reduce their bids without being forced to do so. Also, by articulating clear standards in advance (the target premium in the first year and a target increase in subsequent years), it left up to a plan's managers whether to risk regulation. The whole structure was designed to blunt charges that the board would have great discretion and arbitrary power.

Unfortunately, within the structure as designed, if a plan ever bid less than its costs, it would have had a very difficult time ever obtaining an increase that would enable it to recoup its losses— even if its customers were willing to pay and its price were below the average. As a result, plans would have had strong incentives to play safe and bid high, not low. The risks of the regulatory structure could counteract any incentives to bid low as part of competition. In short, the Clinton plan's automatic premium regulation practically guaranteed perverse results. Regulation, to be responsible, requires some discretion.

Plans, Providers, and the Clinton Cost Controls

There would be no problem, however, if we could be sure that the plans whose premiums were reduced would not lose money or have to significantly reduce the quality of care. Then the cuts would force them to do something that they should have done anyway.

KEEPING COSTS WITHIN REDUCED PREMIUMS. The administration's decisionmakers knew plans might have difficulty meeting a premium target lower than their own bid. They provided some clever, perhaps even sneaky, incentives for plans to do so nonetheless (see the appendix). But if the plans did not, the HSA provided that plans whose premiums were reduced would automatically have their contracted payments to providers reduced as well.

This system might have controlled costs, but consider its implications. Providers who contracted in good faith for one level of payment would be forced to accept a lower amount. Nonnetwork providers would be in the absurd position of receiving lower payments from "noncomplying" plans than from complying plans that could be less expensive. The threat of such a result might make providers more likely to contract with less expensive plans, but expecting providers to guess about (or even understand) such complications is neither fair nor reasonable. If a plan tried to meet the target in some other manner, it could only do more of whatever it was already doing: turn down services through utilization review, pressure its risk-bearing gatekeepers, or, in a group- or staff-model HMO, perhaps make access less convenient. Either way, the mechanical enforcement methods that would reduce premiums to make total costs fit budgets would have perverse or unpleasant effects. Yet the administration could not do without the premium caps, because CBO relied heavily on them in scoring the administration's bill.[66]

Can budgets be made and enforced without these problems at the plan level? I suggest a way in chapter 10, but one point should be made here. The budgeting in the Clinton plan was as extensive as any in the world. Because plans would include all costs, all covered costs would be budgeted. In contrast, in Great Britain pharmaceutical costs are budgeted only for Britons who use fundholders; and they are not budgeted in any other country in this study save, very recently, Germany. Hospital costs are budgeted in many places, but the costs of physician services have only recently been subjected to hard caps in a few places.

A slightly looser U.S. budget system could work, as long as the federal government's own spending, the figure that is subject to Paygo, were credibly limited.

NETWORKS AND CHOICE OF PROVIDER. Within the Clinton plan's budgets, health plans would compete to attract customers. The draft act banned risk-rating in strong language.[67] Regulations would hinder efforts to limit membership to less-risky people through targeted marketing.[68] Once its premiums were determined, a plan could vary its prices only according to the differentials for family type established by the board.

Critics of the Clinton proposal emphasized that competing plans would reduce choice of physician. In fact, their charges were much more true of any managed competition plan than of a mixed plan like the administration's.[69] Every regional alliance would have to offer its members at least one fee-for-service plan. A fee-for-service plan would cover its members "for all items and services included in the comprehensive benefit package that are furnished by any lawful health care provider of the enrollee's choice," and would make "payment to such a provider without regard to whether or not there is a contractual arrangement between the plan and the provider."[70]

They would not be a physician's dream of unregulated fee-for-service medicine, but fee-for-service plans could offer patients substantial choice of physicians. The only exception would be for physicians who practiced exclusively within networks. The administration also required that all network plans, even group- and staff-model HMOs, offer "point-of-service options," separate packages in which, for a higher premium, people could use the network but have the right to pay for care outside the network according to the fee-for-service schedule and the bill's "high" cost sharing.[71]

A non-fee-for-service plan, then, would normally use a limited network of providers. It would pay according to the applicable fee schedule for services provided "out of network" if a customer were traveling outside the plan's service area, or for emergencies. It would have to disclose its utilization review protocols, so customers could compare restrictions.[72]

All of these measures—the encouragement of out-of-network care, the fee schedules to keep it affordable, having most people in the alliances that offered greatest choice of plan, and the protections for particular providers described later in this section—did far more to protect choice than either the Chafee or the Cooper-Grandy plan. The Clinton plan offered more choice than is currently available in most of the country. For example, as a former member of the Kaiser Permanente HMO I could choose to rejoin Kaiser because I would no longer be restricted to plans that my employer offered.

COMPETITION'S EFFECTS ON PARTICULAR PROVIDERS. Access and choice depend not only on insurance but also on the distribution of providers. As is the case in Great Britain, competition risks harm to providers that a system cannot do without. While the United States has some excesses it also has some shortages, such as primary care in the inner city. There is also reason to worry that academic medical centers, crucial parts of the system, could be endangered by health plans' selective contracting.

All of the proposals contained measures to encourage providers to set up shop in neighborhoods that are either unpleasantly urban or rural. The Clinton bill's guarantee that fee-for-service care would survive should have been more important, because fee-for-service payment gives providers a financial incentive to do business where patients have more need on average. But the reasons physicians do not want to work or live in those areas are not simply matters of money.

The draft HSA required that, for the first five years, all networks agree to pay for services from "essential community providers," such as migrant health centers, rural health clinics, and community health clinics.[73] Since the secretary of HHS could choose to define providers in "health professional shortage areas" as "essential," this provision could address the problem of less expensive plans' not having facilities in the areas of greatest need. Yet it inevitably contradicted the basic logic of managed care: if the secretary used her authority broadly, plans could be providing care to a lot of people through providers outside of their networks, making managing themselves much more difficult.

Whether academic medical centers would really be threatened by an environment of competition is a subject of some dispute: on the one hand they have higher costs; on the other, when patients (rather than employers) choose plans, one of the first questions is, what hospital are you affiliated with? Affiliation with the most prestigious centers is a surrogate measure of quality. Nevertheless, given the AMCs' role in research, teaching, and providing care to the poor, plans should err on the side of favoring those institutions.

The administration's bill provided many measures to guarantee business to the AMCs and to subsidize them for some extra costs. It did not include the most obvious measure, direct payment, by a budget, of medical education costs (as in many other countries). But it did provide separate financing for medical residencies and allow some discretionary grants to cover the higher costs of treatment that sometimes are associated with medical education.[74] There is little doubt that policies about the AMCs or medical education require federal action. Not only do states with the lowest incomes have particular problems, but the academic medical centers are concentrated disproportionately in certain states that could not possibly manage the subsidies themselves (for example, Massachusetts).

One more item is related to both costs and access: whether to allow extra billing. The Clinton plan banned it.[75] This ban would have made the development of tiers of providers, with patients sorted among providers according to patients' ability to pay, much less likely. It thus was supported by reformers who wanted more equal care. Physicians, however, objected to the ban on extra billing in the Clinton bill, just as they object in Australia and resisted in Canada. So banning extra billing had political costs.

TYPES OF PLANS. There is no doubt that the administration's central policy designers, just like Cooper-Grandy's, dreamed of a system in which competing group- and staff-model HMOs would provide services to all Americans. Chapter 7 explained why this would be unlikely to occur.

On day one, therefore, most plans that bid to provide care would control costs through third-party managed care and/or risk-bearing gatekeepers. Under these circumstances, the new system might not be simpler or save money on administration. Costs of dealing with utilization review and gatekeepers would be unlikely to decline. Physicians would participate in multiple plans—after all, if they were going to be in only one plan, they might as well join a group- or staff-model HMO. Networks would not pay the same rates as those on the fee-for-service schedule because one of the points of setting up a network is to provide a discount. Physicians then would still have to deal with multiple utilization restrictions and payment schedules.

The new system would save money on administration to the extent that it discouraged risk-rating. But the costs of administering the alliances and subsidies would eat up some of those savings. And the larger administrative costs, those created in hospitals and doctors' offices as the providers dealt with the multiple payers, would hardly be reduced at all.

Within a world of managed care alone, the administration simply could not provide what it promised. Choice contradicts administrative simplification, because the simplest forms of managed care, the group- and staff-model HMOs, restrict care the most. Premium regulation on the dominant forms of managed care would probably lower quality. But the administration's bill, though the administration did not seem to want to admit it, was not simply a managed care plan. It included a regulated fee-for-service sector, which could make a huge difference.

THE FEE-FOR-SERVICE OPTION. The Clinton plan would have created the following delivery system, at the beginning.

Group- and staff-model HMOs could not grow quickly, but they would be able to charge lower premiums or promise the lower cost sharing, and therefore at least maintain market share and probably grow. Back in the rest of the system there would be three, not two, forms of delivery: particular third-party managed care systems, risk-bearing gatekeeper systems, and the fee-for-service world. Within the latter, total spending would be limited not just by the fee schedule but by volume adjustments similar to the current medicare volume performance standards, and medicare-style prospective payment based on DRGs (diagnosis-related groups) for institutional care. The fee-for-service systems would offer fewer hassles and greater choice than the alternatives, and given the volume adjustments and fee schedules, they would also have tools to control costs at least as well.

In a positive scenario, the other forms of managed care would decline, and the system would evolve toward group- and staff-model HMOs competing with a regulated fee-for-service sector. The presence of the fee-for-service system would at least provide increased access and fewer hassles than a world in which open-panel fee-for-service care no longer existed—the current goal of the large American insurers.[76]

A regulated fee-for-service system has one other advantage: we know how to fit it into a budget cap. The institutions, essentially fees with volume adjustments, already exist and have been used in other countries and, in a "soft" form, in medicare. The Health Security Act provided explicitly that fee schedules could be based on prospective budgeting, in which payers and providers agreed on totals for each sector of health expenditures, and payments per service could be adjusted to fit into the budget.[77]

The form of such fee schedules with volume adjustments would be determined in negotiations between a state or alliance and the providers. There is no reason the alliance could not give insurers a large role in negotiating the targets, subject to alliance approval; the result would be defined as "state action" and would not be subject to antitrust law.[78]

The specific provisions in the act might not have allowed payment of different amounts to hospitals, in accord with their different historical and fixed costs. Whether hospitals are budgeted through lump-sum payments or through prospective rate setting, the Australians, British, Canadians, French, and Germans all consider each hospital's unique characteristics and plan payments accordingly. In the United States, in contrast, the purpose of the medicare system of prospective payments and DRGs is to force hospitals with higher costs to find savings, and reward institutions with lower costs. But we already cover some sources of differential costs with special payments, and the HSA included some as well. On balance, the case for allowing payers to negotiate different rates with different hospitals sounds strongest, but the HSA might have included sufficient flexibility to accommodate differences through other payments.

Capital spending limits are another matter. The HSA was virtually silent on that form of cost control. It had detailed provisions for re-orienting physician training from specialization to primary care but did not address issues of physical capacity.[79] Chapter 7 argued that one cannot simply rely on managed competition to control system capacity—unless one is willing to take some grave risks of both under- and overcapacity. A reformed system would require some measures to limit and direct investment.

Yet such regulation is probably not a federal matter. It is not a national decision in any of the federal countries described in this book. The effective markets for capacity are at the state or a lower level, and states must have better information than the federal government about those markets so that there is no technical administrative reason to do capital planning at the national level. Australia, Canada, and Germany also do not see any good policy reason to deny states the right to make their own capacity decisions. If favoring states is acceptable in other countries, it surely makes sense in a huge country like the United States.

Even without any formal procedures for capacity regulation, the Clinton plan might have created incentives that could have caused the states to take action. If the Clinton national health board really did enforce its budgets at the alliance level, that would limit the flow of funds for health care enough that if providers continued their current overinvestment, some of them would get into financial trouble. It is hard to be sure who would take the first steps toward regulation, the states to maintain stability or the hospitals to protect themselves. But it would probably happen. Therefore one might argue that capital regulation does not have to be specified in a national bill. A new financing system for medical education is a more pressing concern. The Clinton proposal had most of what would be needed to control costs in a fee-for-service sector.

For the foreseeable future, good medicine in America will require a viable fee-for-service option, which requires regulation. The Clinton plan recognized this fact; other managed competition plans did not.

Beyond the Clinton Plan

The Clinton administration's Health Security Act was clearly su-perior to either of the managed competition plans. It was more likely to control costs and much more likely to provide universal coverage. Where the other plans seemed less risky, it was only because they were more likely to fail. If implemented, the Cooper-Grandy or the Chafee plan would have reduced choice and increased the dangerous forms of managed care more than the Clinton plan.

But the Clinton synthesis of managed competition and the international standard was not obviously better than the international standard itself. It gained little or no political support by avoiding standard forms of regulation and bureaucracy in favor of its own more original forms: interest groups of all kinds resisted compulsory payments whether they were called taxes or mandates. And the Clinton plan was much harder to explain than, simply, "medicare for all."

Clinton's particular synthesis also involved some real substantive problems. Are the advantages of competition worth the extra difficulties of structuring subsidies? Probably not. Did the administration find an acceptable way of enforcing a budget? I do not think so. On many of the substantive questions posed by the managed competition theory, the Clinton plan, unlike its competitors, made the right choice. But that just guaranteed opposition from the same forces that opposed the international standard.

What, then, can be done? Nothing, unless one accepts that guaranteeing care for all Americans and controlling costs require substantial regulation of some sort. Assuming agreement on the goals of cost control and guaranteed health care, however, there are better and worse ways of regulating, in terms of both substance and politics.

10

Health Care Reform in America

*T*HIS book began by comparing the U.S. health care system with those of six other countries. Today all the others guarantee health care to all citizens, but that was not always true. Each system was created out of political conflict. In some cases elections determined the direction of health care: in Britain in 1945 and in Australia in 1983. In other cases the systems evolved, step by step. In all of these countries the status quo has shaped the reform, so that no two countries' systems are the same. They share fundamental characteristics that seem necessary to ensure universal coverage and better control of costs, yet they differ in many ways.

The United States could itself guarantee health care to all Americans, by choosing aspects of the framework that works in international experience. But doing so has always been difficult for reasons of ideology and interest, and in 1993–94, managed competition added to the obstacles.

Why Reform Is So Difficult

Chapter 6 addressed common assertions that superior American quality and greater American social problems explain other nations' better performance on cost and guaranteed access. They do not. The most telling and appropriate comparison is to Canada, because it is closest to the American level of cost. If given the choice, Americans might accept some of the U.S. system's extra costs, but a substantial part of the difference cannot be justified.

The goal set by President Clinton and other reformers is therefore achievable, as long as one does not define cost control too rigidly. As chapter 9 argued, the standard set in his plan could certainly be met.

251

Why the Goal Is Opposed

Some people oppose the goals of universal coverage and cost control. The reasons for objection go beyond simple self-interest, though that can be a factor.

IDEOLOGY, ENDS, AND MEANS. Any system of social insurance violates some people's belief that individuals must be responsible for their own fate. Supporters of this version of individualism may acknowledge that it has limits: some people are "truly needy" because they are in some way disabled and did not bring their fate upon themselves. But from their perspective, charging for insurance based on individual risk is only fair.[1] To some of them, if there is a policy problem involving cost, the solution is to reduce insurance rather than to expand it. Insurance, after all, allows a person to take less responsibility for his own fate, by reducing the discipline of the market on his consumption.[2] From this same perspective cost control is in fact a dubious goal. If health care is simply a consumption good, then there is no more reason to limit consumption of it than there is for anything else. Those who have the money to buy more should, even if doing so prices others out of the market.

In the health care debate of 1993–94, both advocates and opponents of guaranteed insurance coverage spoke of responsibility. But to one group that meant each person should take care of himself, and whatever happened to him was his own fault. To others, including President Clinton, individual responsibility meant that each person should contribute to the system so that all would be protected.

The kind of radical individualism that would define universal coverage as a bad thing was definitely a minority belief. Otherwise, majorities would not have told pollsters they supported universal coverage.[3] But the same values, applied less strenuously, impeded reform by leading to rejection of any means to that end. A person might define universal coverage as a good idea, as long as it could be achieved without compelling anyone to buy insurance, or to subsidize others, or to accept fee schedules or budgets or capital investment controls, or to accept a payment scheme related to income. All of these measures can be criticized as violations of faith in the market and individual initiative. They are also present in all systems with universal coverage.

Scholars of health care usually discuss ideological orientations in terms of the value of *solidarity*, people in a community standing by each other. The point should not be that some countries have solidarity and the United States does not. If that were true, one would have to wonder how the Australians suddenly gained solidarity in 1983, or had it in 1974 and lost it in 1975. Solidarity is not the term that comes to mind when thinking of relationships between members of the German or French or British industrial and nonindustrial work forces. Pleasant, "homogeneous" Canada has spent much of the past three decades threatening to break apart along lines of language and of regional economic interest. Solidarity cannot be taken for granted in these countries and is not absent in the United States. Social security and medicare are typical solidaristic institutions, and both are extremely popular.

Rather, the United States has a larger political force that is opposed to solidaristic policies than other countries. American conservatism is dominated by the form of individualism described above, while historically the dominant conservative parties in France, Germany, and Japan have been much more accepting of state action, and even conservatives in other English-speaking countries have been more tolerant.[4] Thus American reformers must begin by writing off a large portion of the public, and therefore Congress, as impossible to convince. In seeking to win a large majority of the rest, reformers then must overcome opposition from affected interests.

INTERESTS. Private insurers fear that any form of the international standard would either abolish their line of business or turn it into a form of regulated public utility. Insurers that rely on risk-rating to carve out their markets would have no reason to exist. Insurance agents have as much to lose from reform that would eliminate confusion about insurance policies, and may win more sympathy from legislators and the public.[5] Physicians, hospitals, and pharmaceutical companies object to cost controls when they think the controls might be effective. Any group that would pay more as part of the financing scheme for wider coverage, most evidently "small business" interests, is likely to resist doing so.

Both groups and individuals tend to react far more strongly to the possibility of losing something than to an opportunity to gain something.[6] Therefore the assessments that interest groups make of substantial reform are likely to create a balance of group pressures against that reform. Legislators tend to oppose proposals that impose higher costs on their own districts than on others. If the "losers" from reform had hailed only from conservative areas, that would not have mattered, for interest-group objections would not have added to the ideological opposition. But some wavering Democratic legislators represented areas, such as Omaha, Nebraska, and Hartford, Connecticut, with large concentrations of insurers. Others were from tobacco areas, so objected to tobacco taxes in the Clinton plan, and many of the moderate-to-conservative Democrats whose votes would be needed to pass legislation hailed from districts in which small business, the interest that most vehemently opposed reform, was especially influential.

Some business interests, particularly the large manufacturers in the National Leadership Coalition for Health Care Reform, supported a much larger federal role in health care finance. Both the Clinton and McDermott-Wellstone plans would have reduced costs for large employers that already provided good benefits.[7] Yet business in general did not rally behind the Clinton plan, and the administration's lobbying for the support of big-business organizations met with embarrassing rebuffs.[8]

The Clinton proposal eliminated higher overhead costs for small groups, favored all businesses that paid lower wages, and provided large subsidies for small, low-wage firms. An employer with twenty employees earning an average of $12,000 per employee would have paid $420 per year for each—a very small fraction of the real cost. Nevertheless, small-business organizations were matched only by some Republican legislators in the energy of their opposition to reform. Proprietors of firms that would have benefited would not believe it.[9] The major small business organization, the National Federation of Independent Business, was "fervent" in its opposition to the Clinton plan, which to many members represented "socialism." "I don't care what the subsidy scheme is," its leader declared. "This is the government taking total and complete control."[10] The Chamber of Commerce, which at one point favored an employer mandate, backed off under pressure from small business members.[11]

The small-business worldview rejects government mandates on employers, pure and simple. Big business is not much different.[12] That can be understood in terms of distrust: belief that the government may provide a mandate and subsidy now but get rid of the subsidy later. It can be understood in terms of power: belief that if the government can get away with a mandate on health insurance there will be more mandates on other matters. It can be understood in terms of ideology: seeing the government as the fundamental enemy of business. But however we explain it, this is clearly *not* a matter of material interest that can be compromised by reducing burdens.[13]

In these cases ideology defined interests, so ideology may be viewed as the source of opinion. But the politics involved was interest-group politics: politicians hesitated to anger groups that could deploy financial resources against them, influence the opinions of local media, and bring angry members both to Washington and to rallies in their home districts. Groups used their resources to influence neutral parties. The Health Insurance Association of America was very successful with an expensive ad campaign attacking the administration's proposal. That campaign was so effective that the then-chair of the House Ways and Means Committee, Dan Rostenkowski (D-Ill.), offered to include some substantive concessions in his own proposal in return for the association's ceasing fire with those TV spots.[14]

Thus interest group organization added to the underlying ideological opposition to any version of the international standard means or ends, raising the barrier higher against reform.

FEAR. Ideology and direct interests influence some people, but the average voter has neither direct interests in the provider side of health care nor an ideology that clearly requires opposing national health insurance. For him or her the key question is, how will I be more secure? Fear of losing insurance was a major force in favor of reform. Fear of the consequences of reform was a major force against it.

In 1994 most Americans had insurance. It might not have been very good, but they had it. It might have been insecure, but they had it. Why should they have believed that change would improve their coverage? In order to trust, they would have had to trust the proponents of change, to believe that Bill Clinton (or any other architect of reform proposals) knew what he was doing and had their interests at heart. Or, voters would have had to believe in the theory of change: why change would work.

Trust in both Bill Clinton and the government were none too high, and hardly anyone could explain how the Clinton plan in particular would work. Opponents of reform insisted that any constraints on cost would mean "rationing," with waiting lists and far fewer medical advances. Advocates of reform often seemed to confirm the charge by insisting that the problem was "too much," rather than too expensive, medical care. Those citizens who had good insurance without reform, so who were not the victims of rationing according to insurance status, had to worry that reform would deprive them of access to "the best medical care system in the world."[15]

Even if the United States had the best medical care, cost control would not necessarily have to threaten it. After reviewing the evidence on American and other nations' health care performance, I concluded in chapter 6 that the United States could save substantial amounts without reducing quality. For its lower costs Canada not only had better aggregate statistics, but its performance was comparable in studies of treatment of specific conditions. Canada provided fewer services of some types but more of others, including both office visits and hospitalization. On balance, the evidence is that the average quality of medical care per person in Canada is equal to or higher than that in the United States. But Americans receive their health care through many different systems, some of which offer a better average quality of care than Canada, defined by the extent of benefits and access to specialists. Those Americans, at least, could feel they had something at risk, even if reform did not have to mean they would get less.[16] Others, without good information, could be swayed by scare stories or boasting.

The administration had no obvious way to overcome these fears. It could not argue that other countries had higher quality, because that would mean there was no need for managed competition. Nor did Bill Clinton have a solid governing coalition. The 1992 election was not the kind of decisive triumph that led to the creation of national systems in the United Kingdom and Australia. But elections rarely create coherent legislative majorities in the United States.

INSTITUTIONAL OBSTACLES. Sven Steinmo and Jon Watts have a simple answer to why the United States has so far been unable to pass comprehensive health care reform: the institutions.[17] The constitution created a system that separates the powers and electoral bases of the president and legislators, in which party loyalty is much weaker than in a parliamentary model. It created two equally powerful legislative bodies, the House and the Senate, that are designed to favor different constituencies and so to disagree. On top of that, Congress evolved a committee structure that would make processing health care legislation extremely complex, with multiple roadblocks. These institutions ensure that the House, Senate, and presidency have different electoral bases and therefore represent different public opinions. The legislative process creates innumerable opportunities for obstruction and hostage taking. Under these circumstances, reform of historic dimensions was unlikely to pass without either a very strong popular majority or great party discipline. Nor was the structure of debate likely to help the administration build that popular support.

All of these obstacles have been overcome on various occasions, and some (such as party weakness in the legislature) were not as high in 1994 as they had been a few decades before.[18] Yet these institutional factors greatly raised the odds that at some point in the process the combined forces of ideology and interest and fear would have enough power to derail any proposal that could in fact control costs and provide universal coverage.

Enter Managed Competition

The original Jackson Hole version of managed competition offered to achieve the goals of universal coverage without the standard means, and therefore in theory would have maximized support for reform. Chapters 7, 8, and 9 are the story of why the various iterations of managed competition would not do the job.

SUBSTANTIVE PROBLEMS. Managed competition began with a questionable theory of cause and effect. Its advocates understated the incentives for price competition in the existing markets because they persisted in viewing employees, not employers, as the purchasers. They blithely assumed that plans would seek market share rather than higher margins. They exaggerated the prospects for developing measures of treatment effectiveness that could be used both to make care more efficient and to make patients informed and thus effective consumers. They greatly overstated the effectiveness of existing forms of managed care and the ability to implement the better forms within a short period of time (if at all).

In the end, managed competition's theory of cause and effect was not a theory based on evidence but a leap of faith. The syllogism went something like this: competition is good; competition is hard to make work for medical care; the only approximation of competition that could possibly be created is competition among plans; to make that work certain things would have to come true, so if we set up a system and hope the necessary things come true, competition will work. Equally wishful theories may have shaped policy in the past.[19] But in the era of "pay as you go" (Paygo) rules and the "fiscalization of the policy debate," any reform that involved money would have to be evaluated by the Congressional Budget Office on the basis of evidence, not hope. As we saw in chapter 8, therefore, no plan that relied on institutions of managed competition for its cost controls could claim the savings needed to approach universal coverage.

Moreover, key parts of the theory would be very difficult to implement. Even believers in managed competition's ideal of a tax cap that varies by market and is determined by market competition should pale at the difficulties described in chapter 8 and the appendix. Managed competition also would require a much more complex structure to compensate for individuals' differences in ability to pay for coverage than in any of the other systems described in this book. Partial risk adjustment might be possible, but that too would involve large administrative burdens, and no technology exists that could eliminate incentives for insurers to skim, the cream off the top.

NOT ENOUGH VOTES IN THE MIDDLE. The reasons to believe that managed competition would not work contributed to its political weakness: advocates of the international standard rejected measures that, they believed, would not achieve their goals. Yet managed competition also could not pick up enough votes from skeptics of the international standard unless the theory were compromised so thoroughly as to be nearly worthless.

Managed competition as a theory offered only one new source of revenues to pay for expanded coverage, the tax deductibility cap. The cap was unpopular, could not be implemented, and did not raise enough money. The Cooper-Grandy and Chafee bills could not propose further revenue measures because those would repel the forces, such as small business interests, that they sought to attract. As chapter 8 described, both bills further compromised on fundamental aspects of the theory. If the Chafee compromises were less risky, it was only because they offered even fewer benefits.

The advocates of managed competition hoped to occupy the middle ground; unfortunately for them, that middle was nowhere near a majority. Thus Cooper-Grandy had many fewer House sponsors than either the single-payer plan or the much more limited House Republican proposal.[20] The Clinton administration tried to make managed competition work better by combining it with elements of the international standard. That approach lost managed competition advocates who viewed regulation as a "command and control economy in health care."[21] Those advocates instead tried to forge alliances to the right by diluting their plans. If managed competition were made voluntary enough, perhaps into an even more diluted version than Chafee, it might gain more support on the right—but then it could accomplish very little.

MANAGED COMPETITION AND THE PUBLIC. Nor could managed competition alleviate public fears about the consequences of health care reform. As one analyst reported, "the public does not really understand the technical issues surrounding the health reform debate. Nor should they. . . . [M]ost experts will confess (behind closed doors) that they too are confused about many critical points."[22] Perhaps the best evidence of public confusion was a *Wall Street Journal* poll in early 1994 that showed only 37 percent of respondents endorsing the Clinton plan by name, but 76 percent, a much higher number than for any alternative, supporting a description of the plan without the label.[23] The public was likely to be as confused about managed competition as about other complex theories. But the injection of managed competition into the debate did not offer popular cost controls and could not alleviate public fears.

Polling data did not support the idea that competition was more popular than regulation: asked to choose, a slight plurality favored cost control through regulation over competition at the level of general principle, and the public clearly approved of government regulations of the prices of prescription drugs, physician and hospital fees, and health insurance premiums.[24] Perhaps more important was the association between managed competition and health maintenance organizations (HMOs). Polls ranked "choice of doctor" as a primary consideration in assessing proposed reforms. So did the market, in which systems with point-of-service options grew much faster than systems without them.[25] Managed competition made restriction of choice a more plausible outcome of reform. It also added an extra level of complexity, asking citizens to believe in institutions they had never seen. The Clinton administration then made matters even worse by trying to sell a synthesis that its leaders would not and perhaps could not explain. A confused public understandably chose caution over action.

Long Odds

Comprehensive health care reform is possible in America; it just is not very likely. In 1993–94 there were some favorable circumstances: great concern about the status quo, a president committed to the cause, and a Democratic party in Congress that, while divided on the issue, did want to show that it could govern. Yet ideological and interested opposition to all the necessary measures remained high, and the president's majority in Congress on this issue was ephemeral.

A few interest groups, notably large insurers, preferred managed competition to the international standard. Yet they also could live with the status quo. Managed competition neither won public support nor reduced public fears of the unknown.

Meeting Reform Halfway?

Unable to face that set of political problems, by mid-1994 many in Congress were searching for partial measures—measures that would approach some of the goals of reform but not guarantee success. Senators Daniel Patrick Moynihan (D-N.Y.) and Robert Packwood (R-Ore.) proclaimed that covering 91 percent of Americans would be pretty good.[26] There was a continual search for plans that would not create employer mandates or cost controls from the outset but might "trigger" their creation later. "Hard triggers" would be automatic; "soft triggers" would require a vote.[27] The Chafee bill itself provided one example of triggers: the subsidies that depended on realized savings.

Such measures might be marginal improvements in the existing system, but the odds that any package would do much to control costs or expand coverage were quite low. Yet one partial measure makes a great deal of sense. That approach would be to give states more ability to control costs and provide universal coverage. Later in this section I describe what such a reform would look like and why it would have been a useful step.

"INCREMENTAL" REFORM. Often policy can be improved by moving incrementally: in small steps, so as to see the results before going further and avoid big mistakes.[28] In the health care debate, incremental reforms meant making few changes in the basic institutions of health insurance and causing as little disruption to stakeholders in the existing system as could be managed.

There was a menu of incremental reforms even before the 1993–94 debate. Many were included in the Chafee, Cooper-Grandy, and Clinton plans; most were included in a House Republican proposal, H.R. 3080, sometimes known as the Michel bill after its lead sponsor, House Minority Leader Robert Michel (R-Ill.). Later proposals, such as those introduced by Senator Robert Dole (R-Kan.) and Representatives Michael Bilirakis (R-Fla.) and J. Roy Rowland (D-Ga.), added little to the menu. So the discussion here will again use individual bills, especially the Michel version, as a basis for discussing the components of this approach.

Incrementalism would address some issues as marginal problems, to be met with small amounts of money or by creating an agency with little real power. Thus the Michel bill included new grants to encourage primary care, new definitions in various programs to help rural areas, a new office of emergency medical services, and an office of private health care coverage.[29]

Was the health care system tangled in paperwork? Rather than attack the paperwork at its roots, which were managed care and multiple payment rules, incremental proposals called for standardizing the forms. How this would work without standardizing insurance benefits and administration was rarely explained. But the Michel bill included, for example, requirements that the federal government create standards for data gathering and transmission and standards for magnetized medicare and medicaid health benefit cards.[30]

An incremental bill, like almost all others, could try to encourage the development of outcome measures and treatment guidelines, so as to both improve medical care and give purchasers a better chance to make informed choices. The Michel bill provided for the development of electronic medical data standards and for the development and distribution of comparative value information, all under the authority of the secretary of health and human services.[31]

INCREMENTAL MEASURES TO INCREASE ACCESS. Incremental reform would take small steps to reduce risk-rating and larger ones to limit pre-existing condition exclusions. Insurers would have to guarantee renewal of coverage except for seemingly good reasons, such as beneficiary fraud or nonpayment.[32] Pre-existing condition exclusions would be limited but not eliminated. The provisions in the Michel bill were sufficient to prevent "job lock," as long as the job to which one wanted to move had similar insurance.[33] The bill also required insurers to accept some risks they would have preferred to avoid, either by accepting all applicants during an open-enrollment period, or through mandatory assignment from a pool of high risks.[34]

Requiring plans to accept applicants would accomplish little if they could still charge discriminatory prices. Yet mandating prices definitely interferes with the market. Incremental plans such as the Michel bill therefore would have set only loose constraints on pricing. The Michel bill banned truly egregious increases based on claims experience ("experience rating"), and the substantial increases it allowed would have had to conform to overall limits on variation. Yet the Michel bill allowed rates to vary by "demographic and other similar objective characteristics," including "age, gender, geographic area, family composition, and group size." These measures would only marginally reduce discrimination based on stereotypes about group characteristics; for example, areas could be redlined. The bill also allowed variations by "class of business" within each demographic grouping and between customers within these classes of business. As a result, insurers would have been able to charge one customer up to 62 percent more than another even if they had identical demographic profiles.[35]

Incremental approaches would allow only voluntary alliances. The Michel bill addressed the unpleasant experience with fraud in existing multiple employer welfare arrangements (MEWAs) by providing sixty-one pages of new rules and regulations for those arrangements.[36] If small employers could join such arrangements, they would not be paying the higher administrative overhead costs per capita that are charged to separate smaller employers in the current health insurance market.

Among them, these incremental reforms would have reduced those evils of the status quo that most threaten otherwise economically secure persons: the pre-existing condition exclusions for people who can otherwise afford insurance, and higher administrative overhead charges for small groups. Yet there would still be large price differences, both within and especially among demographic categories, that would make insurance unaffordable for many. Because plans could vary, some pre-existing condition exclusions could still apply even for people who merely changed insurers. Discrimination could occur in marketing as well as price. Taken as a whole, these measures would do little to reduce the economic barriers that made health insurance unaffordable to many Americans.[37]

INCREMENTAL COST CONTROLS. Effective cost control could at least limit the extent to which those barriers rose over the years. Incremental proposals sought savings from an increase in managed care without coercive caps on tax deductibility or mandatory alliances, the centerpieces of the managed competition theory. Instead, the Michel bill eliminated various state requirements that could restrain growth of managed care. For example, states would be forbidden to make utilization reviewers liable for the effects of delayed reviews.[38] Incremental proposals would make it easier to enroll medicare recipients in HMOs or PPOs (preferred provider organizations) and encourage more use of managed care in medicaid. With luck, enrollment of medicaid patients in managed care plans would cost less per patient and enable states to cover more persons, but the incremental approach would provide little or no new money or mandates, so no guarantee of greater coverage.[39]

The Michel and some other incremental proposals claimed health care could be made significantly less expensive by reforming the malpractice system. Many of the same measures as those in the Chafee bill would have discouraged attorneys from representing plaintiffs unless they could claim large economic damages (for example, a young business executive who had been paralyzed).[40] These proposals were anything but incremental from the standpoint of notions of legal redress in America, but the reasons to believe that they would do much about costs, as reviewed in previous chapters, were quite weak.

MERITS AND DEMERITS OF INCREMENTALISM. Most incremental measures would do a little good; most would disrupt existing arrangements only a little; and none threatened the kind of harm that could be caused by Cooper-Grandy's restructuring of the incentives to buy (or avoid buying) insurance. But the relative harmlessness of these approaches did not make them wise.

In other contexts, incrementalism can be a very good thing. In some it is virtually inevitable.[41] But incrementalism is justified by three basic presumptions: that the status quo is broadly acceptable, that it can be maintained whether one likes it or not, and that one has to move in small increments because there is not enough information to judge the effects of larger steps. Each of these assumptions can be questioned in the case of American health care system.

The first is a value question: is the status quo acceptable? For people with good insurance who have no fear of losing it, the status quo is probably fine. But having the highest costs in the world with the greatest access problems among advanced nations is not on its face a good thing. This book argues that the United States could do much better, and if that is true, the current system should not be acceptable.

The second question, whether the status quo can be maintained, is largely a matter of fact. Even a person who accepts the current costs and distribution of coverage might conclude that, if the common estimates about the trend of costs are true, the system cannot be sustained. The issue is why anyone would believe that incremental measures could do more than moderate the dangerous trend—so the system hit the wall in, say, 2004 instead of 2000. In order to believe the system will stabilize without dramatic policy change, one has to believe that managed care will suddenly stabilize costs even without the apparatus of managed competition. As I argue in chapter 7, that is quite improbable. If time is against Americans who seek to control health care costs, incrementalism is not safe.

The third question, whether we know enough to assess nonincremental proposals, is also a matter of fact, with some judgment. Americans do have enough information on which to take larger steps. The rest of the industrialized world has shown ways to universal coverage and substantially better cost control. The road is not easy, but it is much better marked than the road of managed competition, and we can see that other travelers have moved far along it safely.

Americans know how to implement the measures of the international standard because the essential measures involve adopting financial arrangements with which there is extensive experience in America as well. The United States could produce a straightforward adaptation of the international standard by simply expanding medicare. The federal government is entirely competent to collect a payroll tax and to operate a fee schedule with a system of volume adjustments.

Some adaptations would be harder than others. Expanding medicare and leaving most of the administration to the federal government
or its agents would be easier than involving the states, because the
states have very different capabilities. Medicare is already national.
More complex systems, such as all-payer regulation, would be harder
to implement than simpler systems. But there are many examples of
operating such systems; and with care and caution, states could implement their own versions.

Successful implementation of an adaptation that is unique to the
United States—for example, one that created price incentives for individuals—would be less certain. Caution and a slower phasein would
be the cost of trying to do something original. The basic measures of
the international standard, however, would be maintained in any successful reform: the cost controls and a financing system in which the
largest part of the money is collected according to a system of compulsory contributions. Americans know how to do both.

That does not mean the consequences of nonincremental reform
can be calculated precisely. It does mean the directions of effects and
their likely scale are clear. Pursuit of the cost control and coverage
goals stated in the Clinton plan requires no leaps of faith or shots in
the dark. They are modest by international standards, and Americans
can adapt most of the international measures.

Therefore incrementalism in health care reform is neither necessary
nor desirable. But incrementalism, sad to say (or happily for readers
who disagree with the above), is not merely a statement about how to
think about policy. It is also an attribute of political systems. Incrementalism is especially likely when power is fragmented, choices are
complex, and disagreement is rife. Incrementalism is the normal
course of American politics.

In the 1993–94 health care reform debate, incremental proposals
involved one further, particularly deceptive, twist: "triggers." In this
approach, the Congress would enact a set of incremental measures
and "give them a chance to work." If they did not work by a certain
date—defined as coverage being below some standard or inflation
above some standard—then other measures would be taken. Proponents distinguished between "hard triggers," meaning that the gun
would almost definitely go off, and "soft triggers," meaning there
would be more discretion. Yet no trigger could be truly hard: Congress

could always choose not to let it be pulled. Under almost any circumstances a minority could do so, for example by filibustering appropriation of funds to implement the measures.

There is no reason to believe that those who oppose comprehensive reform one year would accept pulling the trigger a few years later. Only when a majority of Americans are uninsured will proponents of the status quo stop arguing that most Americans are doing all right, and even then they will claim that real cost control threatens the quality of care. Using failure to "trigger" reform would require that conditions be even worse than they were in 1994—costs much higher and coverage less widespread. That price for delay is much too high.

Triggers for health care should work no better than they did to "automatically" reduce the deficit, as called for by the 1985 Gramm-Rudman-Hollings Act, one of the greater debacles in the history of American legislation. Failure to achieve the goals of deficit reduction changed no one's mind about how to achieve that goal, or about its desirability.[42] If costs rise even higher, and more people need help to afford insurance, will employers be more willing to pay, or anyone more willing to help their fellow citizens? Of course not. Proposals for triggers are simply a way to allow politicians to avoid admitting that they do not want to control costs and guarantee health care to all Americans. If adopted, a bill with incremental measures and a trigger for more serious action in, say, 2002 would discourage action before then, as opponents of reform argued that the Congress had committed itself to waiting until that date before considering the issue again.

Experimentalism Rather Than Incrementalism: Empowering the States

In 1994 (and at this writing in 1995), only one kind of partial measure was clearly superior to the status quo. The federal government could set the stage for individual states to control costs and create universal coverage within their borders.

Throughout 1993 and 1994, state governments struggled with their own health care reform plans, with minimal success. In state after state, as in Congress, proposals for comprehensive reform were defeated and diluted, because of their sponsors' inability to raise the funds or to agree on ways to control costs.[43] Many of the proposals involved forms of managed competition. Efforts to ensure that small firms could buy insurance, but not necessarily at an affordable price, were common. So were proposals to expand the use of managed care in medicaid and, in theory, thereby expand access, or simply to marginally expand medicaid.[44] Some states had even come close to promising universal coverage, but none, not even the highly publicized examples of Minnesota, Vermont, and Washington state, had the necessary financing.[45]

The states' main problems were political, but the federal government could have helped them out. It could have offered help without requiring participation, just as Canada did in 1964. From the standpoint of advocates of universal coverage, this could not work as well in the United States of the 1990s as in the Canada of the 1960s. The federal government in 1994 had little new money to offer to states—or at least nowhere near as much as Canada could offer to its provinces in 1964. It was a lot easier to reach universal coverage by imitation among ten provinces than among fifty states. The U.S. government could have offered states control of the medicare and medicaid money, but that money was already being spent in those states so would not have offered much possibility of doing something new.

Unlike in Canada, however, the U.S. government could offer to eliminate major obstacles to state action. An American version of the Canadian legislation might provide that if a state enacted legislation that created universal coverage within its borders, according to some rules about portability across borders, with all persons meeting some standard of benefits and comparable access (that is, not full fee-for-service for some and medicaid managed care for others), then the federal government would:

—waive all applicable antitrust laws so as to eliminate any doubt about the legality of creating all-payer bargaining structures between payers and providers. Without these waivers, cost controls could not be implemented in this manner, but instead would require direct state budgeting. The waivers therefore would increase a state's options.

—waive the provisions of the 1974 Employee Retirement Income Security Act that prevented state regulation of self-insurance by corporations. Without this waiver, a state could not bring those systems into a structure of cost control or create the mechanisms for portability across jobs and other necessary provisions.[46]

—hand the state the equivalent of federal medicaid expenditures, according to some formula, and, if the state wished, the medicare money as well. Expecting states to take over medicare would ask too much, but they should have the option. Medicaid long-term care benefits might have to be kept separate.

—provide to the state an extra increment of new funding, for which the logical candidate was a tobacco tax. Tobacco taxes are a public health measure and were popular in the antismoking climate of the 1990s. The federal government could enact a national increase in the tobacco tax and then create a trust fund of collections from each state. As soon as a state met the requirements, the federal government could turn over the balance of the fund plus all future collections. The likely revenue in such a fund would not be huge ($11 billion a year if it were the seventy-five-cent per pack increase proposed by President Clinton), but it would make a difference nonetheless, and be more attractive as it accumulated.[47] The imposition of a national tax means a state does not have to worry that by adopting a levy it will cause employers or customers to flee across state lines; in this case, cigarette taxes would have been raised equally in all states.

—establish the rules under which the Internal Revenue Service and the Social Security Administration would provide to a state the income and payroll information needed to run a system of subsidies.

Within this structure there would be no need for the federal government to impose budgets: costs would be the state's problem. Nor does this approach mandate any particular form of cost control. But it greatly expands state options and, given that state voters would pay if costs rose too quickly, states could be expected to come up with their own adaptations of the international standard. They could even use some of the measures of managed competition, which, if they worked, would finally be good evidence for the theory. But because states could not implement a version of the cap on tax deductibility, advocates would be likely to argue that the theory had never been tried and therefore never disproven.

Incrementalism at its best is a way of learning by doing. The nation would learn more from a few states' taking giant steps than from a form of incrementalism in which the whole nation took small steps. The latter is more likely to tell what will fail; the former is more likely to reveal what will succeed.

The possible "victims" of state action, insurers and self-insured corporations, would protest even allowing states more freedom. Yet they could be challenged by asking if they really wanted the federal government to impose its will on states—a question that also would embarrass most ideological opponents of solidarity. Taxing tobacco would lose a group of votes from tobacco-state Democrats, but that could be an affordable cost for a proposal that would be very hard for anyone besides the conservative core to oppose.

Nor does freeing the states in this way require an either-or choice between forms of incrementalism. The two approaches could easily be combined: national legislation could give states the option to do more. Experience in states could even make triggers more likely to be pulled. If the United States is to go halfway, it ought to combine incremental-ism with experimentalism. A package of modest steps should also give universal coverage and cost control a chance. If only half steps are allowed, they should be designed to make further steps possible.

Getting It Right

A half-step is better than standing still, but state-by-state progress through fifty states could take a very long time. Therefore I cannot say that state-based reform is the best approach to America's health care problems. It is superior only to doing nothing or to taking incremental steps.

National reform seemed foreclosed at the end of 1994. Yet the debate will resume, and at that point all the same questions, of regulation and competition and burdens and benefits, will be addressed again. Even if states go it alone, they will have to answer those questions. I end this book, then, with my answer to President Clinton's question: what kind of combination of competitive ideas with international les-sons would make sense for America? These concluding suggestions are not a complete plan but an approach. A version could be adopted by a state if the federal government freed the states to act, or the federal government could try to create a national system along these lines.

My proposal follows from the basic points of this book. Reform should be based on the international standard, not managed compe-tition. But there are strong arguments for giving the best forms of managed care a chance to flourish. That is easier in the United States than in many other countries because, with its combination of ideo-logical objections and budget pressures, the United States would seem highly unlikely to adopt a plan with as little cost sharing as in Germany and Canada or with benefits as broad as in Germany. Therefore a basic fee-for-service scheme would have some inadequacies—something with which good HMOs could compete.

Reform should be as modest as possible in terms of the behavioral change it requires from caregivers, patients, and payers, and it should establish ways for the system and physicians to work together. There is no way to design cost controls that will make physicians happy. But one of the fundamental tasks in any health care system—whether it be in Australia or Japan, the United Kingdom or France, Canada or Germany—is to create stable and successful arrangements with the medical profession.

In the United States this need takes on an ironic significance. American physicians, historically the most bitter opponents of coverage expansions, are now confused and divided. They are not sure who is the worse enemy—the government or the insurance companies. Universal coverage offers doctors more patients, fewer tough decisions about what to do for the uninsured, and the chance to do more of the work that they trained for. As managed care becomes more pervasive, physicians are becoming more interested in versions of the international standard.[48]

One should not imagine that in 1994 most physicians were in favor of a single-payer system, or even of some other version of the international standard. But the trend was in that direction. The movement was clearest among the leadership of physician organizations, who followed the policy debate more closely than did the membership.[49] That helps explain why the last group anyone expected, the board of regents of the American College of Surgeons, endorsed a single-payer approach on February 4, 1994. Although the board does not represent the majority of surgeons, the leaders were making a plausible judgment of their members' interests.[50]

Nevertheless, even leaders of physicians' organizations that have looked kindly on the Clinton plan do not support a single payer. Above all, they do not want to put all their eggs in the government's basket.[51] A system of all-payer bargaining offers physicians more protections and a clearer voice in the process of cost control.[52] Nor do all physicians have the same opinions about managed care. The founders of Kaiser Permanente believed, correctly, that their institution would attract some physicians and not others; they envisioned a system of alternative delivery systems.[53] The problem for physicians is not the option of working in a Kaiser but the imposition of a wide array of ever-changing rules by competing insurers. These payers keep testing the envelope of regulation in their efforts to save money by squeezing harder—and in the process scare the bejesus out of physicians even if they are able to resist the pressure.[54]

Physicians have every right to a greater voice than anyone else in clinical decisions and any other decision that involves medical judgment. They *should* have the largest say in relative values. They *should* be involved in regulating each other economically as well as clinically. The question is, how far can reformers go to satisfy physicians' concerns about managed care yet still attain the basic goals of reform? The answer is that they can go quite a long way.

Choices within the International Standard

With that in mind, we can consider substantive issues by returning to the themes with which this book began.

All six other countries in this study represent an international standard of health care finance and delivery. All have universal systems based on compulsory participation. All are financed not by individual purchase of insurance for fixed prices, but by contribution schemes in which all payers contribute to a fund in proportion to their incomes and withdraw in proportion to their health care needs. In each, smaller families help larger, wealthier people help poorer, and younger (all other things being equal) help older.[55] They limit costs by combinations of fee schedules for some services and budgets for others. Controls on capital investment further limit the proliferation of expensive technology and limit the cost of using the technology that is available. The question is, what political compromises might be substantively acceptable?

COMPELLING UNIVERSAL COVERAGE. High-income earners in Germany are the only exception to the rule that everyone must contribute according to rules set by the government. Compulsory membership is the necessary companion to guaranteed access. Within any insurance system, if people were guaranteed the right to join whenever they wished, the system would be subject to adverse selection: people would not contribute until they get sick. Compulsory participation can be justified as either a value (called solidarity earlier in this chapter) or a pragmatic calculation. It is already the basis for American social security and medicare, and it must be part of American reform. The only possible exception could be a variation on the German model: that is, people who earn more than the social security income cap could be allowed to buy some other form of insurance if they wished.

American reform could, for example, create a standard benefit package but allow persons who earned more than the amount of income on which social security taxes are collected ($62,200 in 1995) to insure themselves on different terms.[56] This approach could appeal to insurers that would sell these policies, providers who might charge higher prices to those customers, and some persons with high enough incomes, who might believe they were receiving the opportunity to buy "cadillac" health coverage. Ironically, it might also be opposed as inegalitarian, because it would allow people with more money to purchase differently, even if they got a worse deal. Still, this compromise should be considered in any new state or national debate, as long as the threshold is set high enough to ensure that no more than the German proportion of the population can opt out of the main system.

BENEFITS AND INEQUALITY. Within this context of universal and compulsory coverage, all systems provide roughly equal standard benefits, with Japan's varied cost sharing the major exception. Each country has some special populations (undocumented immigrants, veterans, aboriginal populations) who either have special needs beyond the basic system or are not eligible to participate. Each country therefore has some special supplementary programs; the United States does now and will continue to do so. But there is no good excuse for providing a substantially lower than average standard of care to part of the nation. A program that only guaranteed what was perceived to be inferior care would not seem to offer security from risk in return for contributions. Instead it would be viewed as a poor program for poor people. It would be medicaid instead of medicare.

Though the international standard forbids providing explicitly inferior coverage for a minority, it does not prevent care that is better than the norm. Even Canada has private insurance for benefits that are not covered in the public schemes. In Britain some who can afford it pay for private care; in Australia nearly 40 percent have private insurance that provides both some supplementary coverage and greater choice for the same benefits that the public systems provide; in Japan gifts to providers may garner better care or at least better amenities; in France specialists are more accessible to people who can pay more out-of-pocket, and 80 percent of the public has supplementary coverage; in Germany the substitute funds provide slightly more extensive benefits and private insurance pays such high fees that physicians and hospitals are eager to provide (ostensibly) better service. Although the political left in each of these countries does not like those compromises, their health care systems remain much more equitable than the American system.

Once a society decides what must be guaranteed to all, its major concern about extras should be to ensure that they do not threaten the integrity of the universal guarantee. Extra billing is dangerous because it threatens to create a set of doctors who are inaccessible to patients who cannot afford the higher fees. That is especially true in countries, such as the United States, where hospital care involves admission by and separate fees to individual physicians, and where fees are high.[57] Then access to particular hospitals could depend on ability to pay the doctors' extra fees. A system such as Australia's, which allows physicians to charge extra to 40 percent of patients and not to others, provides dangerous incentives to favor the first group. If any favoritism within hospitals is risked, policy should ensure that the group involved is small enough not to threaten access for everyone else.

International practice sets broad parameters for the standard benefit package. Cost sharing is substantial in France and Japan, is limited to ambulatory services in Australia, and barely exists in Canada, Germany, and the United Kingdom. Coverage of pharmaceutical benefits varies widely, though all systems have some coverage at least for persons with lower incomes and for pensioners. Each system with cost sharing limits catastrophic expenses, and all provide unlimited hospital coverage.

Standard benefits in America should at least be more generous than the current medicare package. Its cost sharing is at the high end of the international range, the program does not pay for pharmaceuticals, and the fact that hospital benefits can be used up is, by international standards, shocking. French and Japanese levels of cost sharing could not be justified in the United States, because higher American prices would make the same percentage a greater burden. Any American reform that allows cost sharing must provide extra support to persons with lower incomes.

Within these bounds, the basic benefit package requires political judgments about the trade-offs between cost and coverage. Ultimately politicians must make those choices. They should remember that universal coverage for any set of services increases the political support for cost control because it gives everyone an incentive to control costs rather than try to shift them to someone else. It allows much simpler administration by creating coherent rules. It allows more efficient care within the bounds of the benefit package by allowing persons who would otherwise be uninsured to receive primary care or continuous treatment by appropriate specialists rather than waiting for care until they are so sick that a hospital feels it must accept them as charity cases. For these and many other reasons, universal coverage encourages cost control.

If any forms of cost control were created without universal coverage, their effect would be to eliminate some of the charity care that already occurs. That is why the original Jackson Hole documents called universal coverage a necessity. Both common sense and estimates of the effects of competitive pressures in California support that concern.[58] Americans can reasonably argue about what they want to guarantee to the entire community, at the margin. At the margin, people may have supplemental insurance or pay out-of-pocket. At the margin, costs are relatively low. But excluding any Americans from the core of a benefit package, hospital and physician services, puts them at grave financial and health risk.

The guaranteed level of coverage varies among nations. Who is covered does not. If Americans must choose between narrower benefits for everybody and wider benefits for some, the choice is clear: cover everyone.

CONTRIBUTIONS AND SUBSIDIES—FROM CANADA TO JAPAN. The principle of relating payments to income and benefits to need is already a large part of American health care financing. For all its faults, medicaid is a system in which the larger incomes of other taxpayers fund care for the smaller incomes of the poor. Medicare part A is paid for by a payroll tax. Even group insurance provided through employers often does not charge additional fees for each child.

Among the possible forms of income-related contributions to the health care system, those that are based on employment would require the least change from the status quo. The most sensible American reform would therefore be to mandate employer contributions as percentages of individual payrolls, as France, Germany, and Japan do. The Clinton administration's attempt, with employer mandates, to gain most of the advantages of that method but seem to be doing something else added immense administrative complexity and did not have much political support.[59]

There are many arguments for financing health care through other taxation. Yet in principle, as discussed in chapter 4, a dedicated source of funds seems superior to general revenue financing. Dedicated financing gives everyone a way to relate the money raised to the money spent. It would be difficult to generate large dedicated revenues other than through income contributions; other possibilities, such as tobacco taxes, could yield only supplementary funds.

Some critics of payroll contributions argue that this method of financing inhibits employment by burdening either employers or employees. This argument is plausible, but it begs a few issues and fudges some choices: First, the arguments against employer contributions contradict each other. One says employer payments are offset by lower wages. The other says employer payments are a burden on employers. If employer health care payments simply replace wages, they are not a burden on the employer.[60] The truth is somewhere in between: over the long run perhaps 80 percent of total health care contributions by employers could be derived from lower wages, but in the short run the number might well be lower. As Henry Aaron notes, "Few people other than economists believe this offset, and economists acknowledge that the adjustment process may be slow and painful."[61]

Because both immediately and over the long run a portion of employer contributions for health care is not paid for by reducing wages (but instead with higher prices or lower profits), the effect of employer contributions is to provide some subsidies to workers from customers and investors. Particularly in the case of low-wage workers, that might be significant assistance for the wage earner. Employers therefore oppose required contributions, and employees support them, for obvious reasons. At the same time, the fact that most of the costs would not be borne by employers means that the effect of health care contributions on employment levels is easily exaggerated.

Although the effects of employer mandates on employment have often been greatly exaggerated, some negative effects would still be likely. That is not a sufficient reason to reject employer-based payment, because the effect would be much smaller than advertised and because clever opponents could argue that almost any financing method would reduce employment. Thus a value added tax would reduce sales and ultimately unemployment. *Any* argument that treats *any* payment only as an extra cost to somebody must claim that employment would be reduced. On the other hand, any cost could be viewed as a transfer: for example if employers would otherwise have paid wages, the only question is whether money moves directly from employers to health care providers or stops in an employee's bank account first. Either way, the money that supposedly reduces employment when it is taken from one source pays for some employment when it is used to purchase health care.

The real issues, then, are distributional: arguments about employment are made by employers who do not pay now and who want to avoid paying. The rules about employer contributions can influence whether the contributions are more likely to reduce hiring or to be paid for from wages. If employers were required to pay a percentage of each employee's earnings, for example, they would have no reason to favor part-time employees over full-time, or to prefer paying over-time to hiring new workers. The Clinton plan's approach would have encouraged inefficient restructuring of the labor force into high- and low-wage pools, as some employers sought to minimize their required payments. But employment arguments in general are exaggerated for self-interested effect.[62]

No form of financing is ideal. But, given that the United States already has an employment-based system, advocates of an alternative must show that it is clearly superior. Any alternative to employer payments would be less popular, would favor employers over employees, would threaten to destabilize existing employer contributions (if they were not immediately eliminated), and would be of questionable economic benefit.[63] It would increase the possible windfall benefits and costs of reform, creating further issues of fairness and support. Building on existing institutions makes more sense.

In an ideal world, perhaps called Canada, there is no justification for an insurance system with universal coverage but a series of different payment pools. Nevertheless, they exist in Germany, Japan, and to a lesser extent France. People are segmented according to geography and/or occupational or employer characteristics. These systems create some inequities in contributions and even, in Japan, in coverage. If the members of a group have lower incomes or greater health risks than the average, they have to pay a larger share of income for their insurance.

Each system provides some set of transfers among plans to partially compensate for the distributional effects of having these separate pools. The German reforms of 1992 could eliminate many of the differences among plans in 1996. Nevertheless, they all are examples of political compromises in which some classes of employment are treated differently from others.

These examples are particularly significant in light of the 1994 debate in America over the burden of reform on smaller employers and, conversely, over whether large employers should be allowed to run their own systems. Japan, for example, has a complex and confusing health care financing system that includes: special local regimes (call them alliances) for smaller employers; large subsidies for those alliances from the general revenues of federal and state governments; allowing employers above some size limit to pay for their own schemes, perhaps with different rules about employer and employee shares; and requiring some extra charge to the large employer sector to help the small employer sector. Put in those general terms, Japanese financing institutions do not look so different from the Clinton plan and seem even more like various American "pay or play" proposals. Comprehensiveness is more important than simplicity. If the alternative to complex comprehensiveness is a complex patchwork, as in the United States, the former could be a big improvement.

Reform should not create payment schemes in which some employers contribute much less than others as a percentage of payroll. Allowing small or low-wage businesses (however defined) to pay less would buy almost no political support, would create administrative headaches, and would produce perverse incentives for companies to restructure themselves into high- and low-wage units. The subsidy inherent in an employer's paying a percentage of payroll is generous enough. If employers had difficulty making the transition from paying nothing to paying a fair amount, there are good ways to ease the implementation of new requirements.

First, the government could hold down the minimum wage for two or three years. That would make it easier for employers to compensate for new health care contributions by restraining wages. The workers involved would be mainly part-time young workers, who were not supporting families, or the working poor, who would benefit greatly from having health insurance. Second, reform could include a longer phase-in for certain employers, which would require administrative expenses for only the period of transition. A qualifying employer might, for example, apply in 1998 to be allowed to delay full coverage for two years. The reform might require contributions to cover a sequence of benefits: for example, catastrophic costs in the first year, hospitalization in the second, and full coverage in the third.

The goal should be to ease the transition for small employers from a world in which they fear that higher labor costs from health insurance will put them at a competitive disadvantage, to a world in which those costs are built into all competitors' compensation packages. A gradual transition and relating contributions to earnings are fair ways to implement reform. But further, long-term subsidies are not fair and spend money that could be used in much better ways.

FEE SCHEDULES AND BUDGETS. Within the international standard, costs are controlled by setting fees, making budgets, and imposing controls on investment, not by competition. Competition in Britain may improve the level or distribution of services but is virtually irrelevant to cost control. International experience and common sense show that fee schedules work. Fee schedules for health care have none of the standard flaws of price controls in a functioning market. Rather than adding administrative burdens, they simplify billing, and they do not distort supply and demand in the market, because insurance has already eliminated the price constraints that structure normal markets. Fee regulation does not provide only temporary relief, followed by a burst of hyperinflation once removed, because the fee schedules are not removed. Fee schedules do not generally lead to underprovision of services; indeed, all the arguments about volume adjustments are based on the fact that, if anything, fee schedules lead to provision of more services, as providers try to increase their incomes by doing more instead of charging more.[64]

The right question is not whether to regulate, but how. Multiple insurers that paid according to all-payer agreements would have higher administrative costs than a single-payer system. But those expenses would still be greatly decreased from current American levels, and providers would pay much less to administer their billing and collections. All-payer systems also allow the government to distance itself somewhat from cost control decisions, diffusing political heat.

On balance there is little reason to believe a single-payer system is superior to a well-regulated all-payer approach.

If payers can agree on a budgeting structure for hospitals, that is the most effective tool for controlling their costs. If an all-payer scheme budgeted hospitals, there would be questions about how to allocate expenses among insurance funds, which would require some form of payment per case, as in France. So insurers in any form of all-payer system would pay each hospital according to a fee schedule.

Should the fees be the same for all hospitals in a given area? Most systems allow some differences, either through hospital-specific negotiations or, as in medicare at present, some sort of formula. Some of the sources of different hospital costs could be addressed by financing the educational functions of hospitals separately, but some historical differences would remain. Further, separate financing of medical education requires a national program, to avoid overburdening states, such as Massachusetts, that are centers of medical education. However it is arranged, there must be some way to allow different payments to accommodate hospitals' different tasks; one set fee schedule without adjustments is not appropriate.

Payment rates for all services must vary by region in a nation the size of the United States. If states are acting separately, differences among states will occur as a matter of course. Whether states act separately or as part of wider federal reform, variation within states should be up to the states. In an all-payer bargaining structure large states are almost sure to create something resembling alliances, because effective medical markets are smaller than those states.

States have no need to develop different relative value scales. The Health Care Financing Administration (HCFA) has already done almost all the work: it has increased its consultation with organized medicine, and the AMA has already endorsed using a national scale.[65] Negotiations instead can focus, as in Germany, on conversion factors. If a state and its physicians prefer to work out different relative values, as in Canada, there is no reason why the federal government should prevent that.

The most difficult issue is whether to allow any variation in physician fees. Given standard fees, physicians with better reputations still will earn more, because they will have more business. But physicians clearly object to standard fees, and some patients want to believe that they can get better treatment by paying more.

As discussed above, allowing any extra billing raises serious issues of equity. At a minimum, an all-payer system must, as in Australia, forbid supplementary insurance to cover payment of more than the fee on the fee schedule. If that approach is taken, there should also be separate, extra payments by governments to support outpatient care in the academic medical centers, as a backup to ensure access. A version of the German model, under which only a small portion of the public has the privilege of paying more, is less likely to create risks for ordinary citizens.

SYSTEM CAPACITY AND QUALITY. However funds are raised and bills are paid, every system needs measures to ensure appropriate supply and quality of care through medical education, licensure, quality monitoring, and the distribution of capital equipment.

The health care system is too large and complex to rely on federal regulation to ensure quality. Some matters, such as hospital accreditation, are sufficiently technical that in practice they are likely to remain the province of professional bodies. Others involve such measurement difficulties that they are best determined through close contact that creates a mass of anecdotes and thus a reputation, which is how individuals choose providers and physicians make referrals now; "report cards" would not work nearly as well. The federal government can fund efforts to improve measurements, but one should not expect very useful results for a long time.

Medical education can be addressed only at a national level. Professional graduates move easily across state borders. Medical schools and hospitals should receive appropriate budgets that include grants to cover the tuition of medical students. A system that leaves physicians deeply in debt upon graduation can only increase their feelings of financial insecurity and their belief that they are entitled to high incomes. It is unfair to those physicians who choose less remunerative specialties. Relieving physicians of their debt burden is common throughout the world and should be part of the trade-off for their accepting fee regulation.

Restricting some forms of managed care would automatically reduce the most bizarre aspect of our current malpractice tort system: the fact that physicians can be trapped between fear of lawsuits for not providing services and insurer demands to restrict services. Practice within group- and staff-model HMOs, on the other hand, should be a matter of enterprise, not individual physician, liability. If the point of that model is that it involves collegial decisionmaking, the medical group should be legally responsible as a group.

Since the malpractice system seems poorly designed to ensure quality, restrictions on suits can be justified *as long as they are accompanied by better self-regulation.* The preferred approach of the American Medical Association, putting a cap on pain and suffering damages at $250,000, is too stringent, but a higher cap, say $1 million and indexed to inflation, might be fair. On balance, this choice too should be left to the states, because they should be in a position to give malpractice relief to medical societies that agree to do more in return. It would be interesting to see a few states try some version of the New South Wales approach that was described in chapter 5. Having complaints developed by a government body but judged mainly by medical professionals seems a logical way to bypass most of the obstacles to serious enforcement of professional standards upon individual providers.

Any method to restrict capital investment in health care is bound to be politically contentious. Eventually, however, some measures will be needed. Since the benefits are long-run, however, such measures might be postponed until the rest of a reformed system were created. Any explicit capital regulation would require a joint federal-state structure to implement a system of federal subsidies to poorer states. That in turn would require some national standards as a basis for payment. But within any state the available funds would have to be allocated by a local decisionmaking body. There are too many capital investment decisions for any federal agency to cope with.

BASIC DIRECTION. Many approaches could combine aspects of the international standard to provide universal coverage and better cost control in the United States. This review has suggested choices within the international menu that would be considered compromises by advocates of a single-payer approach but would nevertheless create a much better American health care system.

No reform can succeed without compulsory participation and regulation of costs. All-payer regulation is entirely adequate in place of single-payer regulation. It should accommodate hospitals' uniqueness and pay physicians according to a national relative value scale and local agreements about conversion factors. The federal government should pay for education (including medical students' tuition) and research from separate budgets. Any reform must create a basic, decent system for all Americans, with exceptions only for people to choose more, not to be stuck with less. Some exceptions to fee regulation could be allowed but should be limited.

Financing is best based on employer payments, and individual contributions should be related to income. Financing should be simple, but different pools for different types of employers would be within the bounds of international compromises. Benefits at the low end of the international range would not be ideal but would be acceptable. Certainly universal coverage with less generous benefits is better than more generous benefits with only a hope for universal coverage.

The basic direction of compromise would then be toward financing that is more like Japan's and cost control that is more like Germany's. But what should be done about managed care? American reform should preserve a place for the best forms of managed care, in which they could compete with the rest of the system. The major benefit that reformers could offer to physicians is abolition of the worst forms.

Managed Care and Competition

American health care reform should greatly restrict both third-party managed care and risk-bearing gatekeeper systems. Unless physicians practice in single group- or staff-model HMOs, they should operate under the rules of an all-payer fee-for-service system.

BANNING MOST FORMS OF MANAGED CARE. The Clinton administration's more fervent believers in managed competition dreamed of a system in which competing integrated networks managed by physicians served the public.[66] But, for reasons given in chapter 7, competition would be unlikely to produce that result. It would be more likely to intensify use of third-party management and to displace risk onto individual physicians. The simplest way to prevent that result is to ban those approaches in favor of all-payer bargaining.

All-payer bargaining cannot duplicate the advantages of an integrated group- or staff-model HMO. But almost everything the other forms of managed care do, an all-payer system can do better.

When competing managed care organizations analyze physician billings in order to identify outliers, they make random error more likely by dividing up a physician's activity. By random chance doctors who have an unusually high proportion of a certain billing in one group and a lower figure in another will be branded as bad actors in the first. The reviewers for competing plans are not physicians, and competing plans cannot develop guidelines in cooperation with the physician specialty societies. In all-payer systems they see all of a physician's activity, physicians are reviewers, and no physician has to worry about which guidelines apply to which insurer's patients.

The notion of making gatekeepers bear risk is sweeping American managed care. But when physicians deal with a number of insurers, they are vulnerable to the random variation that comes from having a small group of patients from each source. International versions of gatekeeper approaches are much fairer to physicians because they do not divide up a physician's practice, and they ask him or her to bear only a portion of the risk created by the "ordering pen."[67] Physicians can logically bear some risk as part of a regulated all-payer system, or of a group- or staff-model HMO. Either makes more sense than bearing risk for multiple, competing, managed care organizations.

A regulated fee-for-service system offers patients and providers more freedom of choice than a world of managed care. Physicians have more options for referrals and patients are more likely to be able to go to the doctor who is recommended by friends. A patient who wants to switch does not have to go "out of network" and spend more.

All-payer bargaining also offers superior cost control. Payers have more bargaining power as a group than the average payer does in a system of competition. The providers receive in return a much simpler billing environment, guaranteed payment for all necessary care, and less interference with practice. It is a better system for both sides.

The other forms of managing most physician services could be banned by a few rules. First, insurers should be required to include "any willing provider" unless the plan contracts with providers to work only with that plan.[68] Second, no plan should be allowed to impose risk-bearing contracts except in the context of such an exclusive relationship. Thus plans could maintain closed panels and allocate risk only if each physician in the plan worked only within that plan. Third, the legislation would make some forms of review the responsibility of cooperative organizations rather than individual insurers, and limit the remaining review that insurers could themselves perform.

ALL-PAYER REGULATION AND DIFFERENCES AMONG PLANS. Physician payment within the all-payer sector then would be negotiated and administered much as it is in Germany, although it would likely begin with less powerful volume adjustments and might have more subcategories of types of care.[69] If medicare were folded into the other insurance or allowed to operate as one insurer in the bargaining, the insurers could negotiate hospital budgets. Otherwise, they would negotiate rates of payment with each hospital according to medicare's diagnosis-related group classification. Then hospitals would be paid in the same manner by both private and public payers.

Plans would then compete on efficiency and quality in limited ways. If the system had neither hospital budgets nor volume adjustments to fees, plans would perform utilization review for hospital use. But if payment were made according to rates per diagnosis, the review would not have to focus on what happens inside the hospital, such as length of stay. It would need apply only to admission, so would be much less of a hassle for doctors than the current review system.

Some other, mainly nonphysician, services would benefit from review. The clearest example is mental health benefits, which are especially subject to abuse and can take many forms (for example, inpatient and outpatient care). Rehabilitation is another example. Review of such care should be performed by professionals who monitor reports on patient progress, not by clerks who process hundreds of claims per hour looking for anomalies. In general, review by insurers should be allowed for categories of treatment for which case management by professionals is viable and appropriate. Following this principle, the law could designate a set of services for which review would be allowed, with measures to encourage integrated case management.

Plans also could offer a choice among two or three legally established cost-sharing structures, as the Clinton plan did. Thus plans would differ in their cost sharing, in their management of hospital admissions, and in management of services such as mental health and rehabilitation. These differences would preserve the best applications of utilization review yet eliminate the vast bulk of interference with treatment decisions. All bills for those decisions would go to central payment units in each region. The clearinghouse would bill the insurers and pay the claims. Its records would be the basis for any volume adjustments to fees. Organizations of physicians, based on county or state medical societies, would profile physicians and identify those who made particularly high use of resources or unusual treatment decisions for given diagnoses. The reforms would have to establish the legal structure for that process.

BUDGETING AND THE PLACE OF HMOS. German experience before 1992 shows that cost increases can be strongly restrained (though not enough to suit the Germans) without directly enforceable budgets. Yet some form of target setting is necessary. Germany set targets for premium increases; an American state could set its own targets or budgets. The difficulty would be ensuring that the federal budget is not at the mercy of state-level failures. In Germany this is not a serious issue because the federal government's role in health care financing is very small.

Federal payments could be limited according to a formula and states made responsible for extra costs. Then only inhabitants of each state would have reason to care about that state's costs, and there would be no reason for federal budget setting. If instead the federal government paid some set share of local costs, the federal contribution would depend on state achievements, and then the federal government would need a way to enforce targets.

In either case, a government that wants to be sure that it limits total spending has to limit premiums. If premiums vary, any effort to limit a weighted average of premiums must be inaccurate, and enforcement measures could easily, as in the Clinton plan, have perverse effects. But if most of the intermediate forms of managed care were eliminated, the task of controlling total costs would be much simpler.

There would be three types of plans: fee-for-service with higher cost sharing, fee-for-service with lower cost sharing, and group- and staff-model HMOs. Most of the population that needed to be subsidized would likely be in plans with low cost sharing because they could not afford high cost sharing and the HMOs would probably not be located nearby. If most of the government's subsidies went to the plans with low cost sharing, the government's main task would be to set a maximum premium for those plans. Capping their premiums would leave some doubt about exact government spending, but so would any other set of guarantees. The budget effects would be estimated using formulas that predicted enrollment in the different plans; the governments and their scorekeepers would have to agree on the formulas, but so would they in any system that allowed choice of plans. But unlike trying to target the average, setting the maximum would eliminate all issues of perverse incentives and administrative complexity and establish a clear maximum for subsidy costs.

Plans with high cost sharing would have to charge less than the cap. Depending on their levels of service and efficiency, the cost of some group- and staff-model HMOs might be greater than those of the plans with high cost sharing, and the cost of others might be less.[70] HMOs could also choose whether to offer out-of-network options (except for emergencies, for which allowing use of any provider must be mandatory).

As part of their competition with the fee-for-service sector, anything these HMOs spent to improve their capital plant would have to be offset by savings on operating costs; if they could do so and satisfy customers without raising their premiums, more power to them. The government would only need to ensure that if HMOs used services that had been financed by a state or national capital investment program, they paid a surcharge as a contribution to that capital fund. HMOs thus would compete with each other and the fee-for-service sector on both cost and quality. They could attract business by charging lower premiums for the schedule with low cost sharing. If managed efficiently they might be able to pay for more capital investment, and eventually better facilities, than the regulated system. By making greater use of nonphysician providers, some HMOs might provide care at a lower unit cost that enabled them to reimburse physicians at higher overall rates than the fee schedule. Some thought should be given to allowing them to offer some supplemental benefits. In all these ways, HMOs would have a chance to win the competition with fee-for-service medicine.

Some supporters of managed competition argue that regulation of the sort suggested in this conclusion would have horrible consequences for medical care and that therefore, even if it saved money, it would force individuals to accept lower-quality care. Yet if these advocates' preferred model were in fact a better deal, the competition described here would allow HMOs to prove that they could provide better quality for the same money, or equal quality for less money. And if a regulated fee-for-service system were so bad, that would be revealed by the applications to join the "competing" sector.

The difference between my plan and other models of competition is not in whether competition exists. The difference is in what kinds of plans would compete and how a budget would be enforced. In the model presented here, fee-for-service medicine is set up to be as cost-effective as possible. Managed care is restricted to its best forms. Spending is capped by controlling the *highest* premium but not budgeted to control total premiums. That change would eliminate the perverse effects of the Clinton plan, and the regulated fee-for-service sector and HMOs could compete on equal terms.

Financing Reform

As chapters 7 and 8 explained, however, any reform that seeks to create some price competition among forms of health insurance must overcome obstacles such as the danger that risk competition will displace efficiency competition and the difficulty of combining effective price constraints with adequate income-related subsidies.

RISK ADJUSTMENT. Because HMOs would compete on price with the fee-for-service sector, difficult issues of risk adjustment would remain. The marketing of plans should be restricted to limit bias. Open enrollment through an alliance structure (whether called that or not), combined with limits on other marketing (such as advertising), would be the most effective measures. Premiums would also have to be adjusted for demographic variables.

These measures would not eliminate problems, but the problems would be less severe than in other versions of competition for two reasons. The fee-for-service competitors would not be able to bias enrollments through their selections of providers, because they could not have closed panels. And the group- and staff-model HMOs would have natural catchment areas based on clinic locations and, except in a few places, would be a relatively small part of the market. Thus patient selection by provider selection would be much less of a threat. As HMOs grew, risk selection might become a problem, but that would take some time.

THE RELATIONSHIP BETWEEN SUBSIDIES AND BUDGETS. If the federal government were not at financial risk, it would not have to worry about setting budgets (though it still would need a formula for its payments to states). If employers all paid by the same rules, there would be no need to assess each firm's size and wage level.

Having avoided subsidies to firms, government would only be subsidizing individuals. The subsidy structure could be designed to cover the individual payments for the option with low cost sharing up to some point, such as the poverty line. As the subsidy phased out above that line, recipients could choose which plan to buy. Thus cost-sharing subsidies would be built into the premium subsidies.[71]

In order to budget its subsidy costs, the government would only need to set a maximum premium for the plans with low cost sharing. Those targets then would set the parameters for the fee negotiations among payers and providers, much as currently occurs in Germany. This approach reverses the logic of many proposals in states today, which try to force the subsidized population into managed care plans. Ensuring that acceptable plans are available to the lower-income population is, however, extremely difficult. Both the Cooper-Grandy and Clinton bills provided special provisions in recognition of the fact that the low-income population is not, in fact, likely to be able to join the less expensive HMOs.

THE EMPLOYER SHARE. As in the Clinton design, there would still have to be three flows of funds: from employers, from individuals, and from the governments. Instead of requiring employers to pay a percentage of the "weighted average premium," the employer share would be set at the level needed to pay a set percentage of the cap on premiums for the plans with low cost sharing. Individuals would pay flat fees for the difference between this amount and the plan they chose, so if they enrolled in an HMO or a plan with high cost sharing they would pay less.[72]

The payroll-based flow of funds then would be the percentage of earnings per employee necessary to collect the target amount. Distinctions by family type would add a layer of complication that the Europeans and Japanese have chosen to avoid, in part because they want to encourage family formation. Americans might choose differently, but allowing different premiums according to beneficiaries' ages is not worth the trouble.

What proportion of costs, then, should be collected as part of the employment-based flow of funds? First, the same percentage charges should be applied to some nonemployment income, as it is in other countries. Second, the defined percentage of the premium cap is not the same as a percentage of costs. Seventy-five percent of the cap on lower-cost-sharing, fee-for-service plans, for example, could be close to the Clinton proposal's standard of 80 percent of costs. Deciding on the employer share requires difficult trade-offs.[73]

Many employers would prefer a lower number, and the Clinton standard was quite high by international standards. The equivalent measure in Germany would be for employers to contribute half and employees one quarter of the target premium as a percentage of payroll, and for employees then to pay the balance for the plan that they chose. One compromise would be, as in Japan, to set a minimum but allow employers to pay more as a business expense. If that minimum were less than the average already being paid by employers, however, it would risk encouraging a decline in the average employer share. No matter what the current average might be, lower mandated employer shares would require higher government subsidies. Therefore a higher employer contribution would work better, and any payment difficulties on the part of employers could be addressed by measures such as the phasein described earlier.

INDIVIDUAL SUBSIDIES. A higher employer share would, by the same logic as in the Clinton plan, explained in chapter 9, make subsidizing individuals much easier though not uncomplicated.

Persons whose low incomes are stable would not present a problem: in their case, an application system such as the one in British Columbia, a form similar to the IRS form 1040 EZ, could report the necessary information, and it could be checked against IRS and Social Security Administration payroll data. The difficulty would be with the people whose income changed during the year. Adjustments made too quickly could overpay; adjustments made too slowly could leave needy people unable to afford insurance.

The system proposed here is similar to what the Clinton plan proposed. If each individual were assumed to have 70 or 75 percent of the cost of the plan with low cost sharing paid from the employer account, no family would owe more than 25 or 30 percent of its total premium, and many would owe less. That should be manageable for virtually everyone for a couple of months, if the breadwinner lost his job or were disabled, for example.

Rather than establish more complicated subsidies as a backup, reformers might instead strengthen the role of hospital outpatient clinics as a supplier of later resort. A few extra billions of subsidy to those clinics, conditioned on participation by physicians affiliated with the academic medical centers in the delivery of care on terms similar to those in Australia or France, could prove to be a safety valve against a wide variety of distributional problems.

The Logic of Health Care Reform

The approach described above adapts the international standard methods of cost control and coverage to encourage competition from integrated closed-panel health plans. In order to do so, individuals must have a choice of premium costs, and the basic benefits must be less generous in some plans than in others.

Implementing such a structure in Canada or Germany would be difficult because it would likely involve reducing the benefits of many voters. It is plausible in the United States, however, because of the nation's historic failure to guarantee even decent, never mind generous, health care benefits to all its citizens. In a more fortunate historic circumstance, America also has some good group- and staff-model HMOs and the potential to slowly create more. Thus the system suggested here makes more political and substantive sense in the United States than in the other countries described in this volume.

Whatever approach one prefers, however, all readers of this book should remember that every other advanced industrial country in the world has found a way to guarantee decent health care to all its citizens. Every year of delay is a year of higher costs and further intensification of America's unique private sector bureaucratic interference with medical treatment; and it is a year in which millions of Americans will suffer for the failure of their country to manage what every other nation of remotely comparable wealth and accomplishment has achieved.

The United States faces many policy challenges. On some, such as how to repair the effects of racism, or how to maintain wages in a changing international economy, we really do not know what to do. We have few examples of successful policy.

On health care Americans do not need new theory. International experience reveals the key measures. We can adapt those measures, add some of our own, and create an American system that can make us proud and secure in the new century.

Americans do not need more information. They do need the clarity of understanding necessary to overcome the obstacle course of the political system, the propaganda of entrenched interests, and above all the ideology that says that responsibility is fending for yourself, not standing up for each other.

A song of the 1960s says that "freedom's just another word for nothing left to lose." For a diabetic who cannot afford insulin, or a woman with a breast lump who cannot afford to see a doctor, or a man with a cough who waits until he spits blood to go to the emergency room, all that is left to lose is one's life. That is the freedom offered by current American health care. Modern medicine is too expensive, and the risks too unpredictable, for all but the very richest Americans to fend entirely for themselves.

In a world of intractable problems, it will be a great pity, and a greater shame, if America never does what it can do to guarantee decent health care to all Americans.

Appendix

Technical Aspects of Managed Competition

*T*HIS appendix elaborates on some of the more technical problems with managed competition, with and without budget caps, discussed in chapters 8 and 9. It has two purposes: to strengthen the argument in those chapters about the practical difficulties of designing a health care financing system of that type, and to provide a reference for people who nonetheless decide to try.

Implementing a Cap on Tax Deductibility of Health Benefits

Chapter 8 summarized the difficulties associated with setting and then administering a cap on the tax deductibility of health benefits. It would be relatively easy as a matter of substance, though politically difficult, to set a national cap on tax deductibility. Congress would choose a number, and all employers and employees would use the same number. Unfortunately, the cost of insurance varies substantially across the country, because incomes vary. So a uniform tax deductibility cap could be too high to constrain the cost of premiums in one area and too low to be practical in another.

In any case, the point of managed competition theory is to allow market competition to set the standard, and that means there should be different standards in different markets. A simple version would then have the lowest premium in an area as the "benchmark," because it would represent the lowest price at which the standard benefits could be provided and still meet the established quality standards (if the plan did not meet those standards, it would not have been approved).

Setting the Reference Premium

Unfortunately, the lowest-cost plan might not be generally available—for example, it might be a small health maintenance organization (HMO). Then nonmembers would pay more, not because they elected a more expensive plan willingly but because they could not get into the least expensive plan. It would be hard to imagine a more arbitrary and unfair basis for taxation, which is why the Cooper-Grandy bill provided a standard of availability as well as price.

But defining the right "proportion of eligible individuals" would not be so easy. If it were set too low, many people would not have access to plans at that or a lower price. If it were set fairly high, then in most parts of the country the less expensive forms of care, particularly group- or staff-model HMOs, might not have enough members to qualify. The lowest-priced plan that met the enrollment standard could be an expensive plan, which would eliminate the incentive for savings.

In some areas a number of plans might cluster around a given premium level, so a standard that included one would include a number of others at similar prices. Then the standard would seem fair. In other areas, there might be few other plans near the least expensive one that met the same standard. Then the standard would seem (and be) unfair.

In order to balance the needs for fairness and for a standard that created savings, any regulator therefore would have to make rulings for each coverage area. No plan could delegate that decision to states because the reference rate determines federal taxes; indeed, the IRS might be more than a little upset about an independent organization, such as the Cooper-Grandy health care standards commission (HCSC), having such power to begin with. So the federal regulator would be deeply involved in at least guessing about the structure of the local market, if not trying to structure it. And that raises two further problems.

As Cooper-Grandy was written, an open accountable health plan (AHP) would have had a defined service area, but it need not have included all of the area encompassed by the health plan purchasing cooperative (HPPC).[1] Cooper-Grandy had to accept this because the alternative would have been to require that a plan be available throughout the HPPC area—which would tell the average clinic-based HMO that it had to either expand, which would be hard for all the reasons given in chapter 7, or dissolve, which would be counterproductive and perverse. But a plan then could meet the requirements for the reference plan yet not be geographically available to some people.[2]

Worse yet, it would be too easy to make a mistake in setting the standard. The regulator would have to regulate by price, quality, and membership, but at the time it decided it could know only the price. The regulator might infer quality and membership from previous performance, but it could be wrong. If fewer people signed up for the reference plan than expected, that would be obvious and immediately embarrassing: a public judgment of disagreement with the regulators' notion of acceptability. The regulator (here, the health care standards commission, or HCSC) might also determine at the end of the year that the reference plan had not delivered acceptable quality. Ordinarily, it would be expected to announce that result and impose sanctions. But that would mean admitting that it had based the reference premium on a mistake; worse, it had forced people who recognized the lower quality to pay higher taxes for joining a more expensive plan. The HCSC would also be admitting that other plans had been punished by its mistake.[3] Were it Cooper-Grandy's HCSC or any other human institution, the regulator would hesitate to admit its error—and so to correct it.

This structure for setting the reference premium makes mistakes inevitable because it requires making decisions with only partial information yet also discourages correcting error. Those are not desirable attributes of any system, for any purpose.

The Chafee bill's method for setting its benchmark premiums for tax purposes was much simpler. The bad news begins with a question: how will anybody know the prices of all the plans? According to the bill, "The applicable dollar limit shall be determined annually by the Secretary [of the Treasury], in consultation with the Secretary of Health and Human Services, from information submitted by each State with respect to each HCCA."[4] The text at no point gave the states the authority to require that plans, including those of large, self-insured employers, provide this information on any schedule. That must be inferred. There is no sensible way to figure out what the premium-equivalent for self-insured plans might be.

But assume that states gathered the information far enough in advance for the secretary to analyze it and publish the standards for each coverage area, and that the states in turn distributed the information to their citizens. Now assume that you were the manager of an HMO, and wanted to reduce the chance that your premium would be above the deductible limit. That limit was defined as the average of the cost of the lowest-priced half of the plans in an a given area. For example, if there were ten plans, the limit would be the average of the premiums for the five least expensive plans. If you were a plan manager, you could create another plan, perhaps the same as your own but with a point-of-service option for a 50 percent copayment, with a premium that was 40 percent higher. You might create two extra plans, just to improve the odds.

If all plans did this, the "average premium price of the bottom half" of marketed plans would not represent the prices for the plans that anybody actually purchased. If there were ten plans and each created a more expensive "dummy," so there were twenty plans but only ten that anyone bought, the "average of the bottom half" by Chafee's definition would in fact be the average among the ten plans that anyone joined—a much higher benchmark. This problem could be solved by allowing regulators to identify "fake" plans, but that would give the regulators discretion and power, and the Chafee authors sought to avoid regulation, or at least avoid specifying who would regulate, wherever possible.[5] The problem could be solved by creating some sort of membership standards—but that brings us back to the Cooper-Grandy difficulties.

Managed competition does not eliminate the need for regulation; it just renames regulation (a bad, government thing) as "management" (a good, private sector thing). The catch is that one cannot base a reference premium for tax purposes solely on market signals. Such a decision is fundamentally a regulatory decision, requiring government power, information, and legal standards. Because making the decision requires having information about quality and membership before it is available, mistakes would be extremely likely.

Even so, setting the reference premium might not be as difficult as administering it.

Administering the Tax Cap

Within both the Chafee and Cooper-Grandy bills, the cap on tax deductibility of benefits had to vary not only by health care market but also by family type and by age category. Otherwise people would be taxed for being older or for having children.[6]

In Cooper-Grandy there were four family types. Assuming an average of two HPPC areas per state, and only two age bands, there would be 800 different premiums. For the IRS that would mean 800 different legal deductibles. There would probably be more.[7]

Imagine trying to administer this. I will impose an extra regulation to make it imaginable: any county could be in only one HPPC or coverage area.[8] Then the IRS could add a line for county of residence in the tax return, add a list of all three thousand-plus counties and their HPPCs, and add a schedule with all 800 or more combinations of HPPC and age bracket and enrollment type so people could look up their deductibles. A dozen or so pages later, individuals would compare that table with the account of their employer's contribution on their W2 form, add the amount of their own contribution (from some other record), and compare the total with the allowable amount on the schedule. All of this would be necessary even on 1040EZ. Many mistakes would be made.

Calculating corporate taxes would of course be much more complicated. If (as in Cooper-Grandy) allowable business expenses for health insurance varied by coverage area, family type, and age of employees, then any corporation that spanned boundaries would have to operate under multiple federal tax codes. A firm would be taxed differently for employees who worked in the same plant but lived in different HPPC areas.

In any system a firm, either for its own taxes or to report to its employees, would have to keep track of changing levels of deductibility as employees crossed the age boundaries, got married, had children, the children left home, and so on. If a person lived in one HPPC area but worked in another, and enrolled in an AHP that was available only in the latter, which reference premium would apply? What deductible would be appropriate for couples who were employed in different alliance areas?[9] Rules could be made for all of these circumstances, of course. Figuring them out and enforcing them would be the problem.

Chafee's approach avoided the corporate tax problem, but individual tax administration would have been at least as difficult. Employers would have had to keep track and report; employees and the IRS would have had the burden of filing and checking returns. Chafee's effort to avoid regulating self-insured plans created a further problem. The bill said such employers would provide estimated costs that "to the extent practicable . . . shall be made on an actuarial basis." As the language suggests, in a self-insured structure there would be no way to determine costs per employee.[10] If the employer's package were in fact worth less than the standard the employer might still report that it cost the standard in order to maximize its tax break. How would the IRS audit that?[11]

Conclusion

The cap on tax deductibility is one of the two differences between the theory of managed competition and the existing competition among health insurers in the United States (the other is the limit on risk-rating). Yet the obstacles to implementing that cap would be forbidding. First, the lowest-priced plan in the market would probably not be available to most purchasers. Second, any effort to estimate which plan met any standard aside from price would require regulators to make decisions based on information they did not have, such as quality and enrollment. Third, any attempt to avoid these problems by setting a standard that was not based on customer choices or plan performance, as in the Chafee plan, could easily be distorted by the insurers. Fourth, any market-based tax cap must create hundreds of difference caps and thus huge administrative difficulties for employers, taxpayers, and the government.

Ironically, the administrative difficulty would be much smaller in a smaller country, and a small state would have hardly any problem. But states do not collect federal income tax. The idea of a market-based tax cap makes less sense in the United States than in any other country in this study.

Financing Subsidies

Cooper-Grandy and Chafee both would have expanded coverage through use of means-tested individual subsidies, which require calculating the exact amount of money needed by each applicant according to his or her income. Each bill also sought to limit federal costs to the exact amount saved by various other measures. So the available funds might have been less than needed to cover the promised subsidies.

The Chafee bill's solution to a possible funding shortfall would have been to either reduce the standard benefits (thereby raising taxes for the vast majority of voters) or subsidize fewer people (much more likely). The Cooper-Grandy bill sought to provide more reliable subsidies, and that is why, even though Cooper-Grandy did not promise universal coverage and Chafee did, the former should be considered a much more serious attempt to cover everyone.

Cooper-Grandy would have allowed subsidized families to enroll in any plan and pay only 10 percent of the difference between the reference premium and their plan's premium. Thus if the reference premium were $4,000 and a poor family had a $4,500 policy, it would pay $50 (that is for the poorest families). The government would pay whatever proportion of the reference premium was appropriate given its savings: that is, if it achieved only 80 percent of the target savings, it would pay 80 percent of the reference premium. If the reference premium were $4,000 per year, in this example, the government would pay the insurer only $3,200. Each plan then would take the loss associated with having insufficiently subsidized members. In other words, each plan would "eat" the difference.[12] The plans' other members would have to cover those costs, which would be built into the premiums.

Under these conditions, having members who need to be subsidized is a very bad deal. Cooper-Grandy therefore added a form of risk adjustment; in this case the risk was not that members might be sicker but that they might have too little money. In each area HPPCs would have used their regular contracts with open plans and special contracts with closed ones to collect money from plans with a smaller proportion of people who needed subsidies and send it to plans with greater need. The health care standards commission would then have operated a similar system to move money from more fortunate to less fortunate HPPC areas, "in order to assure the equitable distribution among all AHPs, nationwide, of reductions in premiums and cost-sharing" as subsidies to persons with low incomes.[13]

First of all, this evidently would have involved a lot of bureaucracy for a bill written by people who were trying to avoid creating "big government." But the way this system would operate is a far more significant problem. In principle, all sickness fund systems have subsidies built into the premium structure. In some circumstances the Cooper-Grandy subsidies were more generous than those in the Clinton plan. For example, they included cost-sharing assistance.[14] But the Cooper-Grandy approach had two huge differences from the international models. First, it involved adjustments in a much larger country, among many more plans, with much less stable membership, with a much more complex administrative process. Designing that set of transfers posed such questions as what the HCSC could do if an HPPC that was ordered to send in some money for distribution refused or, more plausibly, dallied. "Developing a national transfer system involving the thousands of AHPs in the country would be an extremely difficult task," the Congressional Budget Office (CBO) reported, "and whether it could be implemented effectively is doubtful."[15]

More important, the subsidies were built into a system of voluntary, not compulsory, membership. Persons who chose to buy insurance for themselves therefore would also have had to choose to subsidize others in a way that people without insurance did not. Therefore some who already might have considered going without insurance because their likely costs were lower than the community rate would be even more likely to do so. That would lead to higher rates as the pool became riskier and then to more people opting out: a version of the "death spiral" that destroyed community rating in the United States, and directly comparable to the pattern that has been driving up rates for private insurance in Australia. Financing the poor through cost subsidies within the charges for insurance is not likely to work unless insurance is compulsory.

Chapter 8 discussed two further problems specific to means-tested subsidies. One problem, the disincentive to work caused by extremely high effective marginal tax rates for the working poor, cannot be solved. Another is the amount of work necessary to administer subsidies.

The latter problem would begin with having to process tens of millions of applications. The system would somehow have to find reliable income data and have some process for correcting hundreds of thousands of errors. Errors would occur because most incomes would not be known until the end of a year. Persons who were temporarily unemployed would have to be subsidized based on a projected annual income that is highly unreliable because no one would know when they would be employed again or at what rates. Somehow the money would have to be directed to the right HPPC areas and plans. As CBO reported on Cooper-Grandy, "It would be difficult for the commission to avoid misdirecting some subsidy payments."[16]

Unless the system were extremely loose, people who lost their jobs would have trouble paying for insurance. Cooper-Grandy required that an applicant's annual income be estimated from earnings over the previous three months. That sounds reasonable, but would mean that if an unemployed breadwinner applied a month after losing her job, her reported income would be two-thirds of her former wages; she would have to be unemployed three months before being eligible for a full subsidy.[17] But the alternative to Cooper-Grandy's approach is no more attractive. A person could be unemployed for a month, get a subsidy, get a good new job, and many months later settle up on her loan from the government—if the government kept good records.

In short, it is hard to design a set of rules for means-tested individual subsidies that seems reasonable. Subsidies that were more generous would risk spending money on people who turned out not to need it; those that were less generous would risk depriving the truly needy. The system could employ enough bureaucrats to do all the work quickly and check it carefully, and for its trouble be accused of creating big government; or it could employ fewer personnel and work more slowly or make more errors.

A system that automatically adjusted contributions to income by charging a percentage of income would be much simpler.

Subsidy Administration in the Health Security Act

Chapter 9 outlined some of the financing of the Clinton administration's Health Security Act. It argued that the bill's approach created, in essence, separate flows of financing.

Of these, the payments by persons who were not employed or only partially employed were especially complex and need not be discussed here. The rules about how much employers would contribute to what I have called the employer account within the alliances are more important, because they involved more money and more controversy.

As noted in the chapter, the plan called for employers to pay 80 percent of the weighted average premium for single individuals, but for couples and families with children, as CBO explained, "an employer's payment would not equal the alliance credit amount because families contain, on average, more than one worker for whom some employer would be paying premiums." Couples were to be in one pool and families with children in another. Thus if the average couple had 1.6 workers, employers would pay only 80 percent ÷ 1.6 for each employee in that class, or 50 percent of the average premium. The system pooled single- and two-parent families so employers would not have incentives to discriminate against single parents.[18]

TABLE A-1. *Estimated Premiums under the Health Security Act*

Unit covered	Total premium	Employer share
Single person	$2,100	$1,680
Married couple	$4,200	$2,315
One-parent family	$4,095	$3,033
Two-parent family	$5,565	$3,033

Source: Congressional Budget Office, *An Analysis of the Administration's Health Proposal.*

CBO's estimate of the size of the resulting premiums and employer payments in 1994 illustrates the effects (see table A-1). One effect of the "employer mandate" in the Clinton plan, then, might have been to lower the premiums paid by employers who provided good family insurance for employees whose spouses worked for firms that did not provide insurance at all. Individual employers would have paid less in a system that required all employers to pay something for all employees than in a system that assumed each employer was paying for entire families.[19]

But many employers would not be able to afford even the required contributions to insurance for low-wage employees. According to the estimates in table A-1, for example, an employer that was required to contribute $3,033 on behalf of a previously uninsured employee making $15,000 per year would be paying more than 20 percent of the employee's wages for insurance.[20] In response to that problem the Clinton plan provided not just the cap of 7.9 percent of payroll on any employer's contributions, but a system of lower caps for firms with fewer than seventy-six employees and average wages below $24,000 (see table A-2). Phasing in (or out) subsidies according to small incre-

TABLE A-2. *Limits on Employer Health Care Payment as Percent of Payroll*
Percent

Average number of full-time equivalent employees	Average annual wages per full-time-equivalent employee				
	$0–$12,000	$12,001–$15,000	$15,001–$18,000	$18,001–$21,000	$21,001–$24,000
Fewer than 25	3.5	4.4	5.3	6.2	7.1
25 to 49	4.4	5.3	6.2	7.1	7.9
50 to 75	5.3	6.2	7.1	7.9	7.9

Source: S. 1957, section 6123, p. 1072.

ments of average income and employment size would reduce the possible advantages to employers of manipulating those figures. A straight drop from 7.9 percent to 3.9 percent at one cutoff point would provide much more incentive to reduce wages or the size of the work force. The disadvantage of the sliding scale is that it requires more precise recordkeeping: more "bureaucracy."

Politically, the plan to give special breaks to smaller, low-wage employers had two further disadvantages: the system would have had to pay for those breaks by doing less for other interests, and the strategy did not buy support from those employers. Instead, once the proposal validated the claim for special breaks, much of the political battle in the first half of 1994 involved how much further to go in reducing employer mandates.

This whole debate ignored the huge subsidies involved in either a simple percentage-of-payroll limit or the Clinton plan. Using the CBO example above, with the cap at 7.9 percent an employer would only contribute $948 per year for an employee with a $12,000 annual wage, which would be far below the standard employer contribution for any family type. Under the Clinton plan, if that employer had fewer than twenty-five employees it would have paid only $468. One hopes that the next administration that proposes an employer mandate at least makes the small business lobbies fight for such extra-special treatment, so that they can be blamed for the extra bureaucracy it creates.

As chapter 9 also discussed, once a set of subsidies is designed, somebody has to administer it. In the Clinton design, each regional alliance would have to keep track of the incomes of individuals who applied for subsidies. It would have to know the number of full-time-equivalent employees, their average wages, and the covered wages for each employee of each employer, according to their family type (the four enrollment categories). Employers would have to report this information on an annual or monthly basis, depending on the datum. There would have to be some sort of clearinghouse process, and continual updating for new hires, persons transferring within a firm, and the like.[21] These information requirements alone would require substantial bureaucracies.

On the basis of this information, alliances would calculate contributions owed (and thus the discounts) for thousands of employers in each area. Because incomes are not known in advance, there would have to be some process of audit and reconciliation, so individuals and employers who paid too much (for instance, more than 7.9 percent of payroll) one year would be charged less the following year, and vice versa.[22] Employer reports would not be adequate because they might not be true and because they would not report nonemployment income. Ultimately, then, there ought to be some way to reconcile decisions to the IRS data base.

Yet the Clinton plan did not change the law to give alliances access to IRS records. Giving that information to semipublic bodies raises questions of confidentiality and proper delegation of state power. Nor did the plan call for doing what might seem obvious, which is to give the IRS the job of running the subsidy system, because it already has the best information. Asked why the IRS did not get the job, one source speculated, "The IRS read Martha Derthick's book." In *Agency under Stress*, Martha Derthick explained what happened when a proud and competent agency, the Social Security Administration, adopted new tasks (administration of supplemental security income and of disability determinations) that were very different from its core task, administering old age and survivors' insurance.[23] The result was a mess. The IRS, which is not used to administering the cash flows from benefit programs, wondered who would audit the system if the IRS ran it and refused to take the job.

There is no good candidate to run the subsidy system. States have access to the IRS data, yet the existing state bureaus (for example, welfare bureaus) experienced with subsidies may be oriented toward rejecting applicants. Further, neither the states nor the alliances would risk their own money in making subsidy decisions. The federal government would pay for all subsidies; state contributions were set at maintenance-of-effort level. This does not seem a good way to protect the federal budget. Yet if the alliances were running the risk-adjustment system, which would be easiest for them because they would pay the plans, perhaps having them allocate other subsidies as well is the best of the bad alternatives.

Administering a Cap on the "Weighted Average Premium"

Chapter 9 argued that the Clinton administration's method of enforcing its budget caps within each alliance area could have had perverse results. This section explains why.

The system relied on a national health board to set premium targets and then to force individual plans to adjust their bids in such a way that the target would be met. The average premium would depend on how many people chose which plans at which prices.

The first issue is, what would make a plan's price "too high"? A plan might cost less than the target average yet be a bad deal for the price, but the Clinton drafters left that judgment to the customers. Instead, they determined that in the first year of the system, no plan that bid below the target premium could fairly be blamed if total spending emerged above that level (if, in essence, too many people chose more expensive plans).

In subsequent years, however, using the target average as the limit is not as logical. If all other plans maintained the same relative premiums, but one less expensive plan raised its price to the average, that alone could raise the total above average. Therefore the bill created a different standard for the second and subsequent years: rather than limiting health plans' bids on premiums, it limited their bids for *increases* over their previous premiums.

Thus when the deadline for "negotiation" was reached and plans' bids became final, an alliance would forward them to the national health board. On the basis of the bids and whatever information the board could develop about how many families would select each plan, the board would guess whether the alliance's weighted average premium would meet the target. If the board thought the weighted average would be too high, it would require premium reductions by those plans it held responsible. In the first year, excess bids would be defined as those above the target premium level. In subsequent years, the target would be defined as the amount premiums could be increased, so excessive bids would be those higher than the targeted increase.

In either case, the board would estimate the total premium reductions needed to meet the target, compare that number with the premiums of the plans involved, and force them to accept the proportional reductions in their bids necessary to hit the target.[24] If the board guessed right about enrollments in plans, spending would fit the alliance budget. If more people than expected enrolled in the more expensive plans, the board would have to correct spending. It would do so by reducing the target increase for that alliance for each of the next two succeeding years.[25]

On a first close look, this approach is very clever. Whether a plan's bid was reduced would be, first, a matter of its managers' choice. Plans that did not bid more than the target would not be in danger. Even if they did bid high, the need for an adjustment would depend on other bids, which were not under the board's control, and on the enrollment estimates, which could be considered a technical procedure. The alliance might even use its own estimates to provoke negotiations that adjusted the totals before the bids reached the board. This sounds as close as one could get to regulation without subjecting the regulated to the willful power of the regulators.

Now consider how premiums would be set in the first year. The national health board would announce a premium target, and the plans would bid—some above the target and some below. The alliance could announce that the board would be likely to enforce a cut. The managers of any plan that bid over the target would know that they were at risk, but they still would have little incentive to bargain with the alliance. Imagine that the "Blue Star" plan bid 110 percent of the target. If other plans reduced their bids by enough, Blue Star might not have to reduce its bid at all. Yet if Blue Star decided to come down to 105 percent, and other plans did not budge, the total might still be too high—and Blue Star, being still over the target, would have to make a second cut! Therefore the threat of cuts by the board is not enough to make any individual plan negotiate with the alliance unless all plans in a similar position agree to a deal. That kind of negotiation is very difficult and unlikely.[26]

Instead, the national health board would receive the bids and make its estimates. If it estimated that premiums would be too high, it would order cuts in the responsible plans. But how would the board make its estimates? It would predict enrollments—by guessing. Just as it would in setting the reference premium in Cooper-Grandy, the regulator would make a judgment based on one thing it did know (the bid) and one thing it did not (enrollment). A plan's premium could be cut, threatening its financial viability and requiring extra cost controls that might dismay its providers and beneficiaries, because the board guessed wrong. This might be only somewhat easier to defend than the consequences of error in Cooper-Grandy, which would force people to pay higher taxes.

How would plan managers respond to this risk? They might decide to keep bids, in the first year, to the target level. But they might instead bid high, on the theory that if your bid is going to be cut, you might as well build in a cushion. This is typical behavior in a budget process.[27] If that strategy were common, the automatic cuts would be even more likely to be needed. And premiums would be set, in this first year, by a series of guesses about what everybody else would do and how the board would estimate enrollments—a random process with less logic than either market competition or the strong alliance role exemplified by the California Public Employees Retirement System described in chapter 8.

That brings us to the second (and all subsequent) years. After the first year, targets would be expressed as allowed increases rather than as totals. If the target in a region for the first year were $4,000, and the board wanted a national increase of 5 percent, and other things such as risk factors were equal, the board would announce that the region could have a $200 increase. If there were no further adjustments from retrospective budget corrections, each plan then would be allowed to bid $200 more than its premium of the previous year.[28]

Imagine, in this example, that a plan (call it DocsPlus) had bid $3,600 (90 percent of $4,000) in the first year. Its managers guessed wrong about its expenses, so DocsPlus lost money. In order to stay in business, it bid $4,000 the following year—still less than the new overall target. If the plan were a good one, it might lose few customers at the higher price. But unless other plans on average asked for less than they were allowed, it could not get the increase! DocsPlus would have bid for a $400 increase when the allowed amount was $200. The board would cut it back, not necessarily to $200, but possibly to that amount. In the limiting case, in which no other plans asked for less than their allowed increase, there would be no way for DocsPlus to raise its bid enough to stay in business![29]

If DocsPlus went out of business, what would happen to its customers? They might have to join more expensive plans. Then total costs would be higher than if DocsPlus had been allowed to exceed the target in order to continue operating. This absurd result follows from having a system without discretion, in which the first year's bids would be distorted by efforts to outsmart the system, and then the relationships among bids would be essentially frozen by enforcement of the cap on allowed increases.[30] The difficulty of correcting upward, if understood, would give plans a further incentive to bid high in the first year.

The administration's decisionmakers knew that plans might have difficulty meeting a premium target lower than their own bid. They therefore provided another automatic backup mechanism, to ensure that plans *could* keep costs within the reduced premiums. Each regional alliance health plan, as part of its contract with any participating provider(s), would include a provision that if the plan were deemed noncomplying by the board and subject to a percentage reduction, payments to those providers would be reduced by the applicable percentage, *plus* an amount to offset estimated increases in volume. Its payments to nonnetwork providers would be cut by a similar proportion.[31]

As mentioned in chapter 9, this approach would have the perverse effect of causing providers to be paid less by some high-priced plans than by some lower-priced plans. It also would introduce extra uncertainty into contracting between plans and providers and require providers to keep track of extra fee schedules (because the over-target plans could not even pay the normal out-of-network prices).

A Machiavellian might suspect that the administration's planners figured that providers' reactions to these measures would be so negative that plans would try hard to avoid overbidding. In fact, the Health Security Act provided a further, exceedingly sneaky, incentive to encourage plans not to bid more than their targets. Once a plan received the board's statement of the needed reduction in its premium, it could choose to accept that as a "voluntary" reduction. If a plan were deemed noncomplying and its premiums reduced involuntarily, the savings would be distributed among all policyholders within the alliance. The plan's own policyholders would pay the original bid and receive only a fraction of the reduction![32] If the plan were to reduce its bid "voluntarily," at least its own policyholders would receive the entire savings.[33]

Rather than make their customers pay extra for services from angry providers who were being paid less, we can assume that most plans would find other ways to keep costs within their targets. But because plans could not change their structures overnight, they would have to use the blunt cost controls at hand: turning down services through utilization review, pressuring risk-bearing gatekeepers, or, in a group- or staff-model HMO, perhaps making access less convenient. Otherwise, plans would go out of business. Under those circumstances, having a large fee-for-service system in place, with its costs controlled through regulatory methods, becomes even more significant. Some plan has to be flexible enough to add large numbers of patients in a year. Yet if it grows quickly, controlling its costs is especially crucial to control of the wider system's expense.

Notes

Chapter One

1. The language is from Victor R. Fuchs, *The Future of Health Policy* (Harvard University Press, 1993), pp. 62–63.

2. See Paul M. Ellwood, Alain C. Enthoven, and Lynn Etheredge, "The Jackson Hole Initiative for a Twenty-first Century American Health Care System," *Health Economics*, vol. 1, no. 3 (1992), pp. 149–68; Alain Enthoven, "The History and Principles of Managed Competition," *Health Affairs*, vol. 12, Supplement (1993), pp. 24–48.

3. See Uwe E. Reinhardt, "Comment on the Jackson Hole Initiatives for a Twenty-first Century American Health Care System," *Health Economics*, vol. 2, no. 1 (1993), pp. 7–14.

Chapter Two

1. For a different way of summarizing the issues, based mainly on the logic of economics, see Henry J. Aaron, *Serious and Unstable Condition: Financing America's Health Care* (Brookings, 1991).

2. For a good example see Louis W. Sullivan, "The Bush Administration's Health Care Plan," *New England Journal of Medicine*, September 10, 1992, pp. 801–04.

3. See Louise B. Russell, *Is Prevention Better Than Cure?* (Brookings, 1986).

4. Joshua M. Wiener, *Sharing the Burden: Strategies for Public and Private Long-term Care Insurance* (Brookings, 1994), p. 6.

5. For a superb review of the peculiar issues related to dental, mental health, and long-term care, see William A. Glaser, *Health Insurance in Practice* (San Francisco: Jossey-Bass, 1991), pp. 313–82.

6. Victor R. Fuchs, *The Future of Health Policy* (Harvard University Press, 1993), p. 166. I have not included Fuchs's entire list because I want to mention only those features that cannot conceivably exist in a health care market.

7. Societies create notions of a "social minimum" of consumption that they seek to guarantee. The United States especially has done so through benefits in kind, such as food stamps and subsidized housing, because some consumption seems more necessary than other.

8. The spending in these programs is generally pay-as-you-go, not a matter of building and earning interest on a fund. But from the individual's perspective the effect is like saving: deposits now provide a secure claim for withdrawals later.

9. For discussion in these terms see Fuchs, *Future of Health Policy*, pp. 207–09. See also Deborah A. Stone, "The Struggle for the Soul of Health Insurance," *Journal of Health Politics, Policy and Law*, vol. 18, no. 2 (Summer 1993), pp. 287–317.

10. Careful proposals for education "choice" require subsidies to equalize purchasing power. See John E. Chubb and Terry M. Moe, *Politics, Markets, and America's Schools* (Brookings, 1990).

11. For a discussion that treats allocation separately, see Richard B. Saltman, "The Role of Competitive Incentives in Recent Reforms of Northern European Health Systems," in Monique Jérôme-Forget, Joseph White, and Joshua M. Wiener, eds., *Health Care Reform through Internal Markets: Experience and Proposals* (Montreal and Washington: Institute for Research on Public Policy and Brookings, 1995), p. 78.

12. Physicians prefer the term balance billing, which implies that the patient is filling in a gap left by the insurer, to extra billing, which implies that the doctor tacked on an extra charge.

13. I use the term outpatient care in this restricted way because whether ambulatory care is provided in separate offices or by hospitals is, in some health care systems, a major influence on who receives what care.

14. For a good review of the reasons for waiting lists in the country that has the greatest problem (in this study), Great Britain, see John Yates, *Why Are We Waiting? An Analysis of Hospital Waiting Lists* (New York: Oxford University Press, 1987). Chapter 6 discusses the pattern of individual physicians' having their patients wait rather than referring them to doctors with shorter lists. It's essentially the same as what we all know about telephones. If six people are divided into three pairs, each living in an apartment with one telephone, there is more likely to be a conflict than if they all lived in the same three-telephone house—because the odds that four will want to make phone calls at the same time are not as high as the odds that one of the three pairs will.

15. There are rare exceptions, such as the Greater Victoria Hospital Society in British Columbia, which I visited. It has few residents in its hospitals and relies on a very experienced nursing staff.

16. After World War I, as hospitals began to attract a middle-class population for relatively straightforward services such as maternity, they particularly wanted to ensure that new customers were comfortable. At that time chronic patients tended to be syphilitic or shell-shock victims, neither of which were popular. Treatment in separate facilities can be humane and appropriate,

as in separate veterans' hospitals that specialize in combat-related problems. But it can also mean that patients with unpleasant chronic problems are treated in underfunded public facilities and the better-off in comfy private ones, and such a class system did develop, in part, in the United States. For a good history of hospitals in America, see Rosemary Stevens, *In Sickness and in Wealth: American Hospitals in the Twentieth Century* (Basic Books, 1989).

17. A letter to the *American Medical News*, December 20, 1993, p. 16, asked, "Mechanics specialize, why not doctors?" It is a good analogy: it is nice to have mechanics who specialize in air conditioning systems or brakes or rebuilding engines, but most of us want a good general mechanic for those times when we don't know whether the problem is the fluids or the timing or the exhaust system.

Chapter Three

1. For alternative descriptions, readers might want to consult Henry J. Aaron, *Serious and Unstable Condition: Financing America's Health Care* (Brookings, 1991); Nancy De Lew, George Greenberg, and Kraig Kinchen, "A Layman's Guide to the U.S. Health Care System," *Health Care Financing Review*, vol. 14 (Fall 1992), pp. 151–69; or Marshall W. Raffel and Norma K. Raffel, *The U.S. Health System: Origins and Functions*, 3d ed. (John Wiley & Sons, 1989).

2. Physician Payment Review Commission (PPRC), *Annual Report to Congress, 1994* (Washington, 1994), p. 10. The data are from Employee Benefit Research Institute, "Sources of Health Insurance and Characteristics of the Uninsured," *Special Report and Issue Brief* 145 (January 1994).

3. Ibid., p. 20.

4. Katherine Swartz, "Dynamics of People without Health Insurance: Don't Let the Numbers Fool You," *Journal of the American Medical Association*, January 5, 1994, pp. 64–66. These estimates are conservative both for reasons given by Swartz and because she started from the March 1992 Current Population Survey.

5. Veterans' services are not included in the standard classifications of sources of insurance for two reasons: they are not insurance, and people are not enrolled in them. All veterans are eligible so do not have to "sign up." But because many of them do not use the services, simply counting the number of veterans would not produce an accurate count of those covered by veterans' services.

6. Also eligible for medicare are some nonelderly disabled. The small proportion of elderly who are not medicare-eligible could purchase its coverage at a rate of $245 per month in 1994. See *Overview of Entitlement Programs—1994 Green Book*, Committee Print 103-27, House Committee on Ways and Means, 103 Cong. 1 sess., p. 123 (hereafter *1994 Green Book*).

7. The balance are insured through employment, of which about a quarter are annuitants of the Federal Employee Health Benefits Program. See *Overview of Entitlement Programs—1993 Green Book*, Committee Print 103-18, House Com-

mittee on Ways on Means, pp. 239, 241. The *Green Book* is the source for the summary of benefits that follows in the text.

8. PPRC, *Annual Report*, p. xxxiii. But for efforts to evade the limit see Elisabeth Rosenthal, "Irked by Medicare Limits, Doctors Ask Elderly to Pay Up," *New York Times*, February 15, 1994, p. B1.

9. See *1993 Green Book*, Committee Print, chart 2 on p. 233, table 10 on p. 240. Note that in 1984, out-of-pocket expenses were over $30 billion, and insurance paid for less than $9 billion in care. The burden may not be quite as heavy as it seems, however, because the elderly tend not to have some other expenses, such as raising children, anymore.

10. See Kaiser Commission on the Future of Medicaid, *Medicaid at the Crossroads: A Report of the Kaiser Commission on the Future of Medicaid* (Menlo Park, Calif., November 1992), pp. xiv and 7. The figures are from 1990.

11. Employee Benefit Research Institute, *Sources of Health Insurance*, table 14, p. 33; these numbers probably overlap slightly.

12. John Holahan, Martcia Wade, Michael Gates, and Lynn Tsoflias, "The Impact of Medicaid Adoption of the Medicare Fee Schedule," *Health Care Financing Review*, vol. 14, no. 3 (Spring 1993), p. 11. For current fee levels see David C. Colby, "Medicaid Physician Fees, 1993," *Health Affairs*, vol. 13, no. 2 (Spring II 1994), pp. 255–64. For a thorough review of medicaid's problems see Kaiser Commission on the Future of Medicaid, *Medicaid at the Crossroads*: "Application forms in some states exceed 30 pages and are often hard to understand, especially for people who are poorly educated or non-native English speakers," pp. 40–41; on provider participation, see pp. 43–45; on benefits, see pp. 19–20.

13. Ibid., pp. 48–49. For a similar assessment see Suzanne W. Letsch, "National Health Care Spending in 1991," *Health Affairs*, vol. 12 (Spring 1993), pp. 94–110. The program was expanded to cover children even if the parents were not eligible for the AFDC (Aid to Families with Dependent Children) program, which has very low, state-set, income thresholds. The dubious state maneuvers involved raising their medicaid payments to hospitals, claiming the federal matching funds, and then taxing (or requiring a "gift" from) the hospitals for the difference. So the federal government pays all the extra money, but medicaid *looks* bigger on state books by the full amount of the extra payment.

14. Calculated from Office of Management and Budget, *Budget Baselines, Historical Data, and Alternatives for the Future* (January 1993), table 8.5, p. 359.

15. Congressional Budget Office, *The Economic and Budget Outlook: An Update* (September 1993), pp. 40–42.

16. There are rare exceptions, the most important being the federal government and some states, which offer much wider choice.

17. Congressional Budget Office, *Reducing the Deficit: Spending and Revenue Options* (February 1993), p. 363. For purposes of distinguishing private from public insurance analysts normally focus on whether insurance is obtained through an employment contract or in the market (private) or by law from a

government agency (public). Thus health coverage for federal employees is considered private even though taxpayers pay for it.

18. The issues in this section are discussed in greater detail but using earlier data in Aaron, *Serious and Unstable Condition*.

19. Some of the smaller firms offer insurance, but many employees are not eligible because they work part time or are excluded by a waiting period because their employment is seasonal. About 40 percent of firms with ten or fewer employees offer insurance to at least some of them. See Stephen H. Long and M. Susan Marquis, "Gaps in Employer Coverage: Lack of Supply or Demand?" *Health Affairs*, vol. 12, Supplement (1993), pp. 282–93; and Congressional Budget Office, *Rising Health Care Costs: Causes, Implications, and Strategies* (April 1991), pp. 71–80.

20. Milt Freudenheim, "Health Insurers, to Reduce Losses, Blacklist Dozens of Occupations," *New York Times*, February 5, 1990, p. A1. The General Accounting Office has issued a series of reports on the problems of the American private insurance market. See, for a short summary, General Accounting Office, *Private Health Insurance: Problems Caused by a Segmented Market*, GAO/HRD-91-114 (July 1991).

21. The cost estimate is from Henry Aaron, "Paying for Health Care," *Domestic Affairs*, vol. 2 (Winter 1993–94), p. 35; family income from Council of Economic Advisers, *Economic Report of the President* (GPO, February 1994), p. 304. Survey data in 1993 suggested an average cost of $436 per month for families and $170 for individuals; Jon Gabel and others, "The Health Insurance Picture in 1993: Some Rare Good News," *Health Affairs*, vol. 13, no. 1 (Spring I 1994), pp. 327–36.

22. A further 7 percent were in families headed by part-time, part-year workers. Employee Benefit Research Institute, "Sources of Health Insurance," pp. 9–10, 12.

23. For further analysis see Diane Rowland and others, "A Profile of the Uninsured in America," *Health Affairs*, vol. 13, no. 2 (Spring II 1994), pp. 283–87; note that they use a mix of 1992 and 1993 Current Population Survey numbers.

24. The story was originally told in Michel McQueen, "Ills of the Nation's Health-Care System Are Pulling GOP into Search for New Cures," *Wall Street Journal*, June 24, 1991, p. A12. The version I tell here is more favorable to the insurance company, as related to me by the press office at the RNC.

25. Survey data are from Gabel and others, "Health Insurance Picture," p. 331; similar figures can be derived from the Foster-Higgins and Bureau of Labor Statistics data summarized inter alia in Employee Benefit Research Institute, "Features of Employer-Sponsored Health Plans," *Issue Brief* 128 (August 1992), pp. 4–9. Some raw data for 1991 can be found in Cathy A. Cowan and Patricia A. McDonnell, "Business, Households, and Governments: Health Spending, 1991," *Health Care Financing Review*, vol. 14, no. 3 (Spring 1993), pp. 227–48.

26. See the data and discussion in Employee Benefit Research Institute,

"Features of Employer-Sponsored Health Plans," pp. 11–15; also Mary Ann Chirba-Martin and Troyen A. Brennan, "The Critical Role of ERISA in State Health Reform," *Health Affairs*, vol. 13, no. 2 (Spring II 1994), pp. 142–56. The preemption of state regulation in ERISA was justified at the time as necessary because the federal government would be insuring those employers' pension plans, so needed a coherent regulatory environment. At the time, self-insurance for health care was rare, and the potential effects of the preemption for health insurance were appreciated by very few, if any, members of Congress.

27. See Ellen E. Schultz, "Beware of Coverage Gaps in Today's Health Plans," *Wall Street Journal*, September 29, 1993, p. C1.

28. Milt Freudenheim, "Health Insurance Data Called Faulty," *New York Times*, October 8, 1993, p. A26.

29. One official told me that Blue Cross/Blue Shield of the National Capital Area had over four hundred (usually slightly) different plans.

30. Schultz, "Coverage Gaps."

31. Among full-time employees in medium and large firms in 1989, only 20 percent were covered without restriction by fee-for-service plans for inpatient surgery; 26 percent for outpatient surgery, 14 percent for testing, and no more than 6 percent for any other category. See Employee Benefit Research Institute, "Features of Employer-Sponsored Health Plans," p. 21.

32. The data go back to 1960, and insurance was less common and extensive before. See Letsch, "National Health Care Spending," p. 103.

33. From 1980 to 1985 out-of-pocket payments fell from 23.8 percent to 22.3 percent, and then by 1991 to 19.2 percent, of personal health expenditures. But over that period incomes rose by 113 percent while out-of-pocket payments rose by 143 percent, so as a share of income, out-of-pocket health spending rose from 2.6 percent to 3.0 percent. These calculations are by the author from Letsch, "National Health Care Spending," p. 101, and from Council of Economic Advisers, *Economic Report of the President* (GPO, February 1992), table B-23.

34. The premium data are from Employee Benefit Research Institute, "Employer-Sponsored Health Plans," table 3, p. 8. The family median income data are from the Council of Economic Advisers, *Economic Report of the President 1992*, table B-28, converted back to current dollars by using the GDP deflator in table B-3. Individual income data, for males and females, yield lower income growth rates. Per capita disposable personal income, table B-5, yields slightly higher.

35. Matthew Holt and others, *Medical Ivory Towers and the High Cost of Health Care: A Comparison of Teaching Hospitals in the United States and Japan* (Palo Alto, Calif.: Asia/Pacific Research Center, Stanford University, 1993), p. 80. Holt and others provide a fascinating analysis of the differences between the Stanford University Hospital Medical Center and the University of Tokyo Hospital operations.

36. The balance sheet for a rural community hospital in my possession

showed that it collected about 60 percent of its charges. It, too, stayed in business.

37. Spencer Rich, "Cutting Waste: No Cure-All For Health Care," *Washington Post*, May 4, 1993, p. A1.

38. Stephanie Lin Bloom, "Hospital Turf Battles: The Manager's Role," *Hospital and Health Services Administration*, vol. 36 (Winter 1991), pp. 590–99.

39. Among other reasons, it is easier to increase productivity for procedures than for cogitation and diagnosis, so the incomes of procedure-oriented specialists are likely to rise more quickly unless relative values are adjusted to compensate for the productivity effect.

40. In June 1993, the AMA endorsed expanded use of RBRVS—sort of. See Harris Meyer, "RBRVS Could Boost Price Competition," and Julie Johnsson, "But Old Medicare Baggage Must Go," both in *American Medical News*, July 5, 1993, p. 1; Julie Johnsson, "Advisory Group Urges HCFA to Plug Gaps in RBRVS," *American Medical News*, July 26, 1993, p. 1.

41. For a discussion of objections to and facts about fee schedules see Joe White, "Paying the Right Price: What the United States Can Learn from Health Care Abroad," *Brookings Review*, vol. 12 (Spring 1994), pp. 6–11.

42. PPRC, *Annual Report*, p. 409.

43. See ibid., p. xxxiv, for the quotation from the PPRC; for a detailed report see chaps. 20 and 21 of the annual report and PPRC, *Fee Update and Medicare Volume Performance Standards for 1995*, 94–1 (Washington, May 15, 1994). For the commission's analysis on the issue of declining medicare reimbursements, see PPRC, *Monitoring Access of Medicare Beneficiaries*, 94-2 (Washington, June 1994).

44. For descriptions of managed care see Peter Kongstvedt, *The Managed Health Care Handbook*, 2d ed. (Gaithersburg, Md.: Aspen Publishing, 1993), and Bradford H. Gray, *The Profit Motive and Patient Care: The Changing Accountability of Doctors and Hospitals* (Harvard University Press, 1991), chap. 11. On the morale of physicians, see the front-page series in the *New York Times*, "Doctors in Distress," February 18–20, 1990; it included: Lawrence K. Altman and Elisabeth Rosenthal, "Changes in Medicine Bring Pain to Healing Profession," *New York Times*, February 18, 1990, p. A1; Lisa Belkin, "Many Doctors See Themselves Drowning in Sea of Paperwork," *New York Times*, February 19, 1990, p. A1; Gina Kolata, "Wariness Is Replacing Trust between Healer and Patient," *New York Times*, February 20, 1990, p. A1. Chapter 7 in this volume discusses the data on costs.

45. OECD, *OECD Health Data: Comparative Analysis of Health Systems*, data base (Paris, 1993).

46. Comparisons are from National Center for Health Statistics, *Health, U.S., 1992* (Hyattsville, Md.: Public Health Service, 1993), pp. 123, 127, 129–33, 158. Note that inpatient surgeries rose substantially for the elderly and fell for other groups, and diagnostic work increased even more quickly for the elderly than for everyone else.

47. For an extensive review of American experience with a variety of cost

controls, see Marsha Gold and others, "Effects of Selected Cost-Containment Efforts: 1971–1993," *Health Care Financing Review*, vol. 14, no. 3 (Spring 1993), pp. 183–216; other articles in the same volume address other parts of the story.

48. The residency is required by forty-six states for American medical school graduates and by all states for graduates of foreign medical schools. Raffel and Raffel, *U.S. Health System*, p. 53; their chap. 2 is the main source for this description of medical education.

49. Data on the work week and debt come from American Medical Association (AMA), Center for Health Policy Research, *Socioeconomic Characteristics of Medical Practice, 1992* (Chicago, 1992), pp. 21, 32, 38; explanations of data in appendixes C and D. Medical residency income ranged from about $23,000 for interns to $29,500 for sixth-year residents in 1987, when the median income for full-time employed males was about $27,200. Residency data are from Raffel and Raffel, *U.S. Health System*, pp. 54–55; author's calculations from Council of Economic Advisers, *Economic Report of the President*, 1992, tables B-3 and B-28. For reports on the horrors of internship, see Robert Marion, *The Intern Blues: The Private Ordeals of Three Young Doctors* (Ballantine Books, 1989).

50. The proportion of practicing IMGs is the author's calculation from National Center for Health Statistics, *Health*, p. 144; the discussion is based on Raffel and Raffel, *U.S. Health Care System*, pp. 64–67, 72, and on a special series of articles by Leigh Page in *American Medical News*, February 21, February 28, and March 7, 1994. Note that Canadian medical school graduates are not considered international; the two countries' training is virtually identical.

51. Figures are from Paul D. Frenzen, "The Increasing Supply of Physicians in U.S. Urban and Rural Areas, 1975 to 1988," *American Journal of Public Health*, vol. 81, no. 9, pp. 1141–47. I have summarized both his rural categories as one (thus my approximations). Then I combined osteopaths with primary care allopaths, from his tables 2 and 4, for the primary care category here.

52. In 1991 the figures were 96.1 office visits per week (for those with office practices) in nonmetropolitan areas, 72.9 in large cities. There was a smaller difference, about 11 percent, in hours spent on direct patient care. Urban physicians made up a bit more of the difference with extra professional activities. See AMA, *Medical Practice, 1992*, pp. 38, 42, 68.

53. Elisabeth Rosenthal, "Shortage of Doctors in Poor Areas Is Seen as Barrier to Health Plans," *New York Times*, October 18, 1993, p. A1.

54. De Lew and others say 33 percent; see De Lew, Greenberg, and Kinchen, "A Layman's Guide," p. 156. Raffel and Raffel say 40 percent; see *U.S. Health Care System*, p. 72. The actual number of general practitioners, family practitioners, pediatricians, and internists combined, in 1990, was 40 percent of physicians in office-based practice: author's calculations from National Center for Health Statistics, *Health*, p. 144. For a good look at issues of definition, see Leigh Page, "Internal Struggle: Internists Debate Whether They Are Really Generalists or Specialists," *American Medical News*, July 26, 1993, p. 5. Data on percentages are from *OECD Health Data*, 1993 data base. Totals for 1988 are given in De Lew, Greenberg, and Kinchen, "A Layman's Guide," p. 156.

55. The average physician spent nearly nine hours conducting hospital rounds per week in 1990, with pediatricians at the average and general and family practitioners at six and a half hours. AMA, *Medical Practice, 1992*, p. 52. Among active certified family physicians, 84.8 percent were reported to have hospital admitting privileges in May 1992. See American Academy of Family Physicians (AAFP), *Facts about Family Practice* (Kansas City, Mo.: 1993), pp. 10–11, 105, 107.

56. The rest are engaged in teaching, administration, research, and other non-patient-care activities. Author's calculations from National Center for Health Statistics, *Health*, p. 144.

57. Absent very good computerization, group practice probably does not create economies of scale in medical record-keeping. In a solo practice, all relevant records may be in one person's reach. In a partnership, junior physicians may well be on salary until, as in a law firm, they become partners. For a full description of the range of groups and payer strategies, see Kongstvedt, *Managed Care Handbook*.

58. The Clinton administration had some useful proposals. For a review of the issues, see Josh Wiener, *Sharing the Burden: Strategies for Public and Private Long-term Care Insurance* (Brookings, 1994).

59. The data are from National Center for Health Statistics, *Health*, p. 153; for a thorough assessment of the importance of the profit motive, see Gray, *Profit Motive and Patient Care*.

60. National Center for Health Statistics, *Health, United States, 1992*, author's calculations from p. 172. Both "physician service" and "all other personal health care" grew more quickly than hospital expenditures. The quotation is from Prospective Payment Assessment Commission, Global Budgeting: Design and Implementation Issues, Report to Congress C-93-01 (July 1993), pp. 26–27.

61. Use of the emergency room for routine care is often called an unnecessary expense, to be eliminated by national health insurance. But emergency room personnel may be fairly cheap—residents are paid a lot less than office-based doctors. And many of those patients might not find their way to a doctor's office even if it were paid for—because of language, transportation, or other problems. Hospitals are on the bus line.

62. William J. Hall and Paul F. Griner, "Cost-Effective Health Care: The Rochester Experience," *Health Affairs*, vol. 12, no. 2 (Spring 1993), pp. 58–69.

63. Stephen H. Long and M. Susan Marquis, "The Uninsured 'Access Gap' and the Cost of Universal Coverage," *Health Affairs*, vol. 13, no. 2 (Spring II 1994), p. 214; they estimate that the uninsured have about two-thirds as many hospital admissions.

64. Rowland and others, "Profile of the Uninsured," p. 286 and cites therein.

65. Swartz, "People without Health Insurance," pp. 65–66 and cites therein.

66. For a good review of regulation of medical education, medical practice,

and hospitals, see Raffel and Raffel, *U.S. Health System*, chaps. 2, 3, and 6. The table on page 45 shows the interlocking relationships among medical education overseers.

67. For figures on the amount of disciplinary action, and one good review of the issues, see General Accounting Office, "Medical Malpractice: Experience with Efforts to Address Problems," Testimony of Lawrence H. Thompson, May 20, 1993, GAO/T-HRD-93-24. For a summary of the survey results, see Peter P. Budetti and Stephanie M. Spernak, "Medical Malpractice," in Stephen M. Shortell and Uwe E. Reinhardt, eds., *Improving Health Policy and Management: Nine Critical Research Issues for the 1990* (Ann Arbor, Mich.: Health Administration Press, 1992), pp. 319–20; the Harvard University study is Troyen A. Brennan and others, "Incidence of Adverse Events and Negligence in Hospitalized Patients," *New England Journal of Medicine*, February 7, 1991, pp. 370–76; Lucian L. Leape and others, "The Nature of Adverse Events in Hospitalized Patients," *New England Journal of Medicine*, February 7, 1991, pp. 377–84. For a general discussion see Raffel and Raffel, *U.S. Health System*, pp. 83–85.

68. Budetti and Spernak, "Medical Malpractice," p. 323.

69. Dr. Brad Cohn, quoted in Brian McCormick, "AMA Demands 'True' Tort Reform before It Backs Clinton Plan," *American Medical News*, December 20, 1993, pp. 3, 27.

70. Budetti and Spernak, "Medical Malpractice," p. 321. Readers in search of good examples of physicians' fears and a wide assortment of the cases that are brought and decisions made should page through issues of the *American Medical News*.

71. Budetti and Spernak, "Medical Malpractice," pp. 327–28.

72. Physicians and hospitals spent $8 billion on insurance in 1990, according to GAO, "Medical Malpractice," p. 4.

73. Lynn Payer, *Medicine and Culture: Varieties of Treatment in the United States, England, West Germany, and France* (Henry Holt, 1988), pp. 124–37; quotes on pp. 128 and 127.

74. One day I heard both comments within ten minutes of conversation with physicians from whom I was receiving treatment.

75. Budetti and Spernak, "Medical Malpractice," p. 325.

Chapter Four

1. For a discussion of the use of the Canadian example in American political debate, see Theodore R. Marmor, "Health Care Reform in the United States: Patterns of Fact and Fiction in the Use of Canadian Experience," *American Review of Canadian Studies*, vol. 23, no. 1 (Spring 1993), pp. 47–64. For an earlier account, see John K. Iglehart, "Health Policy Report: The United States Looks at Canadian Health Care," *New England Journal of Medicine*, December 12, 1989, pp. 1767–72. For a discussion of cultural differences see this book's introduction and conclusion.

2. The provinces are at least as different as American states in economy

and culture. They include the richer western provinces of British Columbia and Alberta; the agricultural provinces of Manitoba and Saskatchewan; Ontario, the largest and with an economy much like that of the American Great Lakes states; Quebec, second largest and French-speaking and not at all sure it wants to be part of the country; and the four small and impoverished maritime provinces of New Brunswick, Newfoundland, Nova Scotia, and Prince Edward Island. The Northwest and Yukon Territories are, as the stereotype would have it, very, very, large, cold, and empty. For a good review of Canadian politics see R. Kent Weaver, ed., *The Collapse of Canada?* (Brookings, 1992).

3. Anne Crichton and David Hsu, *Canada's Health Care System: Its Funding and Organization* (Ottawa: Canadian Hospital Association Press, 1990), p. 28; the authoritative text on development of the Canadian health insurance system is Malcolm G. Taylor, *Health Insurance and Canadian Public Policy: The Seven Decisions That Created the Canadian Health Insurance System and Their Outcomes*, 2d ed. (Kingston and Montreal: McGill-Queen's University Press, 1987). For other summaries, see General Accounting Office, *Canadian Health Insurance: Lessons for the United States* (GAO/HRD-91-90, June 1991); Laurene E. Graig, *Health of Nations: An International Perspective on U.S. Health Care Reform* (Washington: Wyatt Company, 1991), pp. 55–111; "Does Canada Have the Answer?" *Consumer Reports*, September 1992, pp. 579–88; and the series of articles by John K. Iglehart, "Health Policy Report: Canada's Health Care System," *New England Journal of Medicine*, July 17, 1986, pp. 202–08; "Health Policy Report: Canada's Health Care System," *New England Journal of Medicine*, September 18, 1986, pp. 778–84; "Health Policy Report: Canada's Health Care System," *New England Journal of Medicine*, December 18, 1986, pp. 1623–28; "Health Policy Report: The United States Looks at Canadian Health Care," *New England Journal of Medicine*, December 21, 1989, pp. 1767–72; and "Health Policy Report: Canada's Health Care System Faces Its Problems," *New England Journal of Medicine*, February 22, 1990, pp. 562–68.

4. For examples of the numbers see the charts in chapter 2. See also Theodore R. Marmor, "Commentary on 'Canadian Health Insurance: Lessons for the United States,'" *International Journal of Health Services*, vol. 23, no. 1 (1993), p. 47; Gordon H. Hatcher, Peter R. Hatcher, and Eleanor C. Hatcher, "Canada," in Marshall W. Raffel, ed., *Comparative Health Systems* (Pennsylvania State University Press, 1984).

5. Taylor, *Health Insurance*, p. 230.

6. Ibid., p. 328; pp. 239–330 tell the story.

7. The Royal Commission's makeup and report are described in ibid., pp. 341–49. The report was a surprise in part because its chairman was a conservative jurist, Emmett M. Hall. Taylor does not describe the commission's internal deliberations—a pity but perhaps understandable since he was its chief researcher.

8. In the Canadian context of the 1960s, the logical alternatives were profit-making businesses and plans run by the medical profession, neither of which seemed entirely reliable users of public authority.

9. Taylor, *Health Insurance*, pp. 362, 365; see also Canadian Embassy,

"Health Care in Canada," handout dated March 1991. Health care costs are inherently related to local income levels, because less wealthy areas tend to have lower rents, wages, and other costs. The national average thus would be lower than costs in Ontario and higher than costs in the maritimes.

10. Roger Gosselin, "The Quebec Health Care System in the Canadian Context: Impact on Medical Practice," in Marilynn M. Rosenthal and Marcel Frenkel, eds., *Health Care Systems and Their Patients: An International Perspective* (Boulder, Colo.: Westview Press, 1992), pp. 43–61; Gerard de Pourvoirville and Marc Renaud, "Hospital System Management in France and Canada: National Pluralism and Provincial Centralism," *Social Science and Medicine*, vol. 20, no. 2 (1985), pp. 153–66; on cost control see Morris L. Barer, Robert G. Evans, and Roberta J. Labelle, "Fee Controls as Cost Control: Tales from the Frozen North," *Milbank Quarterly*, vol. 66, no. 1 (1988), p. 26.

11. Figures are from the Organization for Economic Cooperation and Development (OECD), OECD Health Data: Comparative Analysis of Health Systems, data base (Paris, 1993) (hereafter OECD 1993 data base). By far the best summary and analysis is Robert G. Evans, Morris L. Barer and Clyde Hertzman, "The 20-Year Experiment: Accounting For, Explaining, and Evaluating Health Care Cost Containment in Canada and the United States," *Annual Review of Public Health*, vol. 12 (1991), pp. 481–518.

12. Quoted in Taylor, *Health Insurance*, p. 448; he describes the whole conflict on pp. 435–62.

13. Carolyn J. Tuohy, "Medicine and the State in Canada: The Extra-Billing Issue in Perspective," *Canadian Journal of Political Science*, vol. 21, no. 2 (June 1988), pp. 267–96.

14. On the importance and near ubiquity of such arrangements see William A. Glaser, "Doctors and Public Authorities: The Trend toward Collaboration," *Journal of Health Politics, Policy and Law*, vol. 19 (Winter 1994), pp. 707–27.

15. Taylor, *Health Insurance*, pp. 422–34; As usual, the stakes and trade-offs in negotiating a new federal-state transfer regime were far more complex than can be explained here, as emphasized in William A. Glaser, "Federalism in Canada and West Germany: Lessons for the United States," NTIS accession number PB 81 152340 (Springfield, Va.: National Technical Information Service, 1979).

16. The British Columbia Health Association estimated the federal contribution figures in real dollars as $C448 per capita in 1986–87, falling to $C401 in 1993–94. British Columbia Health Association, "Figuring Health Care," 1993 ed. (Vancouver, B.C.), graph 5.5. The federal government estimates that its contribution fell from 30.8 percent to 23.5 percent of costs from 1986 to 1993; Policy and Consultation Branch, Health Canada, "National Health Expenditures in Canada, 1975–1993" (Ottawa, June 1994), table 3C.

17. The federal government's financial influence on provinces would be eliminated first in Quebec, because the EPF transfer is defined two ways, as cash and "tax points." One point on the income tax is equivalent to the revenue raised by a 1 percent tax, and legally the federal government is simply serving as a collection agent for the province. Therefore the federal government cannot

withhold tax points as punishment (unlike cash). As a sign of its special status Quebec receives an extra 8.5 points in lieu of cash. As the federal contribution falls, Quebec could be receiving no cash by the end of the decade. For discussion and estimates, see House of Commons, Canada, *The Health Care System in Canada and Its Funding: No Easy Solutions*, First Report of the Standing Committee on Health and Welfare, Social Affairs, Seniors and the Status of Women (June 1991), pp. 14–19, 107–11.

18. Health Canada, "National Health Expenditures," tables 5A and 1A. GDP shares in these figures rose from 9.9 percent to 10.1 percent in Canada and 13.2 percent to 14.4 percent in the United States from 1991 to 1993.

19. Bruce Little, "The $71-Billion System Seeks a Cure," *Toronto Globe and Mail*, April 27, 1992, p. A9.

20. An employer may pay some or all of the premium, though payment of the public premium, unlike payment for private premiums in either Canada or the United States, counts as income. Subsidies are paid on a sliding scale on the basis of net income adjusted for family size. The maximum premium for a family is $72 per month, and there are subsidies for families with incomes below $25,001, so the maximum premium is 3.46 percent of income. See Province of British Columbia, Ministry of Health and Ministry Responsible for Seniors, Medical Services Plan of British Columbia (Victoria), form MISC-71A-04/93, "Premium Assistance Rates," and form HLTH-MSP-0119-150M-05/93, "Application for Premium Assistance."

21. The summary of benefits is from Crichton and Hsu, *Canada's Health Care System*, pp. 35–39, 89; for Pharmacare, British Columbia Ministry of Health and Ministry Responsible for Seniors, "What Is Pharmacare?" brochure PHN116 901.008 (Victoria, B.C., October 1990.)

22. Graig, *Health of Nations*, p. 77.

23. For a comprehensive treatment of methods around the world as of the mid-1980s see William A. Glaser, *Paying the Hospital: The Organization, Dynamics and Effects of Differing Financial Arrangements* (San Francisco: Jossey-Bass, 1987).

24. The standard pattern is known as incrementalism and is fundamental to any repetitive budgeting. For an example of the plaint, see Allan S. Detsky and others, "Global Budgeting and the Teaching Hospital in Ontario," *Medical Care*, vol. 24 (January 1986), pp. 89–94. For a discussion of the general pattern, see Joseph White, "Markets, Budgets, and Health Care Cost Control," *Health Affairs*, vol. 12 (Fall 1993), pp. 44–57. For a review of current decisionmaking, including attempts to reallocate resources in Alberta, British Columbia, and Ontario, see Morris L. Barer, "Hospital Financing in Canada," Discussion Paper HPRU 93:6D (University of British Columbia, Centre for Health Services and Policy Research, April 1993).

25. Frank G. Sabatino, "The Delivery Changes Posed by Canada: A Bilateral View," in Richard J. Umbdenstock and Winifred M. Hageman, eds., *Critical Readings for Hospital Trustees* (Chicago: American Hospital Publishing, 1991), pp. 120–23.

26. Robert G. Evans, "Managing Health Care Reform in Canada" in Monique Jérôme-Forget, Joseph White, and Joshua Wiener, eds., *Health Care Re-*

form through Internal Markets: Experience and Proposals (Montreal and Washington: Institute for Research on Public Policy and Brookings, 1995), p. 221.

27. Jonathan Lomas, Cathy Charles, and Janet Greb, "The Price of Peace: The Structure and Process of Physician Fee Negotiations in Canada," Working Paper 92-17 (McMaster University, Centre for Health Economics and Policy Analysis, August 1992), p. 184. This is by far the most comprehensive source on physician payment arrangements in Canada.

28. Article 13 of the master agreement between the government of the province of British Columbia, the Medical Services Commission, and the British Columbia Medical Association (Victoria, B.C., October 1993).

29. Barer, Evans, and Labelle, "Fee Controls," p. 22; also Lomas, Charles, and Greb, "Price of Peace."

30. W. Pete Welch, Steven J. Katz, and Stephen Zuckerman, "Physician Fee Levels: Medicare versus Canada," *Health Care Financing Review*, vol. 14, no. 3 (Spring 1993), pp. 41–54; Steven J. Katz, Stephen Zuckerman, and W. Pete Welch, "Comparing Physician Fee Schedules in Canada and the United States," *Health Care Financing Review*, vol. 14, no. 1 (Fall 1992), pp. 141–49; Victor R. Fuchs and James S. Hahn, "How Does Canada Do It? A Comparison of Expenditures for Physicians' Services in the United States and Canada," *New England Journal of Medicine*, September 27, 1990, p. 886.

31. AMA, *Medical Practice, 1992*, pp. 132, 137, reports mean 1990 incomes of just under $165,000 and a median of just under $130,000. A Canadian survey reported in Rod Mickleburgh, "Canadian Doctors Feel Less Gloomy, Survey Finds," *Toronto Globe and Mail*, October 23, 1992, p. A12, reported a 1991 mean of $C127,000. That would be about three-quarters of the American median and 60 percent of the mean. See also the comparisons in John K. Iglehart, "Canada's Health Care System Faces Its Problems," *New England Journal of Medicine*, February 22, 1990, pp. 562–68.

32. Lomas, Charles, and Greb, "Price of Peace," p. i.

33. Ibid., pp. 68–69, 120.

34. The Ontario figures are from David K. Peachey, M.D., "Global Expenditure Limits in Canadian Health Care: The Application and The Implication," paper prepared for Robert Wood Johnson Foundation workshop, "Managing the Health Care System Under a Global Expenditure Limit," April 28–29, 1993. Quebec's caps apply only to general practitioners, who receive only 25 percent of average fees once they exceed a quarterly threshold; Lomas, Charles, and Greb, "Price of Peace," reports that this affected 16.8 percent of GPs in 1989–90 (p. 93). The account here updates Lomas and Peachey for subsequent developments in British Columbia, based on my own interviews.

35. See especially the argument in Lomas, Charles, and Greb, "Price of Peace," pp. 167–81; for British Columbia I rely on the texts of the master agreement, interviews in the ministry and BCMA, and documents of the BCMA.

36. The wording is from personal communication about this section, but see also Glaser, "Doctors and Public Authorities."

37. Examples of services that might be delisted—taken off the fee schedule

and therefore not insured—include prenatal ultrasound in British Columbia (unless indicated by symptoms) and tattoo removal in Ontario (which has already been delisted; tattooing itself was never covered).

38. It is common for IMGs to be admitted to practice in rural areas and then to move to the city after a few years—necessitating their replacement by new IMGs.

39. John K. Iglehart says the statistic is 52.5 percent. See Iglehart, "Canada's Health Care System Faces Its Problems," *New England Journal of Medicine*, p. 567.

40. For more, if slightly outdated, information on hospital governance see Hatcher, Hatcher, and Hatcher, "Canada," pp. 95–97. This author's summary information on hospital stays is derived from figures in the OECD 1993 data base and in British Columbia Health Association, *Figuring Health Care* (November 1993), graph 3.6. Since 1985 the rate of decline in the American figures has flattened out, while Canada has been catching up (but because the race is to do less, "catching down" might be the more appropriate phrase).

41. Robert G. Evans and others, "Controlling Health Expenditures: The Canadian Reality," *New England Journal of Medicine*, March 2, 1989, pp. 573–74.

42. For a summary of capital budgeting, see Morris L. Barer, "Hospital Financing," pp. 23–34. Donald A. Redelmeier and Victor R. Fuchs report that, adjusted for population size, there were five times as many MRIs and ten times as many lithotripters in California as in Ontario. See their article "Hospital Expenditures in the United States and Canada," *New England Journal of Medicine*, March 18, 1993, pp. 775–77.

43. For a summary of the developments in Germany, see Detlev Zollner, "Germany," in Peter A. Kohler and Hans F. Zacher, eds., *The Evolution of Social Insurance 1881–1981: Studies of Germany, France, Great Britain, Austria, and Switzerland* (St. Martin's Press, 1982), pp. 2, 17–23.

44. William A. Glaser, *Health Insurance in Practice: International Variations in Financing, Benefits, and Problems* (San Francisco: Jossey-Bass, 1991), p. 18. This is by far the best source for the history, logic, and operations of the sickness fund systems and for a description and analysis of American institutions in that light.

45. While this is conventionally referred to as the world's first national sickness insurance law, William Glaser in personal communication points out that Prussia had one even earlier. Bismarck, like some later reformers, would have preferred government financing but was stymied by a familiar factor, difficulty raising the money, and a less familiar one, workers' suspicion that if they did not pay they would lose control of the funds. Thus the two-thirds worker share.

46. The account in the previous paragraphs summarizes Zollner, "Germany," pp. 24–75. For a history of physician payment see Bradford L. Kirkman-Liff, "Physician Payment and Cost-Containment Strategies in West Germany: Suggestions for Medicare Reform," *Journal of Health Politics, Policy and Law*, vol. 15, no. 1 (Spring 1990), pp. 69–99. For another overview, see Graig, *Health of Nations*, pp. 121–25.

47. Translating that 58,500 DM per year into American terms can only be inaccurate, because prices are different in the two countries, exchange rates vary from day to day, a family may have two income earners, among other reasons. Fifty-eight thousand five hundred DM was about $35,250 in 1991; it was also about 40 percent higher than the average earnings of German workers within the set of industries for which the International Labor Organization reports data. The key point is that the mandatory standard included 80 percent of the population of a rich country.

48. See Eliot K. Wicks, *German Health Care: Financing, Administration, and Coverage* (Washington: Health Insurance Association of America, 1992), pp. 6–8 and 20–26. How high the cutoff seems depends on whether one translates deutschmarks into dollars by exchange rates or by purchasing power parities. Other good recent summaries of the German system include Carol Stevens, "Does Germany Hold the Key to U.S. Health-Care Reform?" *Medical Economics*, January 6, 1992; Graig, *Health of Nations*, pp. 113–60; and J. Mathias Graf v.d. Schulenberg, "The German Health Care System: Concurrent Solidarity, Freedom of Choice, and Cost Control," in Rosenthal and Frenkel, *Health Care Systems and Their Patients*, pp. 83–104.

49. Blue-collar workers with incomes above the threshold were compelled to join a primary fund until the law was changed in 1988. Andreas Ryll, "Bargaining in the German Ambulatory Health Care System," in Fritz W. Scharpf, ed., *Games in Hierarchies and Networks: Analytical and Empirical Approaches to the Study of Governance Institutions* (Boulder, Colo.: Westview, 1993), pp. 5 (n. 6) and 11.

50. Wicks, *German Health Care*, pp. 7–8, 24–25, 28–29; Michael Arnold, *Health Care in the Federal Republic of Germany* (Cologne: Deutscher-Artzte-Verlag GmbH, 1991), pp. 25–29.

51. Arnold, *Health Care in Germany*, p. 24; see also Suzanne Letsch, "National Health Care Spending in 1991," *Health Affairs*, vol. 12 (Spring 1993), p. 103.

52. Jeremy W. Hurst, "Reform of Health Care in Germany," *Health Care Financing Review*, vol. 12, no. 3 (Spring 1991), p. 76; Uwe Reinhardt, "Global Budgeting in German Health Care: Insights for Americans," *Domestic Affairs*, vol. 2 (Winter 1993–94), p. 172.

53. An extensive discussion of sickness fund premium-setting is provided in Glaser, *Health Insurance in Practice*.

54. As usual, figures in sources are similar but not quite identical: see Wicks, *German Health Care*, pp. 22–23, and Arnold, *Health Care in Germany*, p. 27. Note that inequalities in contribution rates relative to income are not the same as differences in absolute premium. Three thousand dollars per year is 15 percent of $20,000 and 10 percent of $30,000; so to the extent rates vary according to income rather than risk, absolute payments could be much more similar than the percentages.

55. Glaser, *Health Insurance in Practice*, p. 124.

56. See the discussion in ibid., pp. 122–23, and the mention in Wicks, *German Health Care*, p. 25.

57. For data on some of these limits, see Markus Schneider, "Health Care Cost Containment in the Federal Republic of Germany," *Health Care Financing Review*, vol. 12, no. 3 (Spring 1991), pp. 87–101. I also benefited from the discussion at a symposium hosted by the Goethe Institut in Boston, Harvard School of Public Health, and Eberhard-Karls-Universität Tubingen, "The German Health Care System: A Model for the United States?" Boston, October 15–18, 1992 (hereafter, Goethe Institut, Boston, 1992). The estimate for over-the-counter pharmaceuticals spending is from that session.

58. On spas, see Lynn Payer, *Medicine and Culture: Varieties of Treatment in the United States, England, West Germany, and France* (Henry Holt, 1988), pp. 90–91 and 96–97 for Germany and 71–73 for France. Payer also discusses psychotherapy, pp. 95–96. For summaries of benefits see Wicks, *German Health Care*, p. 8; Arnold, *Health Care in Germany*, various chapters. Sickness fund payments to spas in 1991 totaled 2.9 billion DM (around $1.9 billion), 1.9 percent of their expenses, according to a handout from Dr. Rainer Hess, Director of the National Association of Sickness Fund Physicians (KBV), "Leistungsausgaben der GKV 1991 und Anteile ausgewählter Bereiche," Goethe Institut, Boston, 1992. The long-term care package was passed in April 1994. Its politics and contents are described in Jens Alber, "Paying for Long-Term Care in a Social Insurance System: The Example of Germany," paper presented at the OECD meeting "Caring for Frail Elderly People: Policies for the Future," Paris, July 5–6, 1994.

59. Glaser, *Health Insurance in Practice*, provides a thorough explanation of both German private insurance and level premiums; the latter are normal in Switzerland as well. Note that if a plan underestimates medical costs all its premiums, whatever the age of entry, will be too low; it therefore will raise them all proportionately. Level premiums therefore are level in principle but change in practice.

60. See Wicks, *German Health Care*, pp. 27–34; Glaser, *Health Insurance in Practice*, pp. 164–72. Eligibility changes, for example, when one's income falls below the threshold. Under those circumstances, a person may pay the private insurer a small fee to preserve the right to return to the private sector without being charged for a higher rate. My thanks to Andreas Ryll for explaining this point. If a sickness fund really wants to, the director of the National Association of Company Sickness Funds told me, it can find a way to let someone back in—but it is the fund's choice.

61. Other aspects of medical governance, such as approval of internship programs and licensure, are in the hands of a separate organization of doctors, the State Chamber of Physicians (Landesärztekammer, or LAK).

62. Wicks, *German Health Care*, p. 39. Private hospitals and private care in public hospitals are paid somewhat differently. Separate day rates are charged to the private insurance. These rates are lower than the rates for sickness funds because they do not include physician fees, which are billed separately and at substantially higher rates (about double) than the sickness funds pay. Private patients also pay extra for amenities such as private rooms. In general, therefore, charges to private patients are about double the norm both in hos-

pital and ambulatory sectors, as described by Schneider, "Health Care Cost Containment," pp. 98–99, and Wicks, *German Health Care*, pp. 31–32.

63. U.S. General Accounting Office, "Health Care Spending Control: The Experience of France, Germany, and Japan," GAO/HRD-92-9 (November 1991).

64. The number of procedures is from Andreas Ryll, "Bargaining in the German Ambulatory Health Care System," p. 8 (n. 10). The examples are from Hurst, "Reform of Health Care in Germany," p. 77. All accounts of the German system include some summary of the physician payment structure; see, for example, Kirkman-Liff, "Physician Payment and Cost-Containment Strategies," and Glaser, *Health Insurance in Practice*.

65. Wicks, *German Health Care*, p. 38.

66. These control doctors also review hospital lengths of stay. Glaser, *Health Insurance in Practice*, p. 364.

67. This account is summarized from Kirkman-Liff, "Physician Payment and Cost-Containment Strategies," pp. 89–91.

68. See the summary in ibid., pp. 76–77.

69. These figures come from Wicks, *German Health Care*, p. 69 (n. 66), and from Hurst, "Reform of Health Care in Germany," p. 82. Note that in 1989 wages for hospital physicians were just more than half those for office-based physicians (compare Wicks, *German Health Care*, n. 68, and Arnold, *Health Care in Germany*, p. 39). Both these sources and the charts supplied by Dr. Rainer Hess of the KBV at Goethe Institut, Boston, in 1992 show relative incomes were falling at least as quickly before as after imposition of the global cap.

70. OECD 1993 data base.

71. Payments rose from 12.2 percent of wages in 1991 to 13.4 percent at the beginning of 1993. See Janet L. Shikles, "1993 German Health Reforms: Initiatives Tighten Cost Controls," T-HRD-94-2 (U.S. General Accounting Office, October 13, 1993), p. 1.

72. See Schulenberg, "German Health Care System," pp. 86–90.

73. Michael Moran, "Across the Wall," in Annabelle May, ed., *Healthcare in Europe*, special issue of *Health Service Journal* (Macmillan Magazines, Ltd., 1993), p. 17.

74. Wicks, *German Health Care*, p. 17; the figure on hospital beds is the author's calculation from Arnold, *Health Care in Germany*, pp. 39 and 43. For the most thorough explanation see Glaser, *Paying the Hospital*, pp. 306–09.

75. Arnold, *Health Care in Germany*, pp. 36–37 and 39; Hurst, "Reform of Health Care in Germany," p. 76. For a view of one practice, see Timothy Harper, "German Medicine—through a Doctor's Eyes," *Medical Economics*, January 6, 1992, pp. 156–59.

76. Glaser, *Paying the Hospital*, p. 308. For figures on hospital staffing see Arnold, *Health Care in Germany*, pp. 36, 40; also Kirkman-Liff, "Physician Payment and Cost-Containment Strategies," p. 73.

77. In other words, regular patients are referred to the hospital. Patients with private insurance may pay extra for referral directly to the "chief of

service." The chief supervises (at least in theory) that patient's care and provides some special attention. But he delegates much of the work to his staff and therefore shares with them the extra fees.

78. This principle applies mathematically only if the chance that any person wants to use a service at a particular time is less than 50 percent. But if the average person were in the hospital more than half the time, who would take care of everyone?

79. The German average in 1987 was 11.5 office visits, nearly one inpatient stay per every five persons, and a 13.1 day average length of stay for acute care. Arnold, *Health Care in Germany*, pp. 35, 40; OECD 1993 data base; and author's calculations.

80. Hurst, "Reform of Health Care," pp. 77–78; Glaser, *Paying the Hospital*, pp. 216–25; Arnold, *Health Care in Germany*, pp. 40–41; Wicks, *German Health Care*, pp. 44–46. The availability of some equipment, such as cardiac surgery units and MRIs, is reported to be much lower in Germany than in the United States; see Dale A. Rublee, "Medical Technology in Canada, Germany, and the U.S.," *Health Affairs*, vol. 8, no. 3 (Fall 1989), pp. 178–81.

81. Reliable data on equipment in office-based practice are hard to come by. I have found no data on the distribution of equipment within offices, but many observers claim those physicians invest heavily.

82. See Reinhardt, "Global Budgeting," pp. 179–85. Another source is Shikles, "1993 German Health Reforms," pp. 1–12. I have also relied on descriptions and explanations provided by a number of participants, including Gerhard Schulte, Director of the Federal Ministry of Health, at the Goethe Institut conference in Boston, October 15–18, 1992, on correspondence with German scholars, and on reports by State Department staff on briefings they received.

83. Andreas Ryll, letter to the author, February 10, 1994.

84. My thanks to Markus Schneider, Marcus Kruse, and especially Andreas Ryll for their efforts to help me understand these measures.

85. See Schneider, "Health Care Cost Containment," pp. 95–96; Payer, *Medicine and Culture*, especially pp. 77–94. The figures are from Dale A. Rublee and Markus Schneider, "International Health Spending: Comparisons with the OECD," *Health Affairs*, vol. 10, no. 3 (Fall 1991), tables on pp. 191–92; pharmaceutical payments in Germany were 16 percent higher using purchasing power and 38 percent higher using exchange rates. Other sources give different numbers but the same story.

86. Stephen D. Moore, "European State-Funded Health Systems Come under Fire for Skyrocketing Costs," *Wall Street Journal*, May 4, 1993, p. A14; Shikles, "1993 German Health Reforms," p. 10.

87. Returning from a conference in Germany in June 1994, my colleague Josh Wiener reported that German policymakers were somewhat embarrassed by the short-term accomplishments of the 1992 reforms; they had not expected such thorough success.

88. Neither liberals nor conservatives, however, should be sure that people

will respond to incentives as the analysts hope. One source comments that only a minority of Germans know what they personally are paying, despite the fact that rates are a political issue!

89. The problem is, what can be measured? One report claims Germany has more of some expensive diagnostic equipment. But Germany provided many fewer bone marrow transplants, which would seem to be a more telling indicator.

Chapter Five

1. Sidney Sax, *A Strife of Interests: Politics and Policies in Australian Health Services* (Boston: George Allen and Unwin, 1984), pp. 54–55. Sax provides a thorough history of Australian medical politics up to the 1984 passage of medicare. For a shorter description, see Colin Burrows, "The Ever-Changing Australian Health-Care System: A Problem of Structure and Ideology," in Marilynn M. Rosenthal and Marcel Frenkel, eds., *Health Care Systems and Their Patients: An International Perspective* (Boulder, Colo.: Westview Press, 1992), pp. 111–35.

2. Neil Henderson and Richard Tate, *Hospital Finance: Understanding the Basics* (South Melbourne: Secretariat and Research Division, Victorian Hospitals' Association Limited, 1991), chap. 2; National Health Strategy, *Hospital Services in Australia: Access and Financing*, Issues Paper 2 (Canberra: National Health Strategy, September 1991), pp. 71–80; interviews.

3. These negotiations become caught up in partisan politics as well, as state governments of one party seek to embarrass national governments of the other. But agreements are made, eventually, since no state can do without the money and no Commonwealth government could afford to have a state drop out.

4. Australian Institute of Health and Welfare, *Australia's Health 1992: The Third Biennial Report of the Australian Institute of Health and Welfare* (Canberra: Australian Government Publishing Service, 1992), pp. 158–61. Pages 92–172 provide a thorough overview of the system. One excellent summary for American readers is Stuart Altman and Terri Jackson, "Health Care in Australia: Lessons from Down Under," *Health Affairs*, vol. 10, no. 3 (Fall 1991), pp. 129–46. For another treatment of Canadian and Australian lessons for the United States, see Peter Botsman, "USACARE: A National Health Insurance Strategy for the USA," report prepared for the Midwest Center for Labor Research (Chicago, January 1992).

For descriptions of Australian medicare, see Medicare (Australia), "What Does Medicare Cover?," brochure MCU 0392 611 (Canberra, March 1992); Health Insurance Commission, "Mediguide: A Guide to Understanding Medicare, 1992," pp. 18–20; National Health Strategy, *The Australian Health Jigsaw: Integration of Health Care Delivery*, Issues Paper 1 (Canberra, July 1991).

5. For example, it can monitor physician practice patterns better than a more fragmented system. Although doctors may bill more than the amount

on the fee schedule, there is no system of private insurer review or argument about fees, because they are allowed to pay only the difference between medicare's payment and the amount on the medicare fee schedule. All extra billing then must be collected directly from the patient—which means fewer administrative costs, and who-knows-what effect on collections!

6. Australian Institute of Health and Welfare, *Australia's Health 1992*, pp. 100–03.

7. National Health Strategy, *Hospital Services in Australia*, p. 131. The broadest package, with extensive dental benefits, for example, cost much more—$1,718.40 per year for New South Wales/ACT Medibank Private Insurance, according to its promotional guidebook, *Select & Save*, October 1992, p. 23.

8. Figures are from New South Wales/ACT Medibank Private Insurance, *Select & Save*, p. 13.

9. National Health Strategy, *Hospital Services in Australia*, pp. 124–25, and interviews.

10. Peter Baulderstone, "Hospital Funding—Dilemmas and Directions," speech delivered to the Combined Regional Workshop, Australian College of Health Services Executives, Canberra (April 1–3, 1992), p. 4.

11. Premium increases from National Health Strategy, *Hospital Services in Australia*, p. 131; enrollment and opinions from Australian Institute of Health and Welfare, *Australia's Health 1992*, pp. 100–02; enrollment trends can be found in Private Health Insurance Administration Council, *Annual Report 1993–94: Operations of the Registered Health Benefits Organisations* (Canberra: Australian Government Publishing Service, 1994), tables 10a and 10b, p. 98. Note that "basic cover," which provided less coverage for private hospital services, declined more steadily from 1985 on. The decline of basic cover may have been more important to public hospital budgets; decline in supplemental cover would be more of a threat to private hospitals.

12. The patient can pay the doctor immediately and bill medicare, receiving a check from the government (or even cash from a local medicare office); or he can delay paying, in which case medicare will send him a check made out to the doctor. The options and exceptions are explained to doctors in Health Insurance Commission, "Mediguide," pp. 47–66.

13. Australian Institute of Health and Welfare, *Australia's Health 1992*, pp. 140–41. For more detail on medical practice, see John Deeble, *Medical Services through Medicare*, Background Paper 2 (Canberra: National Health Strategy, February 1991), and National Health Strategy, *The Future of General Practice*, Issues Paper 3 (Canberra, March 1992).

14. Altman and Jackson, "Health Care in Australia," p. 143.

15. National Health Strategy, *Australian Health Jigsaw*, p. 108. See also Australian Institute of Health and Welfare, *Health Services Bulletin* (May 1992), table 4c, p. 12.

16. National Health Strategy, *A Study of Hospital Outpatient and Emergency Department Services*, Background Paper 10 (Canberra, June 1992), pp. 96–97, 104–05. In personal communication on February 28, 1995, Professor R.B. Scotton, one of Australia's most eminent health economists, argues that voluntary

"bulkbilling" by specialists is more important, and use of the hospital outpatients unit is less so. I don't believe that fits the spending data or my interviews; in any case, the hospital is at worst a crucial backup.

17. Medicare (Australia), "What Does Medicare Cover?"

18. Australian Institute for Health and Welfare, *Australia's Health 1992*, pp. 100–04, 125.

19. "AHA Hospital Brief," Newsletter of the Australian Hospital Association (October 1992), pp. 1, 4; Australian Institute of Health and Welfare, *Australia's Health 1992*, p. 14.

20. One careful study concluded, "There was evidence of preferential access to public hospital care for privately insured patients due to medical misrepresentation of the urgency of their cases." Alan Davis and others, "The Influence of Health Insurance Status on the Organisation of Patient Care in Sydney Public Hospitals," *Australian Health Review*, vol. 14, no. 4 (1991), p. 450.

21. Data comparing public and private hospital volume are in National Health Strategy, *Hospital Services in Australia*, pp. 26 and 107. I was told that a number of private hospitals in Melbourne have opened emergency services, and one Melbourne private hospital does a very large proportion of that area's cardiac surgery. On investment in private hospitals, see *Hospital Services in Australia*, pp. 114–19; also Australian Private Hospitals Association, "Background to the APHA Hospital Financing Policy" (Deakin, ACT, September 1991), pp. 3–4 and 11, which show their greater level of investment, and page 12, complaining about lack of profitability. A biting commentary on public hospital capital financing and an explanation of why the largest private hospital corporation in Australia feels it has an advantage, is provided in Mary Foley, "Capital Funding of Public Hospitals: A Private Sector Perspective," address to the Australian Hospital Association Congress, Canberra, October 30, 1992.

22. Davis and others, "Influence of Health Insurance Status on Patient Care," *Australian Health Review*, vol. 14, no. 4 (1991), pp. 450 and 459–60.

23. The specific rules for bed allocation, according to interviews, vary widely and seemingly unsystematically among hospitals.

24. Gillian Ednie, "A Consumer Perspective on Health Complaints Mechanisms in Australia" (Canberra: Consumers' Health Forum of Australia, November 1992), p. 18.

25. The Complaints Unit has a series of handouts explaining its procedures to providers. In this case the quote is from Complaints Unit, "The Role of the Complaints Unit: The Complaints Investigation Process" (Sydney: New South Wales Department of Health, 1991), p. 2. The following description is based on those handouts and on interviews with leaders of the Complaints Unit and of the New South Wales Medical Association.

26. Complaints Unit, "What Happens When a Complaint Is Made against You" (Sydney: New South Wales Department of Health), p. 2.

27. Two hundred twenty-one were not investigated for reasons such as lack of information or that there was no possible remedy; 62 investigated com-

plaints were referred to another agency; in 121 cases the investigation was terminated along the way; in 436 the complaint was not substantiated. Data are from Complaints Unit, "1991 Statistics" (Sydney: New South Wales Department of Health, 1991).

28. Ednie, "Consumer Perspective," p. 20.

29. For a history, see Yves Saint-Jours, "France," in Peter A. Kohler and Hans F. Zacher, eds., *The Evolution of Social Insurance 1881–1981: Studies of Germany, France, Great Britain, Austria, and Switzerland* (St. Martin's Press, 1982), pp. 93–149, or William A. Glaser, *Health Insurance in Practice* (San Francisco: Jossey-Bass, 1991), pp. 506–11.

30. The most thorough account of medical care politics in France is David Wilsford, *Doctors and the State: The Politics of Health Care in France and the United States* (Durham, N.C.: Duke University Press, 1991); see particularly the chapter, "The Continuity of Crisis: Patterns of Making Health Policy in France, 1978–1990," pp. 118–60. For another account of French developments, see Jean de Kervasdoue, Victor Rodwin, and Jean-Claude Stephan, "France: Contemporary Problems and Future Scenarios," in Jean de Kervasdoue, John R. Kimberly, and Victor Rodwin, eds., *The End of an Illusion: The Future of Health Policy in Western Industrialized Nations* (University of California Press, 1984), pp. 137–66.

31. Victor G. Rodwin and Simone Sandier, "Health Care under French National Health Insurance," *Health Affairs*, vol. 12, no. 3 (Fall 1993), p. 116. Other good summaries include Jonathan E. Fielding and Pierre-Jean Lancry, "Lessons from France—'Vive la Différence'," *Journal of the American Medical Association*, August 11, 1993, pp. 748–56; Glaser, *Health Insurance in Practice*; Laurent Chambaud, "A La Carte," in Annabelle May, ed., *Healthcare in Europe* (Special issue of the *Health Service Journal*) (London: Macmillan Magazines, 1993), p. 47.

32. See Glaser, *Health Insurance in Practice*, pp. 205–07. In most countries some groups were so economically and politically important that pensions were created for them before others. As they became less important over the years, they ran into problems everywhere. In the United States, railroad retirement is separate from social security but subsidized; miners have special coverage for black lung disease.

33. Figures are taken from Fielding and Lancry, "Lessons from France," p. 750, and Glaser, *Health Insurance in Practice*, pp. 103, 120, 123–24. The employment-based contributions to CNAMTS pay for extensive salary maintenance benefits as well as for health care expenses. If one subtracts the cost of those benefits from the contribution rate, and compares the amount used for health care to the total of wages and other benefit contributions, one gets a significantly smaller figure than the percentages in the text suggest: about 11.4 percent of wages-plus-total-social security, using the data current at this writing.

34. These included taxes on cigarettes and hard spirits (not wine), and a surcharge on automobile insurance (for traffic accidents). There was a cycle of government subsidies when the funds were in deficit and fund paybacks when

they were in temporary surplus. Glaser, *Health Insurance in Practice*, pp. 145–46, 196–99.

35. Part of the point was to respond to the argument that charges directly related to employment reduce employment. The tax, created in the late 1980s, was raised from 1.1 percent by a new conservative government. Interviews with Pascal Chevit, counselor for social affairs, Embassy of France, and with Laurent Chambaud, February 2, 1994.

36. Fielding and Lancry, "Lessons from France," pp. 752 and 749; Rodwin and Sandier, "Health Care under French National Health Insurance," p. 128; schedules of benefits and copayments can also be found in French Embassy Press and Information Service, "Facts on France: The French Health Care System" (Washington, March 1992), table F; and Sharon Waxman, "National Health Insurance: Taking the Pulse of the French System," *France Magazine* (Summer 1992), pp. 11–13. It is too early to be sure, but the higher cost sharing is more likely to switch costs onto private budgets than to reduce care, because most people's supplemental coverage (*mutuelles*) pays the difference.

37. French Embassy Press Service, "Facts on France," table F; Fielding and Lancry, "Lessons from France," p. 755. The OECD reports that the French consume three times as many pharmaceuticals as the Germans. Exact figures are unreliable, because of differences in dosage and difficulty comparing drugs of different types, but all sources agree the French consume a lot of drugs; see OECD, *OECD Health Data: Comparative Analysis of Health Systems*, data base (Paris, 1993).

38. Waxman, "National Health Insurance," p. 13.

39. Chambaud, "A La Carte," p. 47, reports that patients are "reimbursed . . . by the sickness fund a few days later."

40. Office doctors do not bill the mutuelle; an increasing number of pharmacies try to attract business by agreeing to do so. A mutuelle that provides its own services works much like an HMO with a point-of-service option—patients may seek medical service anywhere they wish but pay more when they do not use the providers on the mutuelle's panel. But unless it owns a hospital, the mutuelle has little incentive to reduce hospitalization, since it is liable for only a small part of costs. Note that mutuelle premiums are charged as a percentage of salary, so tax deductibility does not favor higher-wage employees.

41. Fielding and Lancry, "Lessons from France," pp. 750–51; Glaser, *Health Insurance in Practice*, pp. 265, 507–10.

42. Glaser, *Health Insurance in Practice*, p. 297.

43. Aide Médicale had expenses of 3.2 billion francs (less than a billion dollars) in 1990. It will not pay the extra charges of "Secteur 2" physicians, described below. My thanks to Pascal Chevit, M.D., counselor for social affairs to the French Embassy, for explanation and statistics.

44. The first figure comes from Fielding and Lancry, "Lessons from France," table on p. 749 and comment at top of p. 752; see also Waxman, "National Health Insurance," p. 11. The following figures are estimates based on Fielding and Lancry's table.

45. Joseph Murawiec, "Experiences in the French Health Care System: Recollections of a Close Friend," in Marilynn M. Rosenthal and Marcel Frenkel, eds., *Health Care Systems and Their Patients: An International Perspective* (Boulder, Colo.: Westview Press, 1992), p. 81.

46. French Embassy Press Service, "Facts on France," sec. III, pp. 2–3; Rodwin and Sandier, "Health Care under French National Health Insurance," pp. 114–15.

47. Ibid., p. 113. Note that the Australian Medical Association would agree, as would every other medical association in this study, save possibly the British. My thanks to Dr. Pascal Chevit for pointing out that translating *la médecine libérale* as "free medicine" would definitely not represent the physicians' position.

48. On the one hand, the funds can tell the doctors, "the government won't allow that"; on the other hand, the funds may figure, "let's agree, we know the government will veto it."

49. Victor G. Rodwin, Harvey Grable, and Gregory Thiel, "Updating the Fee Schedule for Physician Reimbursement: A Comparative Analysis of France, Germany, Canada, and the United States," *Quality Assurance and Utilization Review*, vol. 5, no. 1 (February 1990), pp. 17–20; Rodwin and Sandier, "Health Care under French National Health Insurance," pp. 114, 118; Wilsford, *Doctors and the State*, emphasizes market conditions in his discussion, pp. 153–54.

50. Rodwin and Sandier, "Health Care under French National Health Insurance," p. 129 (n. 29); Fielding and Lancry, "Lessons from France," p. 751 (table 3 shows 41.6 percent of specialists extra-billing in 1990). Fielding and Lancry point out that "some French courts" have interpreted the law's language that extra billing must be charged "with tact and restraint" as limiting the charges to 50 percent above the schedule. Calculating from the data in Fielding and Lancry, 19 percent of physicians in 1990 were specialists who extra-billed. Assuming similar figures in 1993, about 10 percent would be GPs who extra-billed, or just under 19 percent of GPs. Difficulties finding specialists in the big cities have not been measured but are commonly remarked upon.

51. Fielding and Lancry, "Lessons from France," p. 751; private insurance payments could be hidden in the 28.3 percent figure, but private insurance is too small to cover much of it.

52. For information on outpatient units see Victor G. Rodwin and Charles Brecher, "HHC and AP: System-Wide Comparisons," in Victor G. Rodwin and others, *Public Hospital Systems in New York and Paris* (NYU Press, 1992), pp. 11–28, and Rodwin and Sandier, "Health Care under French National Health Insurance," pp. 120 and 130 (n. 39). Note that Aide Médicale pays only the legal cost sharing, so the poor in a large city are especially likely to use the outpatient clinic.

53. Fielding and Lancry, "Lessons from France," p. 752.

54. William A. Glaser, "How Expenditure Caps and Expenditure Targets Really Work," *Milbank Quarterly*, vol. 71, no. 1 (1993), p. 106. For a review of the politics, see Wilsford, *Doctors and the State*, pp. 162–67. This budget orig-

inally focused on input line items. Since 1991 Loi Hospitalier hospitals have been given more flexibility to, for example, move funds among food, staff, laundry and other costs. Supposedly there is more regional "planification" as well, but the wise student of planning is always skeptical.

55. U.S. General Accounting Office, "Health Care Spending Control, The Experience of France, Germany, and Japan" (GAO/HRD-92-9) (November 1991), pp. 44, 47–48; OECD 1993 data base.

56. Rodwin and Sandier, "Health Care under French National Health Insurance," pp. 128, n. 22.

57. Lawrence Malkin, "A Tale of Two Eyes," *New Republic*, September 4, 1989, p. 15.

58. Again, author's calculations from Rodwin and Sandier, "Health Care under French National Health Insurance," data at pp. 120 and 130.

59. Fielding and Lancry, "Lessons from France," p. 749, 751. Remember that cancer costs are 100 percent covered. William Glaser provides one other explanation of the low costs per day: the sickness funds "are very strict" in the rate negotiations with hospitals. See Glaser, *Health Insurance in Practice*, p. 266.

60. Some sessional fees are paid to office-based doctors, but they normally provide outpatient services. Rodwin and Sandier, "Health Care Under French National Health Insurance," p. 130 (n. 33).

61. My thanks to Dr. Pascal Chevit and Laurent Chambaud for this point. There is a committee on private practice in each public hospital, and use of privileges can be controversial, but it is not viewed as a major problem. Hospitals keep about 20 percent of a surgeon's fees in these circumstances, and the surgeon charges a higher fee, as a Sector 2 physician does.

62. William A. Glaser, *Paying the Hospital: The Organization, Dynamics, and Effects of Differing Financial Arrangements* (San Francisco: Jossey-Bass, 1987), p. 233 for the quote; see also pp. 229–36.

63. Ibid., p. 230.

64. See Dominique Jolly and Victor G. Rodwin, "Planning for the Hospitals of AP in Paris," in Rodwin and others, *Public Hospital Systems in New York and Paris*, pp. 182–97, but esp. pp. 191–93. Private hospitals may become even more competitive if the government goes ahead with plans, suggested in early 1994, to eliminate about 24,000 public hospital beds.

65. For a discussion of capital budgeting under these constraints, see ibid. and Catherine Viens-Bitker and others, "The Committee on the Evaluation and Diffusion of Medical Technologies (CEDIT) at AP," in Rodwin and others, *Public Hospital Systems in New York and Paris*.

66. For speculation on how the availability of prestigious doctors in public hospitals might erode in France see Dominique Jolly and Beatrice Majnoni d'Intignano, "Alternative Futures for AP," in ibid., pp. 241–66, but esp. pp. 249–54.

67. For a history of the Japanese medical system, see Margaret Powell and Masahira Anesaki, *Health Care in Japan* (New York: Routledge, 1990), chaps. 1, 2, 4.

68. See the OECD 1993 data base.

69. The best source on the Japanese health care system is Naoki Ikegami and John C. Campbell, eds., *Containing Health Care Costs in Japan* (Ann Arbor: University of Michigan Press, forthcoming 1995). In the text I cite draft chapters from the conferences that helped create that book. Among published materials as of 1993, see Naoki Ikegami, "The Economics of Health Care in Japan," *Science*, October 23, 1992, pp. 614–18; John K. Iglehart, "Health Policy Report: Japan's Medical Care System—Part I," *New England Journal of Medicine*, September 22, 1988, pp. 807–12, and "Health Policy Report: Japan's Medical Care System—Part II," October 27, 1988, pp. 1166–72; Aki Yoshikawa, Norihiko Shirouzu, and Matthew Holt, "How Does Japan Do It? Doctors and Hospitals in a Universal Health Care System," *Stanford Law and Policy Review*, vol. 3 (Fall 1991), pp. 111–37. Also useful is Matthew Holt and others, *Medical Ivory Towers and the High Cost of Health Care: A Comparison of Teaching Hospitals in the United States and Japan* (Palo Alto, Calif.: Asia/Pacific Research Center, Stanford University, 1993); and for a glimpse of patient reactions, see Keidanren Kaikan Hall, *The First Japan-United States Health Care Symposium* (Proceedings, October 9–10, 1989, Tokyo), hereafter, Keidanren, "Proceedings." Also see Research Institute of Social Insurance, *Guide Book of Social Insurance in Japan 1993* (Tokyo: Social Insurance Agency, December 24, 1993).

70. See ibid., pp. 15–29; National Federation of Health Insurance Societies, *Health Insurance and Health Insurance Societies in Japan, 1992* (Tokyo, 1992), pp. 8–13, 66, 67; Ikegami, "Economics of Health Care in Japan," pp. 615–16. Nobuharu Okamitsu, reference materials for seminar, "Making Universal Health Care Affordable: How Japan Does It," presented by the Japan Society, New York, April 30, 1993, table 3. Premiums are charged against wages only, not against Japan's substantial bonuses, so the rates are lower than they seem.

71. The proportion of people in this category is so high because it includes public employees, including workers for government corporations such as the post office and railways. National Federation of Health Insurance Societies, *Health Insurance Societies in Japan, 1992*, pp. 8–9, 12–13, 66.

72. The problems converting other currencies into dollar values are especially severe for yen and dollars. The exchange rate of yen for dollars has been extremely volatile, falling from 250 to 125 over the decade up to 1992. Those rates are particularly deceptive because Japanese prices for most goods are much higher than American. John C. Campbell, who has faced the same problem for *Continuing Health Care Costs in Japan*, suggested I use a rough purchasing power figure of 200 yen per dollar, and I will do that here.

73. The contributions assessments for National Health Insurance are based on assets as well as income because it is easier to hide income than assets, and self-employed people are not renowned for honesty in such matters in any society. See National Federation of Health Insurance Societies, *Health Insurance Societies in Japan, 1992*, p. 66; Yoshikawa, Shirouzu, and Holt, "How Does Japan Do It?" p. 116; Iglehart, "Japan's Medical Care System," p. 811; Nobuharu Okamitsu, "Basic Data of Japanese Health Care System," distrib-

uted at the conference "Making Universal Health Care Affordable: How Japan Does It," sponsored by the Japan Society in New York, April 30, 1993, table titled "Current Condition of the Medical Insurance Scheme" (hereafter, Okamitsu/Japan Society tables).

74. Ikegami, "Economics of Health Care in Japan," p. 615; Okamitsu/Japan Society tables, "Current Condition of the Medical Insurance Scheme," and "Outline of Health and Medical Services for the Elderly."

75. Naoki Ikegami, "Japan's Health Care Delivery and Financing System" (Blue Cross of California, 1991), and the King's Fund, "Health Care in the '90s: A Global View of Delivery and Financing" (Los Angeles: Blue Cross of California, 1991), p. 56. In 1990, government-managed health insurance, society-managed insurance, and national health insurance paid, respectively, 17.3 percent, 23.0 percent, and 25.6 percent of their total benefits in the form of contributions to the scheme for the elderly; the government-managed plan paid 3.5 percent and the society-managed plan paid 5.3 percent for the retired nonelderly. See National Federation of Health Insurance Societies, *Health Insurance Societies in Japan, 1992*, pp. 66–67. See also Research Institute of Social Insurance, *Guide Book of Social Insurance*, pp. 29–37.

76. Yoshikawa, Shirouzu, and Holt, "How Does Japan Do It?" pp. 114–15.

77. See U.S. General Accounting Office, "Health Care Spending Control: The Experience of France, Germany, and Japan," GAO/HRD-92-9 (November 1991), pp. 31–32; Powell and Anesaki, *Health Care in Japan*, pp. 107–11; interviews with staff at the Stanford University Comparative Health Care Policy Research Project; and Toshihiko Hasegawa, "A Comparative Study of Hospital Admission Rates between the U.S. and Japan," in Ikegami and Campbell, *Containing Health Care Costs in Japan*.

78. Keidanren, "Proceedings," pp. 174–77. The ambulance system decides where patients go, and there is little walk-in traffic at hospital emergency rooms. Powell and Anesaki report that there is a shortage of emergency capacity (see *Health Care in Japan*, pp. 175–77), and of course any system that requires driving in Tokyo cannot work wonderfully.

79. Cost sharing for care for low-income elderly is even lower; see Research Institute of Social Insurance, *Guide Book of Social Insurance*, p. 24.

80. Ibid., pp. 24–25.

81. National Federation of Health Insurance Societies, *Health Insurance Societies in Japan, 1992*, pp. 21–22.

82. Ikegami, "Economics of Health Care in Japan," p. 615; Iglehart emphasizes that although questions of equity exist, all the plans "protect their beneficiaries against the prospect of financial devastation by a serious illness" (Iglehart, "Japan's Medical Care System," p. 811). But see Japan Economic Institute, "Japanese Health Care System No Panacea for Ailing U.S. Program," *JEI Report*, 25A, July 5, 1991. The set of limits on cost sharing is very complex; the most a person could possibly pay is about $2,500. Still, that amount would probably be too much for some, even in a country with high savings rates.

83. National Federation of Health Insurance Societies, *Health Insurance So-

cieties in Japan, 1992, p. 25; Naoki Ikegami, "Low Cost through Regulated Fees," *Health Affairs*, vol. 10, no. 3 (Fall 1991), pp. 97–99.

84. Exceptions include abortions, childbirth, plastic surgery, and much dental work. My thanks to John C. Campbell for this point.

85. In Japan medical schools subsidize hospitals, whereas in America the reverse is true. This is possible because, although the national and local government-run medical schools charge low tuitions, tuition to private medical schools is very high (see Holt and others, *Medical Ivory Towers*, pp. 39–40). The argument about fee schedules that follows is largely drawn from Ikegami, "Japanese Health Care," pp. 95–99 and 103–04, but other sources agree.

86. Ikegami reports that 33 percent of doctors were in private practice and 60 percent in hospitals in 1989 (Ikegami, "Japanese Health Care," p. 108, n. 2). Iglehart estimates the average age of doctors in private practice as fifty-eight (see "Japan's Medical Care System," p. 1170).

87. Ikegami, "The Economics of Health Care in Japan," p. 617; for discussion see Ikegami, "Japanese Health Care," pp. 96–99; Yoshikawa, Shirouzu, and Holt, "How Does Japan Do It?" pp. 124–28. On the power of the Japan Medical Association, see Mitsuru Fujii and Michael R. Reich, "Rising Medical Costs and the Reform of Japan's Health Insurance System," *Health Policy*, vol. 9 (February 1988), pp. 9–24.

88. In 1988 Japan had more than 1.9 million hospital beds, including those in clinics (see text and tables in Yoshikawa, Shirouzu, and Holt, "How Does Japan Do It?" pp. 121–25; also see Iglehart, "Japan's Medical Care System," pp. 1169–70). These figures would be far higher than those for other countries even if we excluded the perhaps 20 percent of the total that is devoted to patients with mental problems, which would not be included in the usual statistics from other countries.

89. Yoshikawa, Shirouzu, and Holt, "How Does Japan Do It?" pp. 118, 131–34; Holt and others, *Medical Ivory Towers*, pp. 61–62.

90. For example, affiliation with a medical school positively affects American respondents' choice of hospital for treatment (see Harold S. Luft and others, "Does Quality Influence Choice of Hospital?" *Journal of the American Medical Association*, June 6, 1990, p. 2903).

91. Powell and Anesaki, *Health Care in Japan*, pp. 165–66; Ikegami, "Japanese Health Care," pp. 99, 103–04.

92. Ibid., p. 99; Hasegawa, "A Comparative Study of Hospital Admission Rates."

93. Yoshikawa, Shirouzu, and Holt, "How Does Japan Do It?" p. 129.

94. Holt and others, *Medical Ivory Towers*, p. 105.

95. The intensive care units themselves have an average of only 2.9 beds per national university hospital (Holt and others, *Medical Ivory Towers*, pp. 47 and 90). The New York and Paris public hospitals have an average of thirty ICU and CCU (cardiac care unit) beds (Rodwin and Brecher, "HHC and AP: System-Wide Comparisons," p. 18).

96. Toshiko Hasegawa, "Does the Difference in Surgical Admission Rate

Account for the Difference in Health Expenditure between the U.S. and Japan? Comparative Analysis of Health Expenditure and Medical Care Activity in the U.S. and Japan," National Medical Authority, Kyushu Region, Ministry of Health and Welfare, p. 17. Duplicated.

97. Powell and Anesaki, *Health Care in Japan*, p. 167. See also Keidanren, "Proceedings," pp. 161, 168. I have heard similar comments from a number of friends and colleagues, but those who use the system do like the low prices. I should add that a lack of space and privacy in Japan is hardly confined to the health care system and, given population density, would be hard to avoid.

98. Naoki Ikegami, "Comparison of Pharmaceutical Expenditure between Japan and U.S.," in Ikegami and Campbell, *Containing Health Care Costs in Japan*.

99. Powell and Anesaki, *Health Care in Japan*, p. 174.

100. "Medicinal Madness," *Economist*, March 27, 1993, p. 73.

101. Interview with John C. Campbell, University of Michigan, December 1993.

102. Ikegami, "Japanese Health Care," reports a 52 percent decrease in the prices of pharmaceuticals and lab tests combined from 1981 to 1990; Iglehart, "Japan's Medical Care System," p. 1171, reports a 61.4 percent decrease in drug prices during the 1980s. See also Ikegami, "Comparison of Pharmaceutical Expenditure between Japan and U.S."

103. Iglehart, "Japan's Medical Care System," p. 1171. Interview and conference presentations provide lower more recent numbers, but this author is not sure that they are based on the same definition of total spending.

104. Ikegami, "Comparison of Pharmaceutical Expenditure between Japan and U.S."

105. Powell and Anesaki, *Health Care in Japan*, p. 203. On the politics of fee setting, see Mikitaka Masuyama and John Creighton Campbell, "The Evolution of Fee-Schedule Politics in Japan," in Ikegami and Campbell, *Containing Health Care Costs in Japan*; also Iglehart, "Japan's Medical Care System," pp. 1171–72.

106. OECD 1993 data base; the latest data are from 1988 for Japan and 1987 for Germany.

107. Iglehart, "Japan's Medical Care System," p. 810.

108. See the account in Eiji Yano and others, "Comparing Postgraduate Medical Education at University and Non-university Hospitals in Japan," *Academic Medicine*, vol. 67, no. 1 (January 1992), pp. 54–58; see also Iglehart, "Japan's Medical Care System," p. 1172.

109. Interview with Dr. Kazu Araki, Comparative Health Care Policy Research Project, Stanford University. Resident pay is quite low, especially in the national university hospitals; $10,000 per year would not be unusual (see Yano and others, "Comparing Postgraduate Medical Education," p. 55; Holt and others, *Medical Ivory Towers*, pp. 35–38, 42). Trainees therefore moonlight extensively (which is possible because their hours are not as long as in the United States).

110. The figures are from Iglehart, "Japan's Medical Care System," p. 1170, and Ikegami, "Low Cost through Regulated Fees," p. 98.

111. Ikegami, "Low Cost through Regulated Fees," pp. 93, 104.

112. Ruth Campbell, "The Three-Minute Cure: Doctors and Elderly Patients in Japan," in Ikegami and Campbell, *Containing Health Care Costs in Japan*.

113. Naoki Ikegami, "Waiting Lists in Japanese Hospitals," January 1993. Duplicated.

114. The speech was given on April 9, 1992, at a Northern Virginia Community College meeting on health care reform.

115. As cited in Laurene E. Graig, *Health of Nations: An International Perspective on Health Care Reform* (Washington: Wyatt Company, 1991), p. 216; Henry J. Aaron and William B. Schwartz, *The Painful Prescription: Rationing Hospital Care* (Brookings, 1984), p. 14.

116. For a discussion of the budget process see chapter 1 of Joseph White and Aaron Wildavsky, *The Deficit and the Public Interest: The Search for Responsible Budgeting in the 1980s* (University of California Press and the Russell Sage Foundation, 1991).

117. When administrators behave this way they are often being responsible, because their job is to maximize output, and the money for investment or deferred maintenance might be provided when better budgetary times arrive.

118. See Joseph White, "Markets, Budgets, and Health Care Cost Control," *Health Affairs*, vol. 12, no. 3 (Fall 1993), pp. 44–57.

119. D. Costagliola and others, "Some Key Factors in the Clinical Diagnosis of Non Insulin-Dependent Diabetes: A Multinational Comparison," *Diabete & Metabolisme*, vol. 15, no. 1 (January/February 1989), pp. 51–52.

120. See Robert H. Brook and others, "Diagnosis and Treatment of Coronary Disease: Comparison of Doctors' Attitudes in the USA and the UK," *Lancet*, April 2, 1988, pp. 750–53; the quotation is from Lynn Payer, *Medicine and Culture: Varieties of Treatment in the United States, England, West Germany, and France* (New York: Henry Holt, 1988), p. 103.

121. Ibid., especially pp. 107–13.

122. The Secretaries of State for Health, Wales, Northern Ireland, and Scotland, *Working for Patients* (London: Her Majesty's Stationery Office, January 1989), pp. 100–02.

123. For accounts, see Alan Maynard, "The United Kingdom," in Jean Jacques Rosa, *Comparative Health Systems: The Future of National Health Care Systems and Economic Analysis* (Greenwich, Conn.: JAI Press, 1990), especially pp. 1–11; David Allen, "England," in Marshall W. Raffel, *Comparative Health Systems* (Pennsylvania State University Press, 1984), pp. 197–257; Odin W. Anderson, *The Health Services Continuum in Democratic States: An Inquiry into Solvable Problems* (Ann Arbor, Mich.: Health Administration Press, 1989), pp. 25–45. For current structure, spending, and language I am using Department of Health and Office of Population Censuses and Surveys, *Departmental Report, The Government's Expenditure Plans 1993–94 to 1995–96* (London: Her Majesty's Stationery Office, February 1992).

124. Department of Health, *Departmental Report,* pp. 1, 2 (England), 94 (United Kingdom).

125. Ken Starkey, "Time and the Consultant: Issues of Contract and Control," and Peter Bryden, "The Future of Primary Care," in Ray Loveridge and Ken Starkey, eds., *Continuity and Crisis in the NHS* (Philadelphia: Open University Press, 1992), pp. 59–60 and 65–72; Kevin Grumbach and John Fry, "Managing Primary Care in the United States and in the United Kingdom," *New England Journal of Medicine,* April 1, 1993, pp. 940–45. Statistics also come from Department of Health, *Departmental Report,* pp. 50, 53.

126. Christopher Potter and Janet Porter, "American Perceptions of the British National Health Service: Five Myths," *Journal of Health Politics, Policy and Law,* vol. 14, no. 2 (Summer 1989), pp. 360–61.

127. Bryden, "Future of Primary Care," pp. 67–68.

128. Personal communication from Clive Smee, chief economic adviser to the NHS, April 25, 1994.

129. *Whitaker's Almanac, 1992* (London: J. Whitaker & Sons, 1991), pp. 498–500; on dentists see Potter and Porter, "American Perceptions of the British National Health Service," pp. 359–60. Pregnancy care is another NHS-provided service that anecdotal evidence suggests particularly satisfies patients.

130. Maynard, "United Kingdom," pp. 13–14; Allen, "England," pp. 230–33; Starkey, "Time and the Consultant," pp. 55–58.

131. Howard Glennerster and others, "GP Fundholding: Wild Card or Winning Hand?" in Ray Robinson and Julian Le Grand, eds., *Evaluating the NHS Reforms* (New Brunswick, N.J.: Transaction Books and King's Fund Institute, 1994), p. 74.

132. Margot Jefferys, "Britain's National Health Service under Pressure," in Rosenthal and Frenkel, *Health Care Systems,* pp. 224–25. Private insurance was encouraged during World War II in the United States by the same policy. Maynard estimates that more than 5 million Britons had private insurance in 1987 and spent about 750 million pounds for acute care in 1988, plus some more for geriatric services (see Maynard, "United Kingdom," pp. 20–21). Total NHS spending in the 1987–88 fiscal year was over 20 billion pounds; see Department of Health, *Departmental Report,* p. 94, and Potter and Porter, "American Perceptions of the British National Health Service," pp. 361–62.

133. Maynard, "United Kingdom," p. 21; Graig, *Health of Nations,* pp. 230–32; "Rolling Back the Private Sector," *Economist,* June 6, 1992, pp. 61–62.

134. John Yates, *Why Are We Waiting? An Analysis of Hospital Waiting Lists* (Oxford University Press, 1987), pp. 48–62. See also Margot Jefferys, "Britain's National Health Service in 1986: Comments from a Native User," in Rosenthal and Frenkel, *Health Care Systems,* pp. 237–45. Even Potter and Porter agree that there were substantial differences in waiting times for specialist appointments and treatment: see "American Perceptions of the British National Health Service," pp. 358–59. In one survey, nine out of ten private patients had an outpatient appointment in less than a month, while just under half of the NHS patients did; Jack O'Sullivan, "Private Care 'Is Often No Faster Than the NHS'," *Independent,* August 6, 1992, p. 5.

135. Yates, *Why Are We Waiting?* is a careful yet passionate review. Brook and others, "Diagnosis and Treatment of Coronary Disease," provide a good example of how British physicians would do less than American, but must do less than they wish. Aaron and Schwartz, in *Painful Prescription*, discuss how physicians rationalize limits, but they say "most British doctors would like to deploy more resources than are now available" (p. 102).

136. Department of Health, "The Patient's Charter," leaflet 51-1024 (HMSO, January 1992), pp. 10, 14, 16.

Chapter Six

1. Physician Payment Review Commission, *Fee Update and Medicare Volume Performance Standards for 1995*, 94-1 (Washington, May 15, 1994), p. 9.

2. James D. Lubitz and Gerald F. Riley, "Trends in Medicare Payments in the Last Year of Life," *New England Journal of Medicine*, April 15, 1993, pp. 1092–96, quote p. 1094.

3. Marc L. Berk and Alan C. Monheit, "The Concentration of Health Expenditures: An Update," *Health Affairs*, vol. 11, no. 4 (Winter 1992), pp. 145–49.

4. For a particularly egregious example of this form of analysis see Irwin M. Stelzer, "What Health-Care Crisis?" *Commentary*, February 1994, pp. 19–24.

5. American advocates of managed care are normally less conservative, assuming that if cost controls work, quality will not be affected.

6. For example, in some countries extremely premature and low birth-weight babies are categorized as stillborn because they die soon after delivery, while in the United States they are counted in the infant mortality figures. My thanks to Dr. Paul Parker for this point. Sources that go beyond the basic statistics do adjust for such factors.

7. The WIC supplementary nutrition program was designed to provide medical testing and vouchers for healthy food, but does not provide a comparable level of medical or nonmedical benefits. For a snapshot of WIC's problems, see Lucinda R. Kahler and others, "Factors Associated with Rates of Participation in WIC by Eligible Pregnant Women," *Public Health Reports*, vol. 107, no. 1 (January–February 1992), pp. 60–65.

8. U.S. Congress, Office of Technology Assessment, *International Health Statistics: What the Numbers Mean for the United States*, Background Paper, OTA-BP-H-116 (November 1993), pp. 29–46 (hereafter, OTA, *International Health Statistics*); Korbin Liu and others, "International Infant Mortality Rankings: A Look behind the Numbers," *Health Care Financing Review*, vol. 13, no. 4 (Summer 1992), pp. 105–18. In 1990 the American infant mortality rate was 0.91 per 100 live births; the others ranged from 0.82 in Australia to 0.68 in Canada, 0.46 in Japan. Data from OECD, *OECD Health Systems: Facts and Trends 1960–1991*, vol. 1 (Paris, 1993), p. 69, table 3.2.6.

9. See Joseph White, "Health Care Here and There: An International Per-

spective on American Reform," *Domestic Affairs*, vol. 2 (Winter 1993/94), pp. 205–06. That analysis uses the OECD 1993 data base, which is incomplete for 1990, and which provides life expectancies at ages forty and sixty, not forty-five and sixty-five. I use the OTA figures here because they are more recent. The OTA figures show a superior French performance and seemingly worse Australian performance, but the similarities between the two data sets are far more significant than their differences.

10. See also OTA, *International Health Statistics*, pp. 47–58 and 69–85, and OECD, OECD Health Data: Comparative Analysis of Health Systems, data base (Paris, 1993) (hereafter, OECD 1993 data base). I did a back-of-the-envelope calculation on which no one should rely because the data are rounded in too many ways, but the effort may suggest a better test to someone else. I calculated what male life expectancies would have been in 1989 in the other countries using the American values given by OECD for life years lost as a result of six seemingly social-related causes: ischemic heart disease, cerebro-vascular disease, lung cancer, road accidents, cirrhosis of the liver, and a catch-all category they call "external causes." Even ascribing all these differences to behavior, American life expectancy still remained lower than in Australia, Canada, France, or Japan, and slightly higher than in Germany or Britain. And some of the differences are not simply due to behavior: for example, Americans who cannot afford blood-pressure medicine are more likely than others to die of cerebro-vascular disease.

11. For a treatment of the issues about both access and choice see Health Care Study Group, "Understanding the Choices in Health Care Reform," *Journal of Health Politics, Policy and Law*, vol. 19, no. 3 (Fall 1994), pp. 499–541.

12. For one discussion with data, see James W. Fossett and others, "Medicaid and Access to Child Health Care in Chicago," *Journal of Health Politics, Policy and Law*, vol. 17, no. 2 (Summer 1992), pp. 273–98.

13. Figures are from OECD 1993 data base.

14. Dissatisfaction with these restrictions provided a political base for the "internal market" reforms in Sweden, as described by Richard Saltman in "The Role of Competitive Incentives in Recent Reforms of Northern European Health Systems," and by Clas Rehnberg in "The Swedish Experience with Internal Markets," both chapters in Monique Jérôme-Forget, Joseph White, and Joshua Wiener, eds., *Health Care Reform through Internal Markets: Experience and Proposals* (Montreal and Washington: Institute for Research on Public Policy and Brookings, 1995). As we will see, the British reforms did not really increase patients' choices.

15. Marilynn M. Rosenthal, "Systems, Strategies, and Some Patient Encounters: A Discussion of Twelve Countries," in Marilynn M. Rosenthal and Marcel Frenkel, eds., *Health Care Systems and Their Patients: An International Perspective* (Boulder, Colo.: Westview Press, 1992), p. 334.

16. I am not addressing inequalities in health that are related to socioeconomic variables here, because the measurement problems and range of questions are too great. I hope readers will agree that people with insurance have better access to care than people without it. At the same time, social differ-

ences have an independent effect on health, and where there are large social differences between populations (such as between native Americans and other Americans, or between Australia's aboriginal population and other Australians), those can outweigh the effects of a national guarantee of treatment. Persons interested in further information might begin with the brilliant analysis by Adam Wagstaff, Pierella Paci, and Eddy van Doorslaer, "On the Measurement of Inequalities in Health," *Social Science and Medicine*, vol. 33, no. 5 (1991), pp. 545–57.

17. Foreigners even go to Britain, though not to use the National Health Service. On Arab sheikhs, see Lynn Payer, *Medicine and Culture* (Henry Holt, 1988), p. 103. Readers should also remember that any Arab sheikh who comes to the United States for treatment is not a member of a managed care organization so faces fewer restrictions than many Americans.

18. Conversation with Dr. Pascal Chevit, Embassy of France, and Laurent Chambaud, February 2, 1994.

19. Remarks of Minoru Kishibe from the First Japan-United States Health Care Symposium, sponsored by Keidanren, Tokyo, October 9–10 1989, p. 145.

20. Quoted in Victor Cohn, "The Patient's Perspective," *Washington Post Health*, May 11, 1993, p. 11.

21. Jack Hadley, Earl P. Steinberg, and Judith Feder, "Comparison of Uninsured and Privately Insured Hospital Patients: Condition on Admission, Resource Use, and Outcome," *Journal of the American Medical Association*, January 16, 1991, pp. 374–79. Note, however, that the likelihood of providing care to the uninsured may be reduced as cost controls are improved: Jonathan Gruber, "The Effect of Price Shopping in Medical Markets: Hospital Responses to PPOs in California," Working Paper 4190 (Cambridge, Mass.: National Bureau of Economic Research, October 1992).

22. The OECD data are very spotty. The United States does not lead all countries in all procedures, partly because some procedures can substitute for each other. Thus U.S. physicians performed functional grafts for renal patients less often than physicians in five of the other countries in 1987 (no data for Japan). In 1980 the United States had much lower rates of appendectomy than many other countries and fewer cholecystectomies than Canada (data presented by Nobuharu Okamitsu at seminar, "Making Universal Health Care Affordable: How Japan Does It," Japan Society, New York, April 30, 1993). But the vast majority of comparisons in these and other sources show the United States doing much more surgery.

23. Mark R. Chassin and others, "Variations in the Use of Medical and Surgical Services by the Medicare Population," *New England Journal of Medicine*, January 30, 1986, pp. 285–90; John E. Wennberg and A. Gittelsohn, "Variations in Medical Care among Small Areas," *Scientific American*, April 1982, pp. 120–35; Constance Monroe Winslow and others, "The Appropriateness of Performing Coronary Artery Bypass Surgery," *Journal of the American Medical Association*, July 22/29, 1988, pp. 505–09; John E. Wennberg, Jean L. Freeman, and William J. Culp, "Are Hospital Services Rationed in New Haven or Over-Utilized in Boston?" *Lancet*, vol. 1, no. 8543 (1987), pp. 1185–88.

24. Lucien L. Leape, "Unnecessary Surgery," *Health Services Research*, vol. 24 (1989), pp. 351–407; Australian Institute of Health and Welfare, *Australia's Health, 1992* (Canberra: Australian Government Publishing Service, 1992), pp. 143–47.

25. Alain C. Enthoven, "What Can Europeans Learn from Americans?" in Organization for Economic Cooperation and Development, *Health Care Systems in Transition: The Search for Efficiency* (Paris, 1990), pp. 57–71.

26. Payer, *Medicine and Culture*; Betty Wolder Levin, "International Perspectives on Treatment Choice in Neonatal Intensive Care Units," *Social Science and Medicine*, vol. 30, no. 8 (1990), pp. 901–12.

27. Unlike other "unnecessary" surgeries, caesarean sections probably do not increase risk. Giving birth is one of the most dangerous activities known, and surgery mitigates that risk. But explaining the wide variation in c-section rates remains difficult. In Australia, it is related to the proportion of deliveries in private hospitals. Because the average private hospital does not have residents, I was told that physicians are likely to perform a c-section to avoid being called back to the hospital for the natural birth at an inconvenient time. For data see Australian Institute of Health and Welfare, *Australia's Health, 1992*, p. 147.

28. See Jonathan A. Showstack and others, "Association of Volume with Outcome of Coronary Artery Bypass Graft Surgery," *Journal of the American Medical Association*, February 13, 1987, pp. 785–89, and "The Cardiac Money Machine," *Consumer Reports*, July 1992, pp. 446–47.

29. John Yates, *Why Are We Waiting? An Analysis of Hospital Waiting Lists* (Oxford Medical Publications: 1987). Among other things, waiting lists may be created as a way of budgeting operating theater time, and they may be lengthened through inefficient hospital management, by slacking on the part of specialists, by physicians' adding people to the lists unnecessarily as the volume of throughput increases, and by poor distribution of resources geographically. Yates neatly shows both the plausibility and limits of all these explanations.

30. "Does Canada Have the Answer?" *Consumer Reports*, September 1992, pp. 584–85, 588; Yates, *Why Are We Waiting?*

31. See U.S. General Accounting Office, "Canadian Health Insurance: Lessons for the United States," GAO/HRD-91-90 (June 1991), pp. 60–61.

32. C. David Naylor, "A Different View of Queues in Ontario," *Health Affairs*, vol. 10, no. 3 (Fall 1991), p. 115.

33. This account is based mainly on Steven J. Katz, Henry F. Mizgala, and H. Gilbert Welch, "British Columbia Sends Patients to Seattle for Coronary Artery Surgery: Bypassing the Queue in Canada," *Journal of the American Medical Association*, August 28, 1991, pp. 1108–11, as well as on interviews.

34. Critics of the "medical model" and its emphasis on treating disease rather than producing health would say that different rates of surgery simply mean that Canadian doctors do less but still do too much. From this perspective, none of the evidence cited here is relevant: waits are too long in Canada because too many people are deemed candidates for surgery. By ignoring this argument in the text, I am giving the U.S. health care system the benefit of

the doubt, while perhaps asking for trouble with both the economics and public health professions.

35. The Bush administration claimed that Canadian surgical care was less effective per case than American, misinterpreting data from a comparison of New England and Manitoba. That work concluded Canadian care was at least as good and maybe more successful than American. See Leslie L. Roos and others, "Health and Surgical Outcomes in Canada and the United States," *Health Affairs*, vol. 11, no. 2 (Summer 1992), pp. 56–72.

36. Jean L. Rouleau and others, "A Comparison of Management Patterns after Acute Myocardial Infarction in Canada and the United States," *New England Journal of Medicine*, March 18, 1993, pp. 779–84; Canadian physicians also prescribed fewer drugs such as beta blockers, a practice that would not be associated with Canada's global budgeting for hospitals.

37. Steven J. Katz, Eric B. Larson, and James P. LoGerfo, "Trends in the Utilization of Mammography in Washington State and British Columbia: Relation to State of Diagnosis and Mortality," *Medical Care*, vol. 30, no. 4 (April 1992), pp. 320–28. Steven J. Katz and others, "Delay from Symptom to Diagnosis and Treatment of Breast Cancer in Washington State and British Columbia," *Medical Care*, vol. 31, no. 3 (March 1993), pp. 264–68.

38. U.S. General Accounting Office, "Bone Marrow Transplantation: International Comparisons of Availability and Appropriateness of Use," GAO/PEMD-94-10 (March 1994), summarized on pp. 3–6. The countries included were France, Sweden, Canada, Australia, the United Kingdom, the United States, Denmark, New Zealand, the Netherlands, and Germany—listed here in order of number of transplants per capita per year (p. 21).

39. Ibid., p. 50.

40. U.S. General Accounting Office, "Cancer Survival: An International Comparison of Outcomes," GAO/PEMD-94-5 (March 1994), p. 4. Survival rates after five years for lung cancer were 11.5 percent in the United States and 12.1 percent in Ontario; for colon cancer, 44.3 percent in the United States and 43.1 percent in Ontario; for Hodgkin's, 71.7 percent in the United States and 71.6 percent in Ontario; for breast cancer, 68.7 percent in the United States and 66.0 percent in Ontario (ibid., pp. 19, 22, 25, 28).

41. Roos and others, "Health and Surgical Outcomes."

42. The OECD data show that the United States had a larger proportion of persons age sixty-five and over in 1991 than Australia or Canada, about the same as Japan, and a substantially smaller proportion than France, Germany, or the United Kingdom. On the other hand, the proportion of elderly grew faster in the preceding decade in Australia and Canada than in the United States, much faster in Japan, and more slowly in France, Germany, and the United Kingdom. This looks like a wash. OECD, *OECD Health Statistics*, vol. 2, table A1.1.5, p. 15.

43. Wendy Max and Dorothy P. Rice, "Shooting in the Dark: Estimating the Cost of Firearm Injuries," *Health Affairs*, vol. 12, no. 4 (Winter 1993), pp. 171–85. Note that most firearm-related deaths are not homicides; in 1988 there were 18,169 suicides, 13,645 homicides, 1,501 accidents, and 442 of unknown

intent. The $14.4 billion figure is from *USA Today*, December 29, 1993, p. 3A; in same issue see Lori Sharn, "Shootings, Killings Cost the USA Untold Billions," p. 4A. Another estimate is $3 billion per year; see "Ammo Tax Proposed to Fund Reform," *American Medical News*, December 27, 1993, p. 2.

44. The homicide rate was 10.7 per 100,000 in 1980 and 10.0 in 1990; motor vehicle death rates fell from 23.5 per 100,000 to 18.8. For this and related statistics see National Center for Health Statistics, *Health, United States, 1992* (Hyattsville, Md.: Public Health Service, 1993), pp. 45, 74, 76, 80–81.

45. OTA, *International Health Statistics*, p. 61.

46. Fred J. Hellinger, "Forecasts of the Costs of Medical Care for Persons with HIV: 1992–1995," *Inquiry*, vol. 29 (Fall 1992), pp. 356–65; for background see Hellinger, "Updated Forecasts of the Costs of Medical Care for Persons with AIDS, 1989–93," *Public Health Reports*, vol. 105, no. 1 (January–February 1990), pp. 1–12; and Jesse Green, Gerald M. Oppenheimer, and Neil Wintfeld, "The $147,000 Misunderstanding: Repercussions of Overestimating the Cost of AIDS," *Journal of Health Politics, Policy and Law*, vol. 19, no. 1 (Spring 1994), pp. 69–90.

47. This assumes the 1991 difference in GDP figures of 3.4 percent, which is certainly too low but consistent with previous conservative estimates, and an economy of just under six trillion dollars. For GDP figures see chapter 2, table 2-1.

48. Differences in ward organization are conspicuous by their absence from the comparative health policy literature. It would be interesting to know what the actual distributions are, and how nursing costs differ for two- and four-bed rooms where both exist.

49. The OECD data base figures are coproduced by CREDES in Paris; and one might think the French and U.S. data would match those of Victor Rodwin and Simone Sandier, "Health Care under French National Health Insurance," *Health Affairs*, vol. 12, no. 3 (Fall 1993), p. 111–31, because Dr. Sandier is one of the senior researchers at CREDES; no such luck. Rodwin and Sandier also compare physician income with income figures that include unemployed and part-time workers, which is clearly inappropriate.

50. OECD 1993 data base.

51. Physician calculations are from the reported inflation and earnings figures in American Medical Association Center For Health Policy Research, *Socioeconomic Characteristics of Medical Practice, 1992* (Chicago, 1992), p. 130; because they are based on rounded inflation numbers, there may be a small error. Population figures are from Council of Economic Advisers, *Economic Report of the President* (Government Printing Office, February 1992), p. 330, also author's calculations but from dollar income figures.

52. In 1990, 79 percent of graduates had debts that averaged $46,224. But this amount of debt itself was less than the difference between one year's average income of American and Canadian physicians. American Medical Association, *Medical Practice 1992*, pp. 21, 132. See also Rod Mickleburgh, "Canadian Doctors Feel Less Gloomy, Survey Finds," *Toronto Globe and Mail*, October 23, 1992, p. A12.

53. Of the examples in this study, only the Japanese private medical schools charge substantial fees that the students themselves pay.

54. The standard measure, staff per bed, depends on how much outpatient care is provided. Australian hospitals, which are major providers of outpatient care, have more staff per bed than U.S. hospitals. But whatever the nature of the hospitals, staff per bed has grown more quickly in the United States than in any of the other countries, according to the OECD 1993 data base.

55. Quoted in Frank G. Sabatino, "The Delivery Challenges Posed by Canada: A Bilateral View," in Richard J. Umbdenstock and Winifred M. Hageman, eds., *Critical Readings for Hospital Trustees* (Chicago: American Hospital Association, 1991), p. 122.

56. Victor G. Rodwin with others, "Louis Mourier and Coney Island Hospitals: A Comparative Analysis of Hospital Staffing and Performance," in Victor G. Rodwin and others, eds., *Public Hospital Systems in New York and Paris* (New York University Press, 1992), author's calculations from p. 38.

57. W. Vickery Stoughton, quoted in Sabatino, "Delivery Challenges Posed by Canada," p. 122.

58. Donald A. Redelmeier and Victor R. Fuchs, "Hospital Expenditures in the United States and Canada," *New England Journal of Medicine*, March 18, 1993, p. 777.

59. U.S. General Accounting Office, "Canadian Health Insurance," pp. 64–65; see also *Survey of Current Business*, vol. 72 (May 1992), table 1.1.

60. In estimating the effect of H.R. 1200, the closest thing to a Canadian-model proposal in the American reform conflict, the Congressional Budget Office estimated that direct administrative costs would fall from 7 percent to 3.5 percent of spending over time (current administrative costs are 2 percent in medicare and less in Canada), while hospitals, physicians, and other health professionals would save about 6 percent of their revenues from simplification of their billing systems. Congressional Budget Office, "H.R. 1200, American Health Security Act of 1993," letter, December 16, 1993, p. 7.

61. Robert J. Blendon and others, "Satisfaction With Health Systems in Ten Nations," *Health Affairs*, vol. 9, no. 2 (Summer 1990), p. 188; Robert J. Blendon and Karen Donelan, "Interpreting Public Opinion Surveys," *Health Affairs*, vol. 10, no. 2 (Summer 1991), pp. 166–69.

62. This author was in the audience when the Australian conservative coalition's spokesman (or "shadow minister") on health issues explained, at a speech on December 11, 1992, that the American system in which competing insurance companies strove to avoid risks was entirely unacceptable.

63. See U.S. General Accounting Office, "Canadian Health Insurance," pp. 60–61.

64. A study found that 60,000 claims during a six-month period were made on behalf of patients who held American driver's licenses. See Clyde H. Farnsworth, "Americans Filching Free Health Care in Canada," *New York Times*, December 20, 1993, p. A1.

65. Philip J. Hilts, "Quality and Low Cost of Medical Care Lure Americans to Mexican Doctors," *New York Times*, November 23, 1992, p. A11.

66. The analysis here is conservative, and larger savings could be expected. See the comments of Professors Robert Evans and Theodore Marmor about an estimate of 2 percent of GDP that I provided at a hearing of the Senate Finance Committee in October 1993. Statement of Joseph White, "Experience of Foreign Nations in Controlling Health Care Costs," Hearing before the Committee on Finance, United States Senate, 103 Cong. 1 sess. (1993), pp. 42–43.

67. See chapter 3 and Victor R. Fuchs, *The Future of Health Policy* (Harvard University Press, 1993), pp. 72–77.

68. "Risk and profit" are only 1.1 percent of benefit cost for firms with 10,000 or more employees, and only 1.8 percent for firms of 2,500 to 9,999. The figure rises for smaller groups in part because "insurers commonly retain a higher proportion of small group premiums as reserves, reflecting the greater unpredictability of benefit costs for small groups." Congressional Budget Office, *Rising Health Care Costs: Causes, Implications, and Strategies* (April 1991), p. 78.

69. For the most thorough report of the Rand study, in which over four thousand families were randomly assigned to insurance with difference levels of cost sharing for three to five years and both costs and health outcomes were then evaluated, see Joseph P. Newhouse and the Insurance Experiment Group, *Free for All? Lessons from the RAND Health Insurance Experiment* (Harvard University Press, 1993).

70. The most balanced and thorough analysis of copayment issues that I have seen is Jeff Richardson, "The Effects of Consumer Co-payments in Medical Care," Background Paper 5 (Canberra: National Health Strategy, June 1991). Most American discussion relies on the Rand experiment. But there is plenty of evidence, much of which Richardson reviews. As Richardson points out, the Rand experiment, because it involved only a very small portion of any health insurance market, shows the savings from cost sharing *when providers as a group do not respond by adjusting their behaviors to maintain their incomes.* So the Rand results cannot be extrapolated to entire health care systems.

71. In the case of psychotherapy, this payment could even be seen as the patient's necessary commitment to the process. I'm not saying I believe any of this; only that it is part of the ideology of free-market medicine around the world.

72. For good examples of the argument that balance-billing personalizes the physician-patient relationship, see Greg Borzo, "Health Plans Use Market Muscle to Squeeze Down Physician Pay," *American Medical News*, December 13, 1993, p. 1.

73. Julie Johnsson, "House Supports Wider Use of RBRVS," *American Medical News*, December 20, 1993, p. 3. National conversion factors would provide higher physician incomes in lower-income areas, but that may be impractical unless the financing includes large transfers to those areas.

74. See Michael J. Graetz, "Universal Health Coverage without an Employer Mandate," *Domestic Affairs*, vol. 2 (Winter 1993/94), pp. 79–104.

75. See the series of articles in *Health Affairs*, vol. 13, no. 1 (Spring II 1994).

76. Japan may be an exception, but it does directly budget a large number

of the AMCs. It also is exceptional on many other dimensions that America is unlikely to imitate, such as the very low levels of surgery and intensive care.

77. William A. Glaser, *Health Insurance in Practice* (San Francisco: Jossey-Bass, 1991), p. 251.

Chapter Seven

1. In attributing these bills I am using the common references used in 1994; the bills themselves are discussed in the next chapter.

2. See Richard B. Saltman and Casten Von Otter, *Planned Markets and Public Competition: Strategic Reform in Northern European Health Systems* (Philadelphia: Open University Press, 1992).

3. The adoption of the prospective payment system via diagnosis-related groups for hospital bills in medicare in 1983 was aided by hospitals, which objected to the temporary measures imposed by the Tax Equity and Fiscal Responsibility Act of 1982; see Joseph White and Aaron Wildavsky, *The Deficit and the Public Interest: The Search for Responsible Budgeting in the 1980s* (University of California Press and the Russell Sage Foundation, 1989), pp. 256, 324.

4. These include the large businesses that are members of the National Leadership Coalition for Health Care Reform.

5. A good example of this discussion is Organization for Economic Cooperation and Development, "Health Care Systems in Transition: The Search for Efficiency," Social Policy Studies 7 (Paris, 1990).

6. If focusing on outputs instead of inputs actually aided cost control, that would be a rare event in the history of budgeting. See Joseph White, "Markets, Budgets, and Health Care Cost Control," *Health Affairs*, vol. 12, no. 3 (Fall 1993), pp. 44–57; Aaron Wildavsky, "A Budget for All Seasons? Why the Traditional Budget Lasts," *Public Administration Review*, vol. 38 (November/December 1978), pp. 501–09.

7. When hospitals are paid essentially on a day rate, moving a service such as surgery to the ambulatory sector would allow the provider to charge a price that is higher than the hospital average day rate. This is so because patients who needed that service previously were at the upper end of the charges that were used to calculate the hospital's average rate per day. Hospitals could then lower their day rates, but that, of course, rarely happens. For many references to the problem in the United States, see Peter Kongstvedt, *The Managed Health Care Handbook*, 2d ed. (Gaithersburg, Md.: Aspen Publishers, 1993).

8. On Britain see Henry J. Aaron and William B. Schwartz, *The Painful Prescription: Rationing Hospital Care* (Brookings, 1984); on the uninsured see Jack Hadley, Earl P. Steinberg, and Judith Feder, "Comparison of Uninsured and Privately Insured Hospital Patients: Condition on Admission, Resource Use, and Outcome," *Journal of the American Medical Association*, January 16, 1991, pp. 374–79. The Canadian example is from my interviews.

9. Australian policy analysts whom I interviewed believed that very high

sessional fees in New South Wales—arguably higher than the reimbursement for private care—did not reduce the incentive to do as little as possible during the sessions.

10. There are so many forms of the idea that it may seem unreasonable to declare any one "pure." Designers of the Clinton plan such as Richard Kronick, Paul Starr, and Walter Zelman have their own bona fides in this area. But in part because they were first and in part because they were best publicized, the "Jackson Hole group" (so named because they convened at the Jackson Hole, Wyoming, vacation retreat of longtime HMO promoter Paul Ellwood) were able to define themselves as the source of the real thing, and commentators tended to view them as authorities on the theory. See, for example, Connie Bruck, "Hillary the Pol," *New Yorker*, May 30, 1994, pp. 85–90.

11. See Paul M. Ellwood, Alain C. Enthoven, and Lynn Etheredge, "The Jackson Hole Initiatives for a Twenty-first Century American Health Care System," *Health Economics*, vol. 1, no. 3 (1992), pp. 149–68; Alain C. Enthoven, "The History and Principles of Managed Competition," *Health Affairs*, vol. 12, Supplement (1993), pp. 24–48; for a good summary from a nonsupporter, see Uwe E. Reinhardt, "Comment on the Jackson Hole Initiatives for a Twenty-first Century American Health Care System," *Health Economics*, vol. 2, no. 1 (1993), pp. 7–14; for a summary that expresses the beliefs of some remarkably uninformed supporters, see Jeremy D. Rosner, "A Progressive Plan for Affordable, Universal Health Care," in William J. Marshall and Martin Schram, eds., *Mandate for Change* (New York: Berkley Books, 1993); for a discussion that considers alternatives and is cowritten by a central member of the Clinton administration deliberations, see Alain Enthoven and Richard Kronick, "A Consumer Choice Health Plan for the 1990s," *New England Journal of Medicine* in two parts: January 5, 1989, pp. 29–37, and January 12, 1989, pp. 94–101; for a wide range of analysis see the Supplement to *Health Affairs*, vol. 12 (1993). When I refer to Jackson Hole in this book I refer to the original proposal, "Jackson Hole 1." In 1994 the group produced a watered-down version that violated much of their original analysis. At best it was a concession as a matter of political realism; at worst, it represented the real interests of the group's paymasters, large insurance companies.

12. Coverage must be standard so providers know what to expect and so insurers cannot skew their set of customers through the design of benefits. Plans cannot be allowed to turn down applicants because they would turn down anyone with greater than average risk.

13. From Enthoven, "History of Managed Competition," p. 41. See also Ellwood, Enthoven and Etheredge, "The Jackson Hole Initiatives," p. 160.

14. There are, of course, many other critiques of the model. Among the best are Thomas Rice, E. Richard Brown, and Roberta Wyn, "Holes in the Jackson Hole Approach to Health Care Reform," *Journal of the American Medical Association*, September 15, 1993, pp. 1357–62; three articles in the 1993 Supplement to *Health Affairs*: Stuart H. Altman and Alan B. Cohen, "The Need for a National Global Budget," *Health Affairs*, vol. 12, Supplement (1993), pp. 194–203; Henry J. Aaron and William B. Schwartz, "Managed Competition:

Little Cost Containment without Budget Limits," ibid., pp. 204–15; and Jonathan E. Fielding and Thomas Rice, "Can Managed Competition Solve Problems of Market Failure?" ibid., pp. 216–28; and Reinhardt, "Comment on the Jackson Hole Initiatives." The difficulties of managed competition in operation can be attacked whether one seeks to increase or limit insurance; for a critique from the latter perspective, see John C. Goodman and Gerald L. Musgrave, "A Primer on Managed Competition," Policy Report 183 (Dallas, Tex.: National Center for Policy Analysis, April 19, 1994).

15. Capping and thus reducing tax benefits is part of the model and would free some federal money to pay for new subsidies, but it is not sufficient.

16. See Richard Kronick and others, "The Marketplace in Health Care Reform—The Demographic Limitations of Managed Competition," *New England Journal of Medicine*, January 14, 1993, pp. 148–52. They assume that the best kind of competition is between plans that own their own hospitals—fully integrated systems such as Kaiser Permanente.

17. A tax benefit is worth the most to higher-income workers, and the employers who can best afford larger insurance expenses also pay higher salaries. Therefore, the open-ended subsidy disproportionately favors higher-income workers.

18. For examples of possible figures see Congressional Budget Office, *Reducing the Deficit: Spending and Revenue Options* (February 1993), p. 363. For reasons described in the following chapter, even the CBO figures are likely to be too high.

19. For discussion of this and even more complex issues in HMO pricing, see Stanley B. Jones, "Multiple Choice Health Insurance: The Lessons and Challenge to Private Insurers," Alain Enthoven's comment, and Jones's reply, all in *Inquiry*, vol. 27 (Summer 1990), pp. 161–66 and (Winter 1990), pp. 368–75. Also see U.S. General Accounting Office, "Managed Health Care: Effect on Employers' Costs Difficult to Measure," GAO/HRD-94-3 (October 1993), pp. 12–16.

20. Health care providers often have extra capacity, such as extra beds in hospitals, but by definition, those are not the most efficient, lowest-priced providers that the theory expects to expand.

21. As explained in chapters 4 and 5, these pools are created by statute rather than competition. The German 1992 legislation is designed to largely eliminate the differences by 1996.

22. As an example of perverse incentives: instead of relying on demographics, which predict costs poorly, one could rely on costs incurred in previous years, which predict costs much more accurately. But that strategy would give plans incentives to generate costs for their patients, because those costs would be rewarded by risk-adjustment payments. Good reviews of the problem include Joseph P. Newhouse, "Patients at Risk: Reform and Risk Adjustment," *Health Affairs*, vol. 13, no. 1 (Spring I 1994), pp. 132–46; Wynand P. M. M. Van de Ven and Rene C. J. A. Van Vliet, "How Can We Prevent Cream Skimming in a Competitive Health Insurance Market?" in P. Zweifel and H. E. Frech, eds., *Health Economics Worldwide* (Boston: Kluwer, 1992), pp. 23–46; James C.

Robinson and others, "A Method for Risk-Adjusting Employer Contributions to Competing Health Insurance Plans," *Inquiry*, vol. 28 (Summer 1991), pp. 107–16.

23. Wynand P. M. M. Van de Ven and Frederik T. Schut, "The Dutch Experience with Internal Markets," in Monique Jérôme-Forget, Joseph White, and Joshua M. Wiener, eds., *Health Care Reform through Internal Markets: Experience and Proposals* (Montreal and Washington: Institute for Research on Public Policy and Brookings, 1995), p. 111.

24. Vivian Hamilton, "Discussion of Major Issues in Internal Markets: Risk Selection," in ibid., pp. 158–61.

25. See the complaints of Florence Nightingale, as quoted and updated in Alan Maynard, "The Cost of Care and the Role of Health Delivery Systems," paper presented at a conference sponsored by the Royal Society of Medicine and the University of North Carolina at Chapel Hill, September 8–10, 1993, London, p. 2.

26. Kaiser Permanente, Northern California Region, and Andersen Consulting, *1993 Quality Report Card* and *1993 Quality Report Card Supplement* (Oakland, Calif., 1993), represent a major effort, with 102 measures. Of those, though, I would argue that only thirty-seven of the measurements represent outcomes related to care, and for eight of those there are no benchmarks. Good measurements include incidence of childhood diseases for which immunization is available; hospitalization for somewhat preventable attacks related to cerebrovascular, diabetic, or asthmatic conditions; stage of diagnosis and mortality rates after diagnosis for some cancers; birthweight and infant mortality; and number of necessary appendectomies. Many benchmarks based on current health statistics would make most plans look good, because the benchmarks include the uninsured.

27. Sociologist Daniel Yankelovich, referring among other things to the Pentagon's emphasis on body counts during the Vietnam War, called this "the McNamara fallacy": "The first step is to measure what an be easily be measured. The second is to disregard what can't be measured, or give it an arbitrary quantitative value. This is artificial and misleading. The third step is to presume that what can't be measured easily isn't very important. This is blindness. The fourth step is to say that what can't be easily measured really doesn't exist." Health policy analyses can make all these mistakes, but the first two are more common. See "Adam Smith" (George W. Goodman), *Paper Money* (New York: Dell, 1981), p. 43.

28. For a good review see Linda Oberman, "Grading the Report Cards," *American Medical News*, February 21, 1994, p. 3. See also Linda Oberman, "AMA Panel on Guidelines Sorts Good from Misguided," *American Medical News*, January 10, 1994, p. 1; On hospital data see Linda Oberman, "Data Driving Quality Advance," *American Medical News*, January 17, 1994, p. 2.

29. Quote from Dr. Francis Crosson, and data from a sidebar, in Oberman, "Grading the Report Cards," p. 22.

30. Ron Winslow, "Health-Care Report Cards Are Getting Low Grades from Some Focus Groups," *Wall Street Journal*, May 19, 1994, p. B1; for another

overview see Barry Meier, "Hurdles Await Efforts to Rate Doctors and Medical Centers," *New York Times*, March 31, 1994, p. A1.

31. E. Sam Overman and Anthony G. Cahill, "Market Government, Information, and Health Policy: A Study of Health Data Organizations in the States," paper delivered at the national meeting of the Association for Public Policy Analysis and Management, Denver, Colo., October 30, 1992, p. 1.

32. For another review of managed care, see Julie Kosterlitz, "All Together Now," *National Journal*, November 13, 1993, pp. 2704–08. For a summary by academics who are carefully neutral on the subject of managed competition, see Robert H. Miller and Harold S. Luft, "Managed Care: Past Evidence and Potential Trends," *Frontiers of Health Services Management*, vol. 9, no. 3 (1993), pp. 3–37. For a description of both the variety of plans and how they address many issues, see Peter R. Kongstvedt, ed., *The Managed Health Care Handbook*, especially Eric R. Wagner, "Types of Managed Care Organizations," pp. 12–27. See also "Understanding the Choices in Health Care Reform," Commentary by the Health Care Study Group, *Journal of Health Politics, Policy and Law*, vol. 19, no. 3 (Fall 1994), pp. 499–541.

33. Group Health Association of America, *Patterns in HMO Enrollment* (Washington, June 1993), p. 5. There is an immense literature on this form, which I would call "real" HMOs; one should begin with Harry S. Luft, *Health Maintenance Organizations: Dimensions of Performance* (Wiley, 1981); see also Lawrence D. Brown, *Politics and Health Care Organizations: HMOs as Federal Policy* (Brookings, 1983); for a close look at the prototype, see John G. Smillie, *Can Physicians Manage the Quality and Costs of Health Care? The Story of the Permanente Medical Group* (McGraw-Hill, 1991).

34. See Vernon S. Staines, "Impact of Managed Care on National Health Spending," *Health Affairs*, vol. 12, Supplement (1993), pp. 248–57, and John F. Sheils, Lawrence S. Lewin, and Randall A. Haught, "Potential Public Expenditures under Managed Competition," ibid., pp. 229–42.

35. This is being modified by the addition of point-of-service options, in which a patient may choose to see a physician not on the panel and pay substantial cost sharing. But such arrangements are not yet common aspects of the group- and staff-model HMOs; they are far more common in loosely structured networks. Providing the point-of-service option should make the internal budgeting of the group- and staff-model HMOs very complicated. But given customers' desire for choice, even Kaiser is trying to figure out how to do it.

36. Wagner, "Types of Managed Care Organizations," pp. 18, 19.

37. In a formal sense, the Institute of Medicine reports, few or no utilization review systems would allow a nurse to disallow a treatment; only doctors can do so. Practicing physicians do not see it that way. First, in some systems, review doctors do not speak to the patient's physician but merely consult with the review nurse. Second, given the volume of review, busy physicians are not likely to spend a whole lot of time arguing each case to the point that it is referred to a review physician. Instead, the doctor's office and the review nurse may negotiate a compromise. So from physicians' perspective nurses,

in practice, make them change their treatments. See Bradford H. Gray and Marilyn J. Field, eds., *Controlling Costs and Changing Patient Care? The Role of Utilization Management* (Washington: National Academy Press, 1989), pp. 106–07.

38. For a good example, see David Finkel, "Doctor of the Future," *Washington Post Magazine*, November 21, 1993, p. 10.

39. This is a great simplification. In many systems the contracting physicians form an intermediary unit, an "independent practice association" (IPA), which acts as a conduit for payment from the insurer to its members and bears the risk; from the individual doctor's perspective in a large IPA, however, the difference is not crucial.

40. My thanks to Harold Luft for explaining to me the advantages of large groups within the network.

41. Congressional Budget Office,"Effects of Managed Care: An Update," CBO Memorandum (March 1994), p. 8. The report says health care costs would be reduced by 4.4 percent, of which "about 83 percent of the savings . . . remained after allowing for the offsetting increase in administrative costs."

42. CBO does not refer to "risk-bearing gatekeepers," but the report describes as most efficient those plans that "select cost-conscious providers, maintain an effective network for information and control, place providers at financial risk, and generate a substantial proportion of each provider's patient load." Ibid., p. 21.

43. See Sheils, Lewin, and Haught, "Potential Public Expenditures"; Staines, "Potential Impact of Managed Care on National Health Spending"; and Stephen H. Long and Jack Rodgers, "Perspective: Managed Competition Estimates For Policy Making," *Health Affairs*, vol. 12, Supplement (1993), pp. 229–57.

44. Julie Johnsson, "Integrated Networks Are Expensive—Can Doctors Find the Capital to Compete?" *American Medical News*, June 13, 1994, p. 3. These problems are well understood in the literature. Thus, "It is expensive for staff-model HMOs to expand their services into new areas because of the need to construct new ambulatory care facilities. . . . The limited number of office locations for the participating medical groups may also restrict the geographic accessibility of physicians for the HMO's members. The lack of accessibility can make it difficult for the HMO to market its coverage to a wide geographic area." Wagner, "Types of Managed Care Organizations," pp. 18, 19.

45. This is a prospective version of the contradiction in the British reforms. In Britain, as discussed below, capital is rationed because the government wants to control total costs. In the United States capital would be hard to raise because investors would know that the government wanted to restrain total sales.

46. The Group Health Association of America reports 1990 data for four categories: group models, staff models, network models (which contract with group practices), and independent practice associations (IPAs, which contract with individual physicians). It reports that staff models had the highest op-

erating margins, groups and networks had the next highest, and IPAs had the lowest for every year from 1987 to 1990. Yet IPAs, because they had the lowest need for investments, had the highest rates of return. Group Health Association of America, *HMO Industry Profile, 1992 Edition*, pp. 130, 133, tables 67, 71.

47. See Luft, *Health Maintenance Organizations*, and Smillie, *Can Physicians Manage the Costs and Quality of Health Care?*

48. I would add that I have asked a great many advocates of managed care, including some of the nation's most distinguished experts, about its future in our health care system, and none believe a world of "competing Kaisers" can be created anytime soon.

49. See Alain C. Enthoven, "What Can Europeans Learn from Americans?" pp. 57–71 (quote p. 57), and the response by Robert G. Evans and Morris L. Barer, pp. 80–85 (quotes p. 84), both in OECD, *Health Care Systems in Transition*. I feel confident extending the Evans and Barer comments to Canada, based on both their written work and personal conversations.

50. Author's calculations from Department of Health and Office of Population Censuses and Surveys, *Departmental Report: The Government's Expenditure Plans 1993–94 to 1995–96* (London: Her Majesty's Stationery Office, February 1992), pp. 93–94.

51. For a review of some of the theoretical issues and practical background to the reforms, see Saltman and Von Otter, *Planned Markets and Public Competition*, pp. 22–37. For another account with a certain authority, see Margaret Thatcher, *The Downing Street Years* (Harper Collins, 1993), pp. 606–18. The most thorough assessment as of spring 1994 was Ray Robinson and Julian Le Grand, eds., *Evaluating the NHS Reforms* (New Brunswick, N.J.: Transaction Books and The Kings Fund Institute, 1994). My research assistant Anthony J. Sheehan and I benefited from interviews or conversations with ten participants in or close observers of the reform, some of whom were RHA and DHA executives. Our special thanks to Roger Jennings and Roy Forey of the British Embassy in Washington for their help in these arrangements. They are blameless for the conclusions!

52. Ray Robinson, "Introduction," in Robinson and Le Grand, *Evaluating the NHS Reforms*, p. 1. One participant in the reforms told me evaluation was not necessary because the reforms were not an experiment! But for precedents see John Butler, "Origins and Early Development," in ibid., pp. 14–16.

53. Department of Health, *Departmental Report*, p. 10; these figures are for England only, and 1.4 percent was from "other" receipts, such as land sales. When I refer to RHAs in the text, I include the Scottish, Welsh, and Ulster administrations.

54. There are slightly fewer than two DHAs per FHSA nationwide, but there is no standard for overlap. In March 1994 the government announced that it intended to submit legislation that would merge DHAs and FHSAs.

55. A detailed list of differences between DMUs and trusts is in *NHS Management Executive*, "NHS Trusts: A Working Guide" (London: Her Majesty's Stationery Office, 1991), Annex A.

56. Howard Glennerster and others, "GP Fundholding: Wild Card or Winning Hand?" in Robinson and Le Grand, *Evaluating the NHS Reforms*, pp. 83, 85. See also Peter Bryden, "The Future of Primary Care," in Ray Loveridge and Ken Starkey, eds., *Continuity and Crisis in the NHS* (Philadelphia: Open University Press, 1992), pp. 65–72.

57. Glennerster and others, "GP Fundholding," p. 76; letter from Joan Firth, deputy director of NHS Finance, to Roger Jennings, first secretary for science and technology, British Embassy, Washington, May 27, 1993, answering questions Mr. Jennings kindly posed on my behalf.

58. Bryden, "Future of Primary Care," pp. 68–69; Kevin Grumbach and John Fry, "Managing Primary Care in the United States and in the United Kingdom," *New England Journal of Medicine*, April 1, 1993, pp. 940–45. The focus on inputs as a guarantee of quality here parallels the pattern for American health plans' "report cards."

59. The 95 percent figure was predicted in Will Bartlett and Julian Le Grand, "The Performance of Trusts," in Robinson and Le Grand, *Evaluating the NHS Reforms*, pp. 56–57, and confirmed by Clive Smee, chief economic adviser to the NHS, personal communication, April 24, 1994. The 36 percent figure comes from Alan Maynard, personal communication, May 17, 1994.

60. Most managers probably also believed they would perform better with less oversight. Taking that position also would increase job security: one observer reported that DMU managers, on short-term contracts, were encouraged to apply for trust status by the chairs of the DHA, who are political appointees.

61. Separate practices may merge to hold a fund together. Although doing so might produce coordination problems, because the fund involves a very small number of physicians, coordination is likely easier than in an American managed care network. There has been a steady redefining downward of the minimum practice size for fundholders; it began at 9,000, and in 1994 the British government proposed to lower the figure to 5,000 and to introduce a modified form of fundholding for practices with 3,000 patients and pilot programs in which fundholders would purchase all services. National Health Service, "Developing NHS Purchasing and GP Fundholding" (Heywood, Lancashire: Health Publications Unit, n.d.).

62. Glennerster and others, "GP Fundholding," pp. 75–76, 86; Alan Maynard, "Can Competition Produce Efficiency in Health Care? Lessons from the Reform of the U.K. National Health Service," paper prepared for the jubilee conference of the Dutch/Flemish Association of Health Economics held at Erasmus University, Rotterdam, November 26, 1993, p. 30; Maynard, "Competition in the UK National Health Service: Mission Impossible?" *Health Policy*, vol. 23 (1993), pp. 193–204; Clive H. Smee, "Self Governing Trusts and Budget Holding GPs: The First 2½ Years," draft for conference, "Implementing Planned Markets in Health Systems," Stockholm, September 27–28, 1993.

63. See Maynard, "Can Competition Produce Efficiency?" p. 12; Margaret Whitehead, "Is It Fair? Evaluating the Equity Implications of the NHS Reforms," in Robinson and Le Grand, *Evaluating the NHS Reforms*, pp. 221–22.

Other sources, such as Glennerster and others, "GP Fundholding," pp. 86–91, disagree; the best guess may be that fundholders had more generous budgets in the first year of the reforms, but that changed.

64. Julian Le Grand, "Evaluating the NHS Reforms," in Robinson and Le Grand, *Evaluating the NHS Reforms*, p. 259.

65. National Health Service, *National Health Service and Community Care Act 1990* (London: Her Majesty's Stationery Office, 1990), part I, section 4 (and part II, section 30, for Scotland).

66. Butler, "Origins and Early Development," pp. 21–22.

67. John Appleby and others, "Monitoring Managed Competition," in Robinson and Le Grand, *Evaluating the NHS Reforms*, p. 30. Also see Butler, "Origins and Early Development," pp. 22–23.

68. Maynard, "Can Competition Produce Efficiency?" p. 8.

69. Ibid., pp. 15–16; James Buchan and Ian Seccombe, "The Changing Role of the NHS Personnel Function," in Robinson and Le Grand, *Evaluating the NHS Reforms*, pp. 191–95. Greater discretion over matters such as hotel services preceded the 1990 reforms, with various contracting out initiatives.

70. The passage is from the letter of Joan Firth to Roger Jennings, May 27, 1993, p. 3. Also see Maynard, "Can Competition Produce Efficiency?" pp. 16–17.

71. Bartlett and Le Grand, "The Performance of Trusts," p. 56.

72. Alasdair Liddell and Greg Parston, "Frozen Assets," *Health Service Journal*, May 28, 1992, pp. 18–20.

73. Maynard, "Can Competition Produce Efficiency?" p. 18; also, letter from Joan Firth to Roger Jennings.

74. Liza Donaldson, "The Primary Aim Is to Give Better Care," *Independent*, May 20, 1993, p. 22; Patrick Butler, "Wessex: Preparing for an Earthquake," *Health Service Journal*, May 28, 1992, pp. 29–30; Jane Huntingdon, "At Least We're Talking," *Health Service Journal*, May 28, 1992, p. 17; "In Brief," "Row over Budget Control Jeopardizes Joint Purchasers' Model Marriage," and "Region Rejects HA's White Paper Cash Call," all in *Health Service Journal*, July 16, 1992, pp. 4, 5, 6, 18; and "One Step Beyond" and "The Five Commandments," both in *Health Service Journal*, May 6, 1993, pp. 15, 23–25.

75. My thanks to Professor Robert G. Evans for this point.

76. Department of Health, *Departmental Report*, p. 33.

77. Ibid., pp. 33, 93–94.

78. Le Grand, "Evaluating the NHS Reforms," p. 244.

79. Julian Dobson, "Scalpel-Happy in Waiting List Land," *Health Service Journal*, May 14, 1992, p. 10. The Hawthorne effect refers to a series of famous experiments on increasing worker productivity at Western Electric's plant in Hawthorne, Illinois.

80. Pat Anderson, "Managers Seek More Cash to Cut Trolley Waiting Times," *Health Service Journal*, July 16, 1992, p. 8; David Glasman, "Plans to Guarantee Total Waiting Times Worry Doctors," *Health Service Journal*, May 6, 1993, p. 4.

81. Provisional figures for 1991–93 from Smee, "Self Governing Trusts"; in

personal communication in April 1994 he said the figures were accurate. See also Dee Jones, Carolyn Lester, and Robert West, "Monitoring Changes in Health Services for Older People," in Robinson and Le Grand, *Evaluating the NHS Reforms*, pp. 142, 150.

82. See Smee, "Self Governing Trusts," tables 2 and 3; Bartlett and Le Grand, "Performance of Trusts," pp. 59–63.

83. *Health Service Journal*, August 6, 1992, p. 16.

84. Patients' definitions of acceptable proximity may be different from analysts'. In the example cited, competition was based on market share in an entire DHA. Le Grand, "Evaluating the NHS Reforms," pp. 253–55; Appleby and others, "Monitoring Managed Competition," pp. 43–46; see also the other chapters cited by Le Grand.

85. Alasdair Liddell, "Planning for Area Health Management: National Health Strategy in the United Kingdom," speech at the national conference of the Consumers' Health Forum, Canberra, Australia, December 10, 1992, p. 15.

86. Glennerster and others, "GP Fundholding," pp. 91–96.

87. Le Grand, "Evaluating the NHS Reforms," p. 248.

88. This argument has been made to me most cogently, though not with the same political spin, by Harold Luft. He is not responsible for my implications or objections—or for the exaggerated claims of many supporters of managed competition.

89. Individual plans would have little incentive to subsidize the rest of a hospital by contracting for one service if they could not rely on the others to do so as well.

90. For a superb discussion, see Lynn Etheredge and Stanley Jones, "Managing a Pluralist Health System," *Health Affairs*, vol. 10, no. 4 (Winter 1991), pp. 93–105.

91. The extent to which this agenda was taken for granted by policymakers was illustrated during the seventh game of the 1994 NBA playoff series between the New York Knicks and Indianapolis Pacers. At halftime Senator Bill Bradley (D-N.J.) was interviewed (in his capacity as a famous ex-Knick). At the end of the session, Bob Costas jokingly asked if Pacer guard Byron Scott's "hip-pointer" injury would be covered under the Clinton health care reform proposal. The senator replied that he did not know—was Scott currently in an HMO? Scott would have been covered under the Clinton plan even if he weren't in an HMO—but the public cost control arguments of the administration emphasized delivery efficiencies so thoroughly that the senator's confusion was typical.

Chapter Eight

1. For the text of Cooper-Grandy I am using *Managed Competition Act of 1993*, H.R. 3222, 103 Cong. 1 sess. (1993); for Chafee, *Health Equity and Access Reform Today Act of 1993*, S. 1770, 103 Cong. 1 sess. (1993). Good summaries

also were prepared by the staff of the Physician Payment Review Commission. The official summary of the Chafee bill is Senate Republican Health Care Task Force, "Health Equity and Access Reform Today," press release on September 15, 1993. Of interest also is Robert B. Friedland, Alison Evans, and Sara Okrend, "Senator Chafee's Proposal for Health Care Reform: An Overview of the Administrative Structure," Report by the National Academy of Social Insurance (Washington, 1994). CBO did not publish a report on Chafee; its report on Cooper-Grandy was: Congressional Budget Office, "An Analysis of the Managed Competition Act," A CBO Study (Washington, D.C., 1994). A press packet including a summary of Cooper-Grandy was released on October 6, 1993, by the sponsors. In addition, comparisons of these and other bills were prepared by many sources, including the Kaiser Foundation and the Congressional Research Service.

2. The background and origins of the relevant congressional procedures are in Joseph White and Aaron Wildavsky, *The Deficit and the Public Interest: The Search for Responsible Budgeting in the 1980s* (University of California Press, 1991).

3. For a quick summary see William Schneider, "Selling Americans an Insurance Policy," *National Journal*, February 19, 1994, p. 450.

4. On the norms of budgeting see Joseph White, "The Two-Faced Profession," *Public Budgeting and Finance*, vol. 10, no. 3 (Fall 1990), pp. 92–102.

5. See the analyses in *Health Affairs*, vol. 12, Special Issue (Spring 1993). "Reasonable," here, is a matter of politics and values. In 1993 it meant something like 1998, or early in Clinton's second term. Anything that projected a later date would not help Clinton's reelection campaign and might be postponed indefinitely by Clinton's successor.

6. There is a huge difference, also, between threatening to take existing customers away, and expecting plans to expand in order to win new customers. CalPERS also saved by requiring higher copayments in some HMOs. See General Accounting Office, "Health Insurance: California Public Employees' Alliance Has Reduced Recent Premium Growth," GAO/HRD-94-40 (November 1993), pp. 8–9; Marilyn Chase, "Calpers Tells 18 Health-Care Providers It Expects a 5% Rollback in Premiums," *Wall Street Journal*, October 14, 1993, p. B5; David Broder, "California Agency Offers a Model for Reining in Health Costs," *Washington Post*, May 18, 1994, p. F1.

7. For another account of CBO's situation, see Viveca Novak, "By the Numbers," *National Journal*, February 12, 1994, pp. 348–52. The following CBO reports are worth consulting by anyone interested in managed competition or the considerations involved in making cost estimates: "Managed Competition and Its Potential to Reduce Health Spending" (May 1993); "Estimates of Health Care Proposals from the 102nd Congress," CBO Papers (July 1993); "Behavioral Assumptions for Estimating the Effects of Health Care Proposals," CBO Memorandum (November 1993).

8. One can argue at length about how the economy performed in the 1980s, but there is no doubt that the economic events that David Stockman hoped would prevent massive deficits did not come true; see David A. Stockman, *The

Triumph of Politics (Harper and Row, 1986), and White and Wildavsky, *Deficit and the Public Interest*.

9. Thus Chafee, unlike Cooper-Grandy, included an option for "medical savings accounts," a pet idea of the Cato Institute and the core mechanism in the proposal of Senators Phil Gramm (R-Tex.) and John McCain (R-Az.), the *Comprehensive Family Health Access and Savings Act*, S. 1807, 103 Cong. 2 sess. (1993). For that idea and why it will not work, see Alissa J. Rubin, "Two Ideological Poles Frame Debate over Reform," *Congressional Quarterly Weekly Report*, January 8, 1994, p. 28; Harris Meyer, "GOP Reformers Push Medical IRA Plans," *American Medical News*, January 3, 1994, p. 1; Minnesota Department of Health, Health Care Delivery Systems Division, "Medical Savings Accounts: A Feasibility Study for the Minnesota Legislature" (February 1994); and Joseph White, "Medical Savings Accounts and Health Care Reform," January 1995.

10. McDermott-Wellstone, sponsored by Representative Jim McDermott (D-Wash.) and Senator Paul Wellstone (D-Minn.), was the "single-payer" plan, a mix between the Canadian approach and medicare for everyone. The House bill was *American Health Security Act*, H.R. 1200, 103 Cong. 1 sess. (1993), and the Senate bill was *American Health Security Act*, S. 491, 103 Cong. 1 sess. (1993).

11. In Cooper-Grandy states could agree to form interstate HPPCs in order to consolidate a metropolitan statistical area, in accordance with rules established by the HCSC. *Managed Competition Act of 1993*, H.R. 3222, section 1101, pp. 33–40. Chafee's "Health Care Coverage Areas" are in *Health Equity and Access Reform Today Act of 1993*, S. 1770, section 1403, pp. 116–17.

12. *Managed Competition Act of 1993*, H.R. 3222, pp. 63–64.

13. Tax-deductibility is in *Health Equity and Access Reform Today Act of 1993*, S. 1770, section 2002, pp. 147–51.

Qualified general access plans are described in ibid., sections 1101–22. Qualified large employer plans are defined, somewhat, in sections 1201–02; but while there is a process to certify the former (section 1402), there is only a process to decertify the latter (section 1207); that this is not accidental seems confirmed by the language of section 1402. *Health Equity and Access Reform Today Act of 1993*, S. 1770, sections 1101–22, 1201–02, 1207, 1402, pp. 27–57, 67–70, 72–76, 116.

14. *Managed Competition Act of 1993*, H.R. 3222, p. 168. Section 1102, p. 40, concerns contracts with AHPs; section 1103, p. 46, covers contracts with small employers; relevant definitions are in section 1701, p. 160.

15. This is part of the requirement to "offer" insurance, see *Health Equity and Access Reform Act of 1993*, S. 1770, sections 1405, 1004, pp. 118, 24–26; but for an employee residing in another HCCA, the employer would still have to allow payroll deductions but would only have to provide "information regarding how to obtain information on qualified health plans offered to residents of that HCCA" (p. 24).

16. An employer could offer (while still making no contribution to) only one standard package plan but would also have to offer one "catastrophic"

plan, covering only expenses above a large (say, $3,000) deductible. The Chafee bill included the odd provision that employees "may" vote on which plan the employer "offers" according to rules to be prescribed by the secretary of labor. Ibid., section 1203, p. 71. Imagine 2,000 employees organizing to vote on which plan their employer should let them pay for.

17. Ibid., sections 1141 and 1404, pp. 57–60, 117.

18. Ibid., section 1405, p. 118, says states must give information to groups and employers and to eligible individuals *upon request*. Section 1143, p. 63, says groups must provide information provided to them; if this does not mean provide all the information they get from the state, then it could allow providing almost none of it, so be meaningless. Section 1142, pp. 60–63, says groups must contract with plans that wish to contract with them, but plans can be offered if they are not parties to such an agreement.

19. See the following articles in *The Wall Street Journal*: John H. Emshwiller, "Firms See More Fraud Risk in MEWA Health Coverage," December 9, 1993, p. B2; Robert Tomsho, "Health Benefit Scams Are Alleged to Take a New Form," January 10, 1994; Albert R. Karr, "U.S. Moves on Health-Insurance Firms It Says Often Renege on Worker Claims," April 1, 1994, p. B2; for a somewhat more favorable but still mixed (and mistitled) report, Eugene Carlson, "Mixed Reviews For Health Plan Like Clinton's," October 26, 1993, p. B1.

20. For a report on state experience see Harris Meyer, "Voluntary State Models Net Small Coverage Gains," *American Medical News*, March 21, 1994, p. 1. In Florida 23,000 out of a possible 2.7 million had been covered; in California for a new program the Legislative Research Office estimated 100,000 out of 4 million will be covered (40,000 were covered at the time of the report).

21. *Managed Competition Act of 1993*, H.R. 3222, section 2009, p. 195.

22. The health care standards commission would have to figure out how this rule could be applied to self-insured ("closed") plans. The relevant tax provisions are in ibid., sections 1001–03, pp. 15–22. The tax itself is a deductible business expense. The bill did intend to delay implementation for employers with a union contract for two years or the length of the contract, whichever was shorter (see p. 21). CBO reports that it would be in employees' interest, on average, for employers to buy the insurance rather than pay the wages: CBO, "An Analysis of the Managed Competition Act," pp. 10–12.

23. *Health Equity and Access Reform Today Act of 1993*, S. 1770, section 2001, pp. 138–40.

24. Henry J. Aaron, testimony to the Committee on Education and Labor, U.S. House of Representatives, March 3, 1994, p. 7.

25. Richard Kronick, "A Helping Hand for the Invisible Hand," response to Alain C. Enthoven and Sara J. Singer, "A Single-Payer System in Jackson Hole Clothing," *Health Affairs*, vol. 13, no. 1 (Spring I 1994), p. 99.

26. Robert Pear, "Taxing Health Benefits Gets Poor Reception at Hearing," *New York Times*, April 27, 1994, p. A15.

27. *Managed Competition Act of 1993*, H.R. 3222, section 1204, pp. 69–72. Chafee also had some regulations of insurance marketing, such as a ban on

financial incentives to brokers to avoid selling to riskier groups. *Health Equity and Access Reform Today Act of 1993*, S. 1770, sections 1111, 1112, 1162, pp. 30–39, 65.

28. *Managed Competition Act of 1993*, H.R. 3222, sections 1205, 1306, and 1102(d), pp. 72, 82–84, 126–27. Thus an HPPC could require that a plan in one service area expand into an adjacent, underserved area (section 1402, p. 140).

29. The restrictions mentioned in the previous paragraph are "additional requirements of open AHPs," while the definition of a closed AHP is simply one that by "structure or law" is limited to "one or more" large employers. Ibid., sections 1208, 1701, pp. 81, 165.

30. The reader should note that there are obvious errors in the draft of the version of the bill from which I worked, which leads to some doubt about what the authors *said*, never mind *meant*. When I consulted with an aide involved with the negotiation and drafting of the Chafee bill, he commented that he had no idea why these provisions were in the bill. On the other hand, another aide remarked that the limit of variation of basic rates across age bands, described in the previous paragraph, was considered a mistake, though perhaps one that should be preserved, by some of the drafters.

31. *Health Equity and Access Reform Today Act of 1993*, S. 1770, pp. 52, 118.

32. Ibid., section 6001, pp. 477–82.

33. Ibid., section 6021, pp. 490–544. Persons who think only the Clinton plan was complicated should note that the Chafee bill required fifty-three pages to create the framework to implement its medicaid managed care.

34. *Managed Competition Act of 1993*, H.R. 3222, section 2101, pp. 196–99.

35. For purposes of budget-process scorekeeping the formula does not have to be accurate; it just has to be the same one CBO would use to estimate state contributions for its estimate of costs under current law.

36. CBO, "Analysis of the Managed Competition Act," p. xiv. The report reviews the administrative and market-behavior difficulties in the plan on pp. 40–45.

37. Henry J. Aaron, "Jim Cooper's Pointless Plan," *New York Times*, February 13, 1994, section 4, p. 15. He used the example of a premium of $5,500, which is realistic in much of the country and would create even higher marginal penalties for each extra dollar of earnings.

38. *Health Equity and Access Reform Today Act of 1993*, S. 1770, section 1003, pp. 9–24, esp. p. 11.

39. Cooper-Grandy gave this job to the health care standards commission. In an interview, one of the bill's authors claimed that states would do the job. But the bill does not require them to, it is hard to see why they would accept the responsibility without a really large bribe, and allowing states to determine eligibility for a program in which the federal government provides all the money is not prudent. Chafee gave responsibility to the secretary of health and human services.

40. Cooper-Grandy automatically included aid to families with dependent children (AFDC), supplemental security income (SSI), foster care, and adop-

tion program beneficiaries, all referenced in *Managed Competition Act of 1993*, H.R. 3222, section 2008, p. 190.

41. *Health Equity and Access Reform Today Act of 1993*, S. 1770, section 1003, pp. 10, 14–16. To give this proposal its due, if savings were realized more quickly, subsidies could be increased more quickly.

42. In other words, if the tax code collects 30 percent of income on average, and health care gets 30 percent of the collections, health costs are 9 percent of income.

43. A good example from other fields would be the belief that making public transit accessible to the handicapped would not require making hard choices because we would invent a new kind of bus; see Robert A. Katzmann, *Institutional Disability: The Saga of Transportation Policy for the Disabled* (Brookings, 1986). Consider also the notions that "smart bombs" will only hit combatants, and that automakers could meed mandated fuel efficiency standards if they only tried hard enough.

44. Physician supply provisions are in *Managed Competition Act of 1993*, H.R. 3222, Title III, pp. 213–26; see esp. pp. 218–21; and *Health Equity and Access Reform Today Act of 1993*, S. 1770, sections 5101–02, pp. 450–64.

45. For Cooper-Grandy's malpractice limits see *Managed Competition Act of 1993*, H.R. 3222, Title V. The Chafee quote is from *Health Equity and Access Reform Today Act of 1993*, S.1770, section 4023, p. 297.

46. For the Cooper-Grandy provisions see *Managed Competition Act of 1993*, H.R. 3222, sections 2201–08, pp. 199–208. For the Chafee provisions see *Health Equity and Access Reform Today Act of 1993*, S. 1770, sections 5102, 6131–39, pp. 462–64, 560–74; also summarized in Senate Republican Task Force, "Health Equity and Access Reform Today," p. 20.

47. In Cooper-Grandy the proposed benefits would take effect unless both the House and Senate vetoed the proposal within a short time period; in Chafee both chambers had to approve the benefits. See *Managed Competition Act of 1993*, H.R. 3222, section 1302, pp. 104–19, and *Health Equity and Access Reform Today Act of 1993*, S. 1770, sections 1311–15, pp. 98–114.

48. *American Health Security Act*, S. 491, section 303, pp. 37–42.

Chapter Nine

1. Bill Clinton, "The Clinton Health Care Plan," *New England Journal of Medicine*, September 10, 1992, pp. 804–07; all quotes from p. 805.

2. Alain C. Enthoven, "Commentary: Measuring the Candidates on Health Care," in ibid., pp. 807–09, quote p. 809.

3. Quotes are from the transcript of "Democratic Presidential Candidate Bill Clinton Address on Health Care," Merck Pharmaceuticals, Rahway, N.J., September 24, 1992, pp. 11, 10.

4. As much as four hundred pages of the Clinton Health Security Act (HSA)—most of Title III and all of Titles V, VII, and X—is taken up by matters that could be plugged into many other structures with minor modifications.

5. The following account is based, first, on the text of the Health Security Act, as introduced by Senator George Mitchell (D-Me.) and others in the Senate on November 22, 1993, *Health Security Act*, S. 1757, 103 Cong. 1 sess. (1993). Readers might also consult the 316-page summary distributed in early November. The earliest summary was the September 7 "working group draft," but significant changes were made between that draft and the bill as introduced. I have also consulted the Physician Payment Review Commission's staff analysis of the HSA and summaries comparing all bills from the Kaiser Commission on the Future of Medicaid, "Health Reform Legislation: A Comparison of Major Proposals" (Menlo Park, Calif., January 1994) and from Melvina Ford and others, "Summary Comparison of Major Health Care Reform Bills," CRS Report for Congress 94-71 EPW (Congressional Research Service, January 6, 1994). The best published source without doubt is Congressional Budget Office, "An Analysis of the Administration's Health Proposal" (February 1994).

6. Thus Ira Magaziner told a Republican congressional aide of my acquaintance that all the bill's savings were from competition, not the cap, and Hillary Rodham Clinton managed to give a speech at Brookings also without claiming any reliance on the caps. When true believers in managed competition attacked the administration for its caps they were being equally inconsistent, since if competition would work the caps could do no harm.

7. The basic provisions were in *Health Security Act*, S. 1757, section 1322, pp. 132–38.

8. Alain C. Enthoven and Sara J. Singer, "A Single-Payer System in Jackson Hole Clothing," *Health Affairs*, vol. 13, no. 1 (Spring I 1994), pp. 81–95.

9. For a review of the reasons, see Joe White, "Paying the Right Price: What the United States Can Learn from Health Care Abroad," *Brookings Review*, vol. 12 (Spring 1994), pp. 6–11. For an example of an analysis by an administration official, see Paul B. Ginsburg and Kenneth E. Thorpe, "Can All-Payer Rate Setting and the Competitive Strategy Coexist?" *Health Affairs*, vol. 11, no. 2 (Summer 1992), pp. 73–86.

10. Walter A. Zelman, "The Rationale behind the Clinton Health Care Reform Plan," pp. 9–29, and Richard Kronick, "Perspective: A Helping Hand for the Invisible Hand," pp. 96–101, both in *Health Affairs*, vol. 13, no. 1 (Spring I 1994).

11. *Health Security Act*, S. 1757, sections 1311–13, pp. 121–31, defines corporate alliances, how they could be set up, and how they could be terminated. Section 1202 established the geographic requirements.

12. The HSA would tax employer-provided insurance for supplemental benefits beginning in 2004. A comprehensible summary of tax changes is provided in CBO, "Analysis of the Administration's Health Proposal," pp. 12–13.

13. Although employers would not have contributed exactly 80 percent exactly for most employees, their total contribution would have paid 80 percent of the employees' total costs.

14. Richard Kronick argued that at a marginal effective rate of 28 percent,

many persons would choose to keep seventy-two-cent dollars rather than buy insurance that cost more than the employer's required contribution: Kronick, "A Helping Hand," p. 99. But it is very unlikely that any plan would have cost less than 80 percent of the average. Neither the Chafee nor Cooper-Grandy plan would have yielded a tax deductibility cap at the lowest available premium, so their caps for the same population of plans would have been above the 80 percent level. If we wish to compare the incentives for economy in the Clinton plan with those in Cooper-Grandy or Chafee, therefore, it is more plausible to compare the Clinton plan's incentives with those of a tax cap at 90 percent of the average. In this comparison, an employee who chose a plan that cost 90 percent of the average could receive seventy-two-cent dollars for the difference between that plan and the minimum plan if he chose the latter in the Clinton scheme, but would have no incentive to choose a cheaper plan within the other schemes.

15. *Health Security Act*, S. 1757, sections 1201–24, pp. 97–118.

16. Ibid., sections 1221–24, pp. 109–18.

17. In relying on a commission with staggered political appointments and a chairman appointed by the president, the governing structure of the Clinton national health board was similar to those of the Cooper-Grandy health care standards commission and the McDermott-Wellstone American health security standards board.

The national health board, with the assistance of various advisory commissions, would set standards for grievance procedures, create and oversee a variety of quality management and improvement programs, develop licensing standards for institutions, set rules for information systems and privacy, and so on. These measures are not central because, however useful they may be, they either take over tasks that were already being done elsewhere (licensing), or involve functions whose effects would be very hard to predict (disseminating information), or involve activities that are likely to have very little result for a long time (developing treatment protocols). They were not controversial because they would affect hardly anyone immediately; thus these measures were in one way or another part of most bills' incremental menus.

18. The budget-setting process is in *Health Security Act*, S. 1757, sections 6001–03, pp. 984–1000.

19. Ibid., sections 1541–45, pp. 279–86.

20. The basic powers are in ibid., sections 1503, 1505, pp. 259–62, 263–64. The process of approving state plans, punishing states, or replacing state with federal operation are at sections 1511–14, 1522–23, pp. 264–74, 275–78.

21. Ibid., sections 1384, 6131, 6021, 6022, pp. 203–05, 1084–86, 1020–21, 1021–24.

22. Ibid., sections 1001, 1006, 1011, pp. 14–15, 18–20, 21–25. The board would define answers for questions such as how to categorize orphans and families with divorced parents.

23. Ibid., sections 1012, 1013, pp. 25–30, 30–32.

24. Ibid., section 1116, p. 53; the key question was, is abortion a service for pregnant women?

25. Ibid., sections 1117–19, pp. 63–65.

26. The summary of benefits is in ibid., section 1101, pp. 32–34; details on clinical preventive care are in section 1114, pp. 38–46.

27. Ibid., section 1115, pp. 46–63, quote p. 58.

28. Ibid., sections 1125, 1126, 1141, pp. 71, 71–73, 90–92.

29. Exceptions included 50 percent copayments for nonresidential mental health services and no copayments for the list of preventive care services. The basic deductible was $200 for an individual and $400 for a family; there were separate deductibles for mental health, pharmaceutical, and dental benefits. The benefit options are defined in ibid., sections 1001–1162, pp. 32–95.

30. By the same token, a person in a plan with low cost sharing who chose to go out-of-network for services would have paid the price of the plan with high cost sharing. The main differences were in deductibles.

31. CBO, "Analysis of the Administration's Health Proposal," p. 2.

32. Health Security Act, S. 1757, section 1371, pp. 183–86.

33. Ibid., sections 4003, 6115, pp. 684–85, 1058.

34. Ibid., section 4001, pp. 674–81. If approved, the state would receive medicare funds for the elderly in a lump sum from the federal government. This is also the section of the bill that would transfer funds to states to incorporate the medicare population into a single-payer system.

35. Thus the asset limits and monthly personal needs limits for nursing home care would be made slightly less stringent. There were other modest changes as well. Ibid., sections 4211–13, pp. 809–14.

36. Ibid., section 4222, pp. 818–25. As states set up their alliances and came into the system, the acute-care portions of medicaid would be closed down; see section 4201, pp. 807–09.

37. A good summary is CBO, "Analysis of the Administration's Health Proposal," pp. 6–7 for benefits and 13–15 for cuts. Key provisions were in Health Security Act, S. 1757, sections 2001–05, pp. 343–87, for increases and 4103–04, 4111–19, 4134–35, 7131, pp. 754–60, 762–92, 801–05, 1116–25, for cuts.

38. The benefit would have had a $250 deductible, a 20 percent coinsurance requirement, and a limit on out-of-pocket payments of $1,000. The HSA would have made this benefit more affordable by demanding rebates from the pharmaceutical firms. They naturally protested, but by international standards they were doing well to avoid a basic price list. See CBO, "Analysis of the Administration's Health Proposal," p. 6; the provisions are in Health Security Act, S. 1757, sections 2001–04, pp. 343–79. New benefits would also include home infusion drug therapy; see section 2005, pp. 380–87.

39. This cap was credible because it was defined in terms of the division of a fixed pool of money among states, rather than as a limit on spending generated by a program that creates entitlements for individuals. Examples from the past include general revenue sharing and Title XX social service block grants.

40. CBO, "Analysis of the Administration's Health Proposal," pp. 6–7;

Health Security Act, S. 1757, sections 2101–09, pp. 389–425; definition of disability at 2103, pp. 398–407; cost sharing at 2105, pp. 408–09; budgets at 2109, pp. 415–25; entitlement at 2101, pp. 389–90. Eligible persons would either have severe cognitive and mental impairments or need assistance with three out of five basic activities of daily living (eating, using the toilet, dressing, bathing, and getting in and out of bed).

41. *Health Security Act*, S.1757, section 4032, pp. 704–05. Whether extra billing was banned already under existing law was subject to some dispute; see Elisabeth Rosenthal, "Irked By Medicare Limits, Doctors Ask Elderly to Pay Up," *New York Times*, February 15, 1994, p. B2.

42. Ibid., sections 9001–04, pp. 1277–85.

43. The self-employed were to contribute to the "employer" account themselves.

44. A good short explanation of the financing is in CBO, "Analysis of the Administration's Health Proposal," pp. 27–33.

45. The actual range might well have been less, but the average would still have been 20 percent.

46. The formula for the individual subsidies was quite complicated, but its intent was to ensure that everyone with any income over $1,000 who was not an AFDC or SSI recipient paid something. No family with an income under $40,000 per year would have to pay more than 3.9 percent of its income. The measures to calibrate contributions from persons who had income but were not employed, or were employed only part-time, or were self-employed, were extremely complex, but at least they existed. See *Health Security Act*, S. 1757, section 6104, pp. 1030–42, esp. pp. 1035–40; sections 6111–13, pp. 1047–55; section 6126, pp. 1081–84.

47. Ibid., section 6123, pp. 1071–72.

48. Alice M. Rivlin, David M. Cutler, and Len M. Nichols, "Financing, Estimation, and Economic Effects," *Health Affairs*, vol. 13, no. 1 (Spring I 1994), p. 46.

49. *Health Security Act*, S. 1757, section 6114, pp. 1055–58.

50. If the retiree health benefits were better than the standard package, the employer might maintain supplemental coverage. If they were worth more than 80 percent of the basic premium, the retiree would be worse off than before.

51. *Health Security Act*, S. 1757, section 6124, pp. 1075–80.

52. The quote is from CBO, "Analysis of the Administration's Health Proposal," p. 12; see that source and also *Health Security Act*, S. 1757, sections 7111–13 (tobacco), pp. 1094–1106; 7141 (chapter S and partnerships), pp. 1125–28; 7142 (state/local), pp. 1128–32; 7201–02 (cafeteria), pp. 1133–39. Previously only state and local employees hired after April 1, 1986, had to pay medicare payroll tax.

53. On the self-employed, see *Health Security Act*, S. 1757, section 7203, pp. 1139–42. This provision was also in the Cooper-Grandy, Chafee, and incremental bills, except that the Clinton bill did not allow the self-employed person

to deduct more for herself than for any of her employees. On long-term care, see S. 1757, sections 7701–04, pp. 1171–92. For figures on extra revenue, see CBO, "Analysis of the Administration's Health Proposal," table 2.2, p. 29.

54. If we wanted to compare how American health care would have been paid for in the Clinton plan with how it is financed in other countries, we would want to assess contributions to the whole system, not just to the alliances. Employers would pay percentages of payroll for medicare and a larger, not-quite-percentage, for the alliances. Individuals would pay percentages of payroll for medicare, and premiums for medicare part B and for alliance health plans. Both (but individuals to a much greater extent) would contribute through general taxation, mainly at the federal but also at the state level.

55. Bureau of National Affairs, *Health Care Policy Report*, May 23, 1994, pp. 901–02; Sharon McIlrath, "Scandal, Gridlock Dog Reform," *American Medical News*, May 23–30, 1994, pp. 1, 21.

56. States could also create reinsurance systems. On the risk adjustment formula see *Health Security Act*, S. 1757, sections 1541–45, pp. 279–86; on reinsurance see section 1203, pp. 101–05; on payment to plans, section 1351, pp. 174–78; on some of the complexities of administering the individual subsidies, sections 1343, 1371–75, 6111–15, pp. 148–63, 183–99, 1047–58, to be discussed below.

57. Zelman, "Rationale behind the Clinton Plan," p. 19.

58. *Health Security Act*, S. 1757, sections 1321, 6004, pp. 131–32, 1000–04, have the basic provisions; the quote is from page 1001. If an alliance could get all the plans into one bargaining session and negotiate all premiums at once, in order to create a structure that would avoid sanctions from the national health board, then negotiations would be meaningful. But that would really be a negotiation among the plans; the alliance would have little to offer.

59. Uwe E. Reinhardt, "The Clinton Plan: A Salute to American Pluralism," *Health Affairs*, vol. 13, no. 1 (Spring I 1994), p. 175.

60. Stuart Altman, "Health System Reform: Let's Not Miss Our Chance," in ibid., p. 78.

61. Henry J. Aaron, "Sowing the Seeds of Reform in 1994," in ibid., p. 60.

62. Jack Hadley and Stephen Zuckerman, "Health Reform: The Good, the Bad, and the Bottom Line," in ibid., p. 117.

63. Note that the administration's plan did not exactly require that increases per capita be held to the consumer price index (CPI) throughout this period. The targets were CPI plus 1.5 percent in 1996, plus 1.0 percent in 1997, plus 0.5 percent in 1998, CPI alone in 1999 and 2000.

64. *Health Security Act*, S. 1757, section 6001, pp. 984–89.

65. Ibid., section 1011, pp. 21–25, defines these classes.

66. Thus, "the limits on the growth of health insurance premiums and the reductions in the medicare program would hold down health spending." CBO, "Analysis of the Administration's Health Proposal," p. 26. CBO did assume that premiums would begin at a higher base than the administration did.

67. "No plan may engage in any practice that *has the effect* of attracting or

limiting enrollees on the basis of personal characteristics" (author's emphasis). *Health Security Act*, S. 1757, section 1402, p. 226.

68. The relevant provisions are in ibid., sections 1402–04, pp. 226–32.

69. A highly publicized example is Elizabeth McCaughey, "No Exit," *New Republic*, February 7, 1994, pp. 21–25.

70. *Health Security Act*, S. 1757, section 1322, pp. 133–34.

71. Plans would not, however, be forced to offer the point-of-service option in their basic packages; they only had to offer a choice of packages, and they might price the one with a point-of-service option so high that few persons chose it. Ibid., section 1402, p. 229, has the key provision, that an HMO "may charge an alternative premium."

72. Ibid., sections 1406, 1408–14, pp. 234–37, 239–41.

73. Ibid., sections 1431, 1432, pp. 249–51, 252–55.

74. The financing of residencies was related to regulation of the supply of residencies in order to decrease specialization. The text allowed $5.8 billion in 1999; ibid., sections 3033–34, pp. 519–26. The text allowed $3.7 billion in 1999; sections 3101–04, pp. 548–58.

75. Ibid., sections 1406, 4032, pp. 234–37, 704–05.

76. On June 14, 1994, Travelers' and Metropolitan Life announced a merger of their health insurance operations, so that they could move from open panels to closed ones.

77. *Health Security Act*, S. 1757, section 1322, p. 137.

78. The negotiation procedures are in ibid., pp. 134–36.

79. Ibid., sections 3001–74, pp. 504–48.

Chapter Ten

1. Thus a blind person would deserve help; an alcoholic, even if he had drunk himself blind, might not. See Deborah A. Stone, "The Struggle for the Soul of Health Insurance," *Journal of Health Politics, Policy and Law*, vol. 18, no. 2 (Summer 1993), pp. 287–317, for a good discussion of the nature of insurance that relates it to the question of solidarity raised below.

2. This was in fact the right-wing position in the American debate in 1993–94, as represented most explicitly by the many proposals to replace insurance with medical savings accounts. MSAs were included as options in the Chafee bill, *Health Equity and Access Reform Today Act of 1993*, S. 1770, 103 Cong. 1 sess. (GPO, 1993); in the House Republican leadership bill, *Affordable Health Care Now Act of 1993*, H.R. 3080, 103 Cong. 1 sess. (GPO, 1993); and in the bill sponsored by Senator Don Nickles (R-Okla.) and based on ideas from the Heritage Foundation, the *Consumer Choice Health Security Act of 1993*, S. 1743, 103 Cong. 1 sess. (GPO, 1993). But MSAs were the main proposal within the bill cosponsored by Senators Phil Gramm (R-Tex.) and John McCain (R-Az.), *Comprehensive Family Health Access and Savings Act*, S. 1807, 103 Cong. 2 sess. (GPO, 1994).

3. Polling data continually showed large majorities in favor of universal coverage; for an example from early 1994 in which 82 percent said it was "very important," see Adam Clymer, "Poll Finds Public Is Still Doubtful over Costs of Clinton Plan," *New York Times*, March 15, 1994, p. A1. In mid-1994 the figure was 78 percent strongly or somewhat in favor: David S. Broder and Richard Morin, "Poll Finds Public Losing Confidence in Clinton, Economy," *Washington Post*, June 28, 1994, p. A4.

4. For a summary of arguments about ideology, parties, and the growth of the welfare state, see Harold L. Wilensky and others, "Comparative Social Policy: Theories, Methods, Findings" (Berkeley, Calif.: Institute of International Studies, 1985). The argument over whether it is the strength of the right, the left, or catholicism that makes most difference misses the point: the right is less of an obstacle to expansions if the left is strong or the right is catholic. Also see David Vogel, "Why Businessmen Distrust Their State: The Political Consciousness of American Corporate Executives," *British Journal of Political Science*, vol. 8, no. 1 (January 1978), pp. 45–78.

5. For an example see Michael Weisskopf, "The Personal Touch Is Their Best Insurance," *Washington Post*, March 22, 1994, p. A8.

6. David Truman, *The Governmental Process: Political Interests and Public Opinions* (Knopf, 1957).

7. Large employers that supported the Clinton and McDermott-Wellstone plans provided good benefits and were already paying more than their share of costs. Some of the more controversial measures, such as coverage of early retirees, would have helped millions of Americans who did not have coverage from those employers. And the help to large employers was limited by other measures, such as the 1 percent payroll tax on corporate alliance employers and the extra contributions for seven years from large employers with a riskier population.

8. On business interests in general, see Vogel, "Why Businessmen Distrust Their State." On business interests in health care, see Lawrence D. Brown, "Dogmatic Slumbers: American Business and Health Policy," and Cathie Jo Martin, "Together Again: Business, Government, and the Quest for Cost Control," both in *Journal of Health Politics, Policy and Law*, vol. 18, no. 2 (Summer 1993), pp. 339–57 and 359–93. For a good account of the administration's effort and failure to win support, see Hilary Stout and Rick Wartzman, "Why Clintons' Effort to Woo Big Business to Health Plan Failed," *Wall Street Journal*, February 11, 1994, p. A1. Some of the big business organizations involved did have direct material interests in defeating reform—most evidently, insurance companies.

9. Eugene Carlson, "Small Firms Don't View Clinton's Health Plan Kindly," *Wall Street Journal*, November 12, 1993, p. B2.

10. Rick Wartzman and Jeanne Saddler, "A Fervent Lobbyist Rallies Small Business to Battle Health Plan," *Wall Street Journal*, January 5, 1994, p. A1.

11. Jeanne Saddler and Kevin G. Salwen, "U.S. Chamber of Commerce Splits Again over Issue of Health Insurance Mandate," *Wall Street Journal*, February 17, 1993, p. A3; for a similar story see Jeanne Saddler, "Group

Withdraws Support for Clinton Health Program," *Wall Street Journal*, March 17, 1994, p. B2.

12. A poll of top executives found that they were much more opposed than the public to the Clinton plan. Louis Uchitelle, "Executives Balking at Clinton Health Plan," *New York Times*, May 10, 1994, p. D1.

13. For further examples of business attitudes see Frank B. McArdle, "How Would Business React to an Employer Mandate?" pp. 69–73, and Sylvester J. Schieber, "Employer Coolness Toward Clinton Plan Mandates," pp. 105–07, both in *Health Affairs*, vol. 13, no. 2 (Spring II 1994).

14. Hilary Stout, "Rostenkowski Offers Health Compromise If Insurance Group Suspends Opposition," *Wall Street Journal*, May 17, 1994, p. A22.

15. In an NBC News special forum on health care reform, broadcast on June 21, 1994, Senator Robert Dole (R-Kan.) spoke of the need to preserve "the best health care system" and Senator George Mitchell (D-Me.) referred to "the best and highest quality of care in the world for those Americans who have access to it." Quotes taken from tape of program.

16. Note that this definition of quality might not be accurate, but for political purposes voters' beliefs about quality, not analysts' beliefs, are what is relevant. Reform need not mean these beneficiaries would get less, because in the Clinton plan, for example, differences among plans could mean greater choice for those who paid more. Further, supplemental benefits are indeed supplemental—that is, they could be covered by separate insurance.

17. Sven Steinmo and Jon Watts, "Why Comprehensive National Health Insurance Fails in America," *Journal of Health Politics, Policy and Law* (forthcoming 1995).

18. For good reviews of the effects of institutional structure from both a comparative and historical perspective, see R. Kent Weaver and Bert A. Rockman, eds., *Do Institutions Matter? Government Capabilities in the United States and Abroad* (Brookings, 1993); David Mayhew, *Divided We Govern* (Yale University Press, 1991); David Rohde, *Parties and Leaders in the Post-Reform House* (University of Chicago Press, 1991); Charles O. Jones, *The Presidency in a Separated System* (Brookings, 1994); and *The Federalist Papers* (Johns Hopkins University Press, 1981).

19. Deinstitutionalization of mental patients comes to mind.

20. Cooper-Grandy was *Managed Competition Act of 1993*, H.R. 3222, 103 Cong. 1 sess. (GPO, 1993); the single-payer plan was *American Health Security Act of 1993*, H.R. 1200, 103 Cong. 1 sess. (GPO, 1993); the House Republican plan was *Affordable Health Care Now Act of 1993*, H.R. 3080, 103 Cong. 1 sess. (GPO, 1993).

21. David B. Kendall, "Health Care Price Controls: A Cure Worse Than the Disease," Progressive Policy Institute Policy Briefing, June 9, 1994, p. 2; Jeremy D. Rosner, "A Progressive Plan for Affordable, Universal Health Care," in Will Marshall and Martin Schram, eds., *Mandate for Change* (Berkley Books, 1993); Alain C. Enthoven and Sara J. Singer, "A Single-Payer System in Jackson Hole Clothing," *Health Affairs*, vol. 13, no. 1 (Spring I 1994), pp. 81–95.

22. Marc L. Berk, "Perspective: Should We Rely on Polls?" *Health Affairs*,

vol. 13, no. 1 (Spring I 1994), pp. 299–300. For other analyses of public opinion see, in the same issue, Robert J. Blendon and others, "The Beliefs and Values Shaping Today's Health Reform Debate," pp. 274–84, and Lawrence R. Jacobs and Robert Y. Shapiro, "Public Opinion's Tilt against Private Enterprise," pp. 285–98.

23. Hilary Stout, "Many Don't Realize It's Clinton's Plan They Like," *Wall Street Journal*, March 10, 1994, p. B1. Forty-eight percent saw "a great deal of appeal" or "some appeal" in the description of the Chafee bill; 34 percent were for Cooper-Grandy and 31 percent for McDermott-Wellstone. Such responses clearly could be affected by question wording, but the pollsters were a team of one Democrat and one Republican, so any bias was probably inadvertent. The June 26, 1994, poll reported in Broder and Morin, "Poll Finds Public Losing Confidence," found 78 percent supporting universal coverage, 75 percent supporting federal price controls, 72 percent supporting an employer mandate, and 61 percent in favor of "a program in which people paid more money to choose their own doctor, and less money if they went to an assigned doctor." But only 42 percent approved of the Clinton health plan, though 49 percent judged it better than the status quo.

24. Blendon and others, "Beliefs and Values," pp. 276–82; Jacobs and Shapiro, "Public Opinion's Tilt," pp. 294–96.

25. Group Health Association of America, *Patterns in HMO Enrollment* (Washington, May 1994), pp. 35–36.

26. Robert Pear, "A Go-Slow Plan on Health Gains Support in Congress," *New York Times*, May 5, 1994, p. B14.

27. There were too many versions to describe here, and the legislative history of health reform in 1994 should be left to others. One example of such discussion is a proposal Senator Bill Bradley (D-N.J.) made in early June; see Ruth Marcus and Dana Priest, "Clinton Won't 'Declare Defeat' on Universal Health Coverage," *Washington Post*, June 22, 1994, p. A4. Another is the back-and-forth between Senator John Breaux (D-La.), Senator Bob Packwood (R-Ore.), and administration officials described in Bureau of National Affairs, *Health Care Policy Report*, June 20, 1994, pp. 1063–64.

28. The classic statements of the case for incrementalism are Charles E. Lindblom, "The Science of Muddling Through," *Public Administration Review*, vol. 19, no. 2 (Spring 1959), pp. 79–88; David Braybrooke and Charles E. Lindblom, *A Strategy of Decision: Policy Evaluation as a Social Process* (New York: Free Press of Glencoe, 1963); and Aaron Wildavsky, *The Politics of the Budgetary Process* (Boston: Little, Brown, 1964).

29. *Affordable Health Care Now Act of 1993*, H.R. 3080, sections 1401, 1411, 1501–02, 1521, 1108, pp. 134–36, 137–46, 146–51, 157–60, 59–61.

30. Ibid., sections 2101–15, 2131–35, pp. 247–61, 267–75.

31. Ibid., sections 2111–24, pp. 254–67.

32. Ibid., section 1013, pp. 16–17; the bill did allow nonrenewal for "noncompliance with plan provisions," which might be hard to define. In addition to the bill text, I also consulted the Leader's Task Force on Health press handout from September 15, 1993.

33. Exclusions could not be applied to pregnancy or to problems at birth, or last more than six months, or apply to a condition that had not been diagnosed or treated within three months of beginning coverage under the plan. If a person moved from one plan to another within an interval of less than sixty days (six months if he left the first plan because he lost his job), and the condition would normally be covered under both plans, an exclusion could not apply. *Affordable Health Care Now Act of 1993*, H.R. 3080, sections 1011–12, pp. 13–16. Somewhat stronger limitations were included in other bills, such as Chafee and Cooper-Grandy.

34. On enrollment, see ibid., section 1101, pp. 27–30. States were encouraged to create reinsurance systems to complement the risk provisions; see ibid., section 1106, pp. 51–54.

35. An insurer could not raise its charge to an employer by more than its increase for new business within that class plus 15 percent; of course, it could do that for a few years in a row. Ibid., section 1105, p. 51. When first implemented, the intracategory variation could be 80 percent, falling to 62 percent after three years. Section 1104, pp. 46 and 50, gives provisions; the 62 percent figure is a calculation by the author based on the bill's text.

36. Ibid., sections 1211–41, pp. 68–129.

37. The Michel bill's major measure to increase subsidies was to extend 100 percent tax deductibility for insurance premiums directly to individuals rather than allowing that treatment only for business expenses. This provision favored persons with higher incomes, both because taxpayers with higher marginal tax rates would receive larger subsidies and because people with low incomes still would not be able to afford insurance. Ibid., sections 1301–02, pp. 129–34.

38. Ibid., sections 1201–04, 2501–04, pp. 64–67, 331–47. This was not a good idea. A more defensible provision was the elimination of state minimum benefit requirements.

39. The Michel bill had no new money nor mandates. See ibid., sections 2401–02, pp. 317–27, for medicare; section 1601, pp. 174–83, for medicaid.

40. Other measures included a requirement for preliminary alternative dispute resolution (ADR). Whoever appealed a finding from ADR would be at risk for court costs and have to post bond for those costs. Ibid., sections 2001–33, pp. 213–40.

41. The classic case is federal budgeting. For an argument as to why it persists in spite of criticism, why it should persist, but also the conditions that make budgetary incrementalism more or less likely, see Joseph White, "(Almost) Nothing New under the Sun: Why the Work of Budgeting Remains Incremental," *Public Budgeting and Finance*, vol. 14, no. 1 (Spring 1994), pp. 113–34.

42. For an account of Gramm-Rudman-Hollings, how it worked, and why its central provisions were repealed in 1990, see the paperback edition of Joseph White and Aaron Wildavsky, *The Deficit and the Public Interest: The Search for Responsible Budgeting in the 1980s* (University of California Press and the Russell Sage Foundation, 1991).

43. This account is based on just a quick sampling of reports from "Update: Health Reform," *American Medical News*, April 11, 1994, p. 6; April 25, 1994, p. 18; May 9, 1994, p. 9; June 13, 1994, p. 9; and from Bureau of National Affairs, *Health Care Policy Report*, May 23, 1994, pp. 921–23; June 13, 1994, pp. 1038–42; June 20, 1994, pp. 1086–87.

44. Among the states with proposals related to managed competition were Florida, Illinois, Minnesota, Missouri, Illinois, Washington, and Wyoming. Among the states with proposals to make it easier for small firms to buy insurance were Colorado, Kansas, Nebraska, New Hampshire, and South Carolina. Hawaii, Kentucky, Oregon, Rhode Island, and Tennessee all had received waivers to expand the use of managed care as of June 1994, while Florida, Massachusetts, Ohio, and South Carolina were discussing such applications with the Health Care Financing Administration. New Mexico, New Hampshire, and Rhode Island had enacted other expansions. Ibid.

45. In Minnesota legislation was signed on May 10, 1994, but it only created a commission to come up with a funding device. Florida's effort died in a Senate committee on June 9. Vermont's governor Harold Dean gave up on May 13. Washington had passed legislation that might approach universal coverage around 1999, but the financing was still uncertain and depended on a waiver of the federal ERISA law, a difficulty discussed below. Bureau of National Affairs, *Health Care Policy Report*, May 23, 1994, pp. 919, 922.

46. For a good summary of reasons see Mary Ann Chirba-Martin and Troyen A. Brennan, "The Critical Role of ERISA in State Health Reform," *Health Affairs*, vol. 13, no. 2 (Spring II 1994), pp. 142–56.

47. Congressional Budget Office, "An Analysis of the Administration's Health Proposal" (February 1994), p. 29.

48. Janice Somerville, "Single Payer Referendum Set," *American Medical News*, May 16, 1994, p. 3.

49. For a statement of the dilemma faced by leaders of the American Medical Association, see Harris Meyer, "Medicine at the Crossroads," *American Medical News*, December 13, 1993, pp. 1, 32–33; see also Harris Meyer, "Support for Employer Mandate Softened," *American Medical News*, December 20, 1993, pp. 1, 21.

50. Sharon McIlrath, "Surgeons Back Single Payer," *American Medical News*, February 28, 1994, pp. 1, 29, 31. For an argument that the surgeons' board was right but that many other physicians should disagree, see Robert A. Berenson, "Do Physicians Recognize Their Own Best Interests?" *Health Affairs*, vol. 13, no. 2 (Spring II 1994), pp. 185–93.

51. McIlrath, "Surgeons Back Single Payer," esp. pp. 29, 31.

52. The AMA's "four main points" for reform included "greater physician involvement in the system" and "antitrust relief to offset the domination of medical decision-making by giant corporate interests." Lonnie R. Bristow, "Rx for Victory: Medicine Must Go for the Glory," *American Medical News*, February 28, 1994, pp. 18–19.

53. John G. Smillie, *Can Physicians Manage the Quality and Costs of Health*

Care? The Story of the Permanente Medical Group (McGraw-Hill, 1991); see, for example, the comments of founder Sidney R. Garfield on p. 55.

54. For example, in April 1994 Blue Cross of Rhode Island announced tentative guidelines suggesting that patients be discharged from hospitals within two days of a caesarean section, twelve hours of a vaginal delivery, or two days of an above-knee amputation. Greg Borzo, "R.I. Doctors Face 'Absurd' Inpatient Limits," *American Medical News*, March 21, 1994, p. 1. Even if not implemented, such proposals disconcerted doctors.

55. Because income tends to be correlated with age, the subsidy from young to old in an income-related system is reduced by the difference in incomes.

56. They might choose, for example, to buy "catastrophic" coverage and pay out-of-pocket for other expenses.

57. Extra billing is inherently a bigger problem in Canada and Australia than in France and Germany also, but in Canada fees are lower and in Australia the admitting physicians also do some salaried work in the hospital and are therefore accessible.

58. Paul M. Ellwood, Alain C. Enthoven and Lynn Etheredge, "The Jackson Hole Initiative for a Twenty-First Century American Health Care System," *Health Economics*, vol. 1, no. 3 (1992), p. 160; Alain C. Enthoven, "The History and Principles of Managed Competition," *Health Affairs*, vol. 12, Supplement (1993), pp. 41–42; Jonathan Gruber, "The Effect of Price-Shopping in Medical Markets: Hospital Responses to PPOs in California," Working Paper 4190 (Cambridge, Mass.: National Bureau of Economic Research (October 1992).

59. Even the Congressional Budget Office, while not quite calling the mandates a tax, treated the proposal as a governmental rather than market approach. CBO, "Analysis of the Administration's Health Proposal," chap. 4. For reactions, see Steven Pearlstein and David Broder, "Clinton and the Analysts: A $133 Billion Difference of Opinion," *Washington Post*, February 9, 1994, p. A4; Hilary Stout and David Rogers, "CBO Disputes Cost Estimates in Health Plan," *Wall Street Journal*, February 9, 1994, p. A3; see also Director Reischauer's concerns about that reaction: Robert D. Reischauer, "Don't Let This Chance Go By," *Washington Post*, February 11, 1994, p. A25. CBO's "ruling," one should note, was not a ruling at all: it was advice that the program should be treated as governmental in principle. CBO did not declare the contributions were in fact government receipts because the alliance spending was not government spending. It neither entered the treasury nor was appropriated. The principle involved, also, would not be believed in any country with a sickness fund system. Those countries do not insist on classifying all transactions as either "governmental" or "private market" because, as explained in chapter 4, the origins of sickness funds are emphatically in neither category.

60. For a good example of both arguments see Michael J. Graetz, "Universal Health Coverage without an Employer Mandate," *Domestic Affairs*, vol. 2 (Winter 1993–94), pp. 79–104. And compare Victor R. Fuchs, "The Clinton Plan: A Researcher Examines Reform," *Health Affairs*, vol. 13, no. 1 (Spring I

1994), pp. 104–05; and Stuart Altman, "Health System Reform: Let's Not Miss Our Chance," ibid., pp. 73–74. For a longer treatment of many issues in which various aspects of employer financing are addressed, see Henry J. Aaron, *Serious and Unstable Condition: Financing America's Health Care* (Brookings, 1991).

61. For an example of use of the 80 percent estimate see Alice M. Rivlin, David M. Cutler, and Len M. Nichols, "Financing, Estimation, and Economic Effects," *Health Affairs*, vol. 13, no. 1 (Spring 1 1994), pp. 30–49, esp. p. 44. The quote is from Henry J. Aaron, "Sowing the Seeds of Reform in 1994," in ibid., p. 68.

62. For excellent reviews of these issues see Karen Davis and Cathy Schoen, "Universal Coverage: Building on Medicare and Employer Financing," *Health Affairs*, vol. 13, no. 2 (Spring II 1994), pp. 7–20, and Alan B. Krueger and Uwe E. Reinhardt, "Economics of Employer versus Individual Mandates," ibid., pp. 34–53.

63. The *Consumer Choice Health Security Act of 1993*, S. 1743, sponsored by Senator Don Nickles, took the straightforward road of basically eliminating employer payments. The provisions for ensuring that employers replaced insurance contributions with wages in the first year were well thought out. But after the first year, the dynamics that make both employers and employees believe that wages plus health benefits adds to more than wages would still have been in place.

64. For a thorough statement of the argument, see Joseph White, "Paying the Right Price," *Brookings Review*, vol. 12, no. 2 (Spring 1994), pp. 6–11. For a thorough review of American experience with fee regulation, to complement this book's report on international cases, see Marsha Gold and others, "Effects of Selected Cost-Containment Efforts: 1971–1993," *Health Care Financing Review*, vol. 14, no. 3 (Spring 1993), pp. 183–225.

65. Julie Johnsson, "April Medicare Rule Set to Complete RBRVS," *American Medical News*, February 28, 1994, p. 1; also Julie Johnsson, "Doctors to Be Given a Say in RBRVS 5-Year Review," ibid., p. 29.

66. For a good example, see the comments of Ira Magaziner in "Cooper Backers Eye Individual Coverage Rule," *American Medical News*, March 14, 1994, p. 10.

67. For example, German doctors bear risk for pharmaceutical costs; the British general practitioner (GP) fundholders, who must combine the equivalent of three GP practices, still are not responsible for the vast majority of hospital expenses.

68. Hospitals would not need exclusive contracts because a closed plan's physicians would in any case only refer to hospitals where they had privileges.

69. Given the proliferation in the United States of radiology and other diagnostic and treatment centers, which bring costs outside the hospital, creating separate caps for such items seems necessary.

70. Therefore those persons who were subsidized only to purchase plans with high cost sharing could reduce their own expenses by joining an HMO. In fact even the poorest should have the right to choose the HMO coverage.

71. If the low cost-sharing still seemed unaffordable to the very poor, another program could be set up for them.

72. The proposed Dutch version of managed competition has a similar design. See Wynand P. M. M. Van de Ven and Frederik T. Schut, "The Dutch Experience with Internal Markets," in Monique Jérôme-Forget, Joseph White, and Joshua Wiener, eds., *Health Care Reform through Internal Markets: Experience and Proposals* (Montreal and Washington: Institute for Research on Public Policy and Brookings, 1995), pp. 99–101.

73. For example, if the cost of the most expensive plan were 110 percent of what the weighted average would have been in the Clinton plan, 75 percent of the most expensive plan would be 82.5 percent of the putative average. The two are identical if the regulated highest premium in this proposal were just under 107 percent of the target the board would have set in the Clinton structure.

Appendix

1. *Managed Competition Act of 1993*, H.R. 3222, 103 Cong. 1 sess., section 1208, pp. 82–83.

2. This problem cannot be avoided by allowing small coverage areas, because doing so would let states isolate unpopular and expensive populations.

3. A plan's price is raised by making part of it subject to tax. The point is to provide "incentives" for persons to choose lower-priced plans: that is, to reduce the plan in question's business. That sounds like punishment to me.

4. *Health Equity and Access Reform Today Act of 1993*, S. 1770, 103 Cong. 1 sess., section 2001, p. 139.

5. There are just too many other examples of vagueness about regulations in the bill to avoid this conclusion—unless one wants to conclude that the drafters were entirely inept.

6. The family type and age distinctions could be avoided by charging community rates, but then the charges to the young and the childless would be too high. They could also be avoided with a general revenue-based or percentage-of-payroll premium system, but that would be the international standard, which these plans were designed to avoid.

7. Florida, for example, created eleven alliance areas in its state legislation. A more likely figure for age bands is three—say, 18–35, 36–50, 51–65.

8. Because this would call for the federal government to limit state flexibility, the idea might be politically unpalatable. But since the alternative would be to list towns or zipcodes or include detailed maps in every tax packet, any of which would kill a forest or two, I hope readers will see the logic of using county boundaries.

9. The language in H.R. 3222 does not enable one to conclude whether persons' deductibles would be calculated based on residence or place of em-

ployment. *Managed Competition Act of 1993*, H.R. 3222, section 1106, pp. 56–58.

10. *Health Equity and Access Reform Today Act of 1993*, S. 1770, section 2001, p. 141. Incurred illness costs could not be used because then the sick would be taxed.

11. In fact, the taxation of benefits in the Chafee scheme was made even more complex by its medical savings accounts (MSA) option. This is not relevant to the main argument, fortunately. But any system with a mix of MSAs and insurance must keep track of the sum of two amounts, the MSA deposits and the insurance premium; it therefore could not be audited as easily as the current common form of tax-free savings, the Individual Retirement Account (IRA). For the provisions see ibid., section 1301, pp. 89–97.

12. Mark Regan, "A Quick 'N' Dirty Comparison of Three Bills' Subsidy Systems," National Health Law Program, December 9, 1993.

13. The quote is from *Managed Competition Act of 1993*, H.R. 3222, section 1102e, p. 45; other relevant sections are 1205(c), p. 76, and 2001–09, pp. 170–96.

14. Ibid., sections 1202(c), p. 66, and 2003, pp. 172–75, establish the cost-sharing assistance; it would have been available to families with incomes at or below twice the poverty level and paid directly by the HCSC to plans.

15. Congressional Budget Office, "An Analysis of the Managed Competition Act," A CBO Study (1994), pp. 43–44.

16. Ibid., p. 41.

17. *Managed Competition Act of 1993*, H.R. 3222, section 2006, p. 182.

18. CBO, "Analysis of the Administration's Health Proposal," pp. 9, 10.

19. This description has ignored complicated matters such as treatment of part-time employment or what happens when one adult works for a regional alliance employer and his or her spouse for a corporate alliance employer. One of the reasons the Clinton bill was so long was that it had answers for such questions.

20. The employee could be eligible for a subsidy for the poor and also the bill's cap on employee contributions at 3.9 percent of income.

21. *Health Security Act*, S. 1757, sections 1602, 1603, 1604, pp. 303–14, 314–15, 315–16.

22. Ibid., section 1602, pp. 303–14.

23. Martha Derthick, *Agency under Stress: The Social Security Administration in American Government* (Brookings, 1990). Those Americans who think of the IRS as a less competent agency would hardly be making a case for giving it the job of running health insurance subsidies.

24. Imagine that the target for a region is $4 billion. In the first year plans expected to include half of the population (net of all adjustments) might be below their target, for a total of $1.8 billion. The other plans in this example would have premiums totaling $2.4 billion, so the total, $4.2 billion, is too high. The difference of $0.2 billion would have to be taken from the plans that caused it, so out of their $2.4 billion. Their premiums would be reduced by .2

divided by 2.4, or 8.33 percent. *Health Security Act*, S. 1757, sections 6000, 6004, and 6011, pp. 982–83, 1000–04, and 1012–17, contain the provisions.

25. Ibid., section 6003, pp. 995–1000.

26. If the drafters in the administration had understood the federal budget process, they would have recognized that this dynamic, in which nobody will settle unless everybody settles, is exactly what happened when the Gramm-Rudman-Hollings Act threatened "sequesters" in all appropriations bills if the total were too high. In that case, though, the appropriations committees could organize the necessary omnibus package, called a continuing resolution, because they controlled the process. Alliances in the Clinton plan would not. See Joseph White, "The Continuing Resolution: A Crazy Way to Govern?" *Brookings Review* (Summer 1988), pp. 28–35.

27. Actually, "highballing" makes more sense in this context than in ordinary budget processes, because the overseer, here the board, has no discretion and therefore cannot impose extra cuts out of irritation with the strategy.

28. Because the allowed increase is the dollar amount, not the percentage, a cheaper plan could get a larger proportional increase and a more expensive plan a smaller one. "Asymptotically," a senior congressional budget official expressed in wonderment, "in a hundred years all premiums would be equal." In a modest way, however, the approach in the bill responds to the criticism that I make below. The relevant language is in *Health Security Act*, S. 1757, section 6011, p. 1016.

29. If all other plans asked for exactly $200 increases, DocsPlus would be responsible for the entire excess in the weighted average. It would be cut back by enough to eliminate the excess—the full amount of its own excess bid. If DocsPlus tried to strategize by asking for a $600 increase instead of $400, it would be cut by $400 instead of $200.

30. They would not be frozen completely because the adjustment is in whole dollars rather than percentages, so plans would move closer together over time. Note that the board still might make mistakes in guessing enrollment; in practice it would probably assume that each year's proportions would be the same as the previous year's and adjust for errors by allowing increases or decreases to the targets in the following year, through the retrospective correction system.

31. I have highlighted this provision so heavily because it is so stunning; the language is in *Health Security Act*, S. 1757, section 6012, pp. 1017–20.

32. Ibid., section 6105, pp. 1042–44

33. The "voluntary" reduction is discussed in ibid., section 6004, pp. 1003–04.

Index

Aaron, Henry, 208, 240, 275
Academic medical centers (AMCs). *See* Hospitals
Accepting assignment. *See* Fees
Accountable health plans (AHPs), 203, 205, 213, 293. *See also* Health care reforms, U.S.
Accreditation Council for Graduate Medical Education, 56
Acquired immunodeficiency syndrome (AIDS), 149, 150, 154
Administration. *See* Clinton health care plan; Health care reforms; individual countries
AFDC. *See* Aid to families with dependent children
AHPs. *See* Accountable health plans
Aide Médicale, 106. *See also* France
AIDS. *See* Acquired immunodeficiency syndrome
Aid to families with dependent children (AFDC), 38, 231, 237
Alcohol consumption, 135
Alliances. *See* Chafee Health Equity and Access Reform Today Act; Clinton health care plan; Cooper-Grandy bill; Health care reforms, U.S.; Managed competition
Alternative medicine, 27
Altman, Stuart, 97, 240
Ambulatory care: Australia, 93, 94, 96; Britain, 123; France, 106, 108; Germany, 79, 81, 83, 87, 97, 148; United States, 52–53, 55, 147. *See also* Hospitals; Physicians
AMCs (Academic medical centers). *See* Hospitals
American College of Surgeons, 270
American Medical Association (AMA), 53, 158, 279, 281

American Medical News, 158
Andrews, Mike (D-Tex.), 200
Arbitration, 69–70
Association of Sickness Fund Physicians (Kassenärztliche Vereinigung or KV; Germany), 78, 79, 81
Atwater, Lee, 42
Australia, 4–5; access to care, 156; cost sharing, 96, 156, 273; fees and fee schedules, 7, 92, 94, 96–98, 157, 160, 280; finance and benefits, 93–94; health care budgeting, 7; health care costs and spending, 93–94; health care delivery, 98–99; history of the health care system, 91–92; hospitals, 92–93, 94, 95, 97–100, 123, 248; insurance, 92, 93, 94, 95–96, 97–98, 99, 102, 272; malpractice, 99–102; pharmaceuticals, 94, 99; physicians, 92, 93, 94, 96, 97, 98, 99, 106, 137, 139, 160, 161, 273; political factors, 91, 93–94, 96, 98; quality of care, 99, 100; technology and equipment, 98, 99; universal health insurance, 4, 5. *See also* International factors and comparisons; International standard; Medicare (Australia)
Australian Hospital Association, 96

Barer, Morris L., 185
BCMA. *See* British Columbia Medical Association
Benefits. *See* Insurance; individual countries
Bilirakis, Michael (R-Fla.), 261
Blue Cross/Blue Shield, 45, 62, 181. *See also* Insurance
Boston City Hospital (Boston, Mass.), 53–54

381